Third Edition

Practical Nurse
Nutrition Education

ALBERTA DENT SHACKELTON, B.S., M.S., M.Ed.

Formerly Associate Professor of Nutrition
Douglass College, Rutgers University

W. B. SAUNDERS COMPANY • PHILADELPHIA • LONDON • TORONTO

W. B. Saunders Company: West Washington Square
Philadelphia, Pa. 19105

12 Dyott Street
London, WC1A 1DB

833 Oxford Street
Toronto, Ontario M8Z 5T9, Canada

Practical Nurse Nutrition Education   ISBN 0-7216-8112-3

Print No.:   9   8   7   6   5   4

PREFACE

Any nurse, practical or professional, in any area she serves — hospital, clinic, industry, school, home, or with a community health organization — faces a challenging opportunity *and* responsibility to play a role in the nutritional improvement of many persons.

This third edition of *Practical Nurse Nutrition Education* continues to provide up-to-date, concise, and easy-to-follow basic principles of nutrition and their application in all nutritional areas for the student in practical and vocational nursing during the preclinical and clinical periods.

The format and organization of the previous edition have been retained, including the unique workbook-type arrangement, providing space for the student to record results of activities and problems. The subject matter is divided in three sections, further divided into units and unit parts, and presented in answer to topical questions. The subdivisions are followed by lists of terms to understand, selected study questions, and nurse- and patient-centered activities, some of which have been enlarged. The expanded list of supplementary readings in current references, bulletins, and other pertinent publications at the end of each part permits additional reading assignments by the instructor to meet the range of interest and background experience of students. Newer developments in nutrition are included as well as new tables and charts in line with the 1970 table of food composition of the U.S. Department of Agriculture and the 1968 Recommended Dietary Allowances.

Section One, Normal Nutrition, introduces the nurse briefly to nutrition terms and orients her thinking to the importance of good nutrition for herself and to the role she will play nutritionally in patient care as a member of the nursing team. It initiates for her a nutritional evaluation of her own food and nutrition habits to be continued as she progresses with nutrition study. It then deals with the relation of food and nutrition to health; the various nutrition guides; essential nutrients for good nutrition — functions, food sources, daily recommended dietary allowances, and use by the body; foods in the Four Basic Food Groups — nutritional contributions, use, selection, and preparation principles and combinations into meals; family diet plans; special nutritional needs at various stages in the life cycle; public health and community nutrition programs for nutritional betterment, and food fads and fallacies.

Increased coverage is given in Unit One to food habits and the state of nutrition in the American population, and what is being done to improve them; in Unit Two, to saturated and unsaturated fats and cholesterol, and newer mineral and vitamin developments, with the addition of those for which dietary allowances appear for the first time in the 1968 Recommended Dietary Allowances. A nutritive evaluation of a basic foundation diet plan has been added to Unit Three. Unit Five, Public Health and Community Nutrition, has been rearranged to cover laws and regulations to provide greater consumer protection in the food supply and to include more detail regarding aims, types, and activities of various community programs to aid in solving community nutrition problems. The area of adolescent nutrition has been slightly revised with new food guides, and the diet habits of older persons reviewed at greater length.

Section Two, Therapeutic Nutrition, deals with the application of the basic principles of normal nutrition to the feeding of persons with certain pathological conditions. The modification of a normal diet is emphasized as the basis for planning a diet for corrective or curative purposes. Normal diet modifications, with foods allowed and foods to avoid, and diet plans for various groups of related diseases are presented. A form for a clinical conference on patients receiving therapeutic diets is included. The parts dealing with atherosclerosis and cardiac and hypertensive disorders have been revised, and current diet lists on fat- and cholesterol-controlled diets and sodium-restricted diets of the American Heart Association have been included. The section on miscellaneous disorders has been rearranged and made more inclusive.

The individual instructor will, of course, adapt the sequence of subject matter to meet the time allowances and facilities of her own teaching situation. It is suggested that the Introduction and Units One, Two, Three, and Five be presented in the preclinical period to provide the basic knowledge and to allow development of attitudes and skills essential to clinical learning experiences. Unit Four, Parts 1, 2, and 3 may be most effective when the nurse is gaining experience on obstetric and pediatric services. Theory of therapeutic nutrition may be taught during the preclinical period but it should be well integrated also during the entire clinical period.

Section Three, Food Preparation and Service, includes simple food preparation activities (geared to complete meals) to illustrate basic principles of food preparation and service for normal diets and for therapeutic diets. All may be food demonstrations conducted by the instructor, if time and facilities do not permit students' individual or group participation. A "Note to Instructor" at the beginning of the section indicates sources of suitable recipes and specialized food preparation procedures. When neither food demonstration nor practice is possible, food models may be used to demonstrate nutritionally adequate (and well-planned in all other respects) meals for a day, at which time food preparation principles for nutrient retention and palatability may be discussed. Food preparation Lessons 1 to 7 correlate with Section One, Unit Three, Part 1; Lesson 8 with Unit Three, Parts 2 and 3; and Lesson 9 with Section Two.

In the Appendix will be found a revised list of current references and a list of sources of nutrition materials, height-weight tables for men and women, growth charts for boys and girls, Canadian dietary standards, and a food composition table for the short method of dietary analysis.

An index is an entirely new feature of this edition, which should add to the book's usefulness.

For permission to quote from or adapt certain published materials the author is deeply grateful to the publishers, authors, governmental departments at various levels, and organizations—scientific, professional, educational, health, and industrial —credited in footnotes throughout the book. She wishes to express her appreciation also to nutrition instructors who used the previous edition of the book for their helpful comments and suggestions in preparing this revision.

ALBERTA DENT SHACKELTON

CONTENTS

Section Three   Food Preparation and Service

Appendix

Section One

NORMAL NUTRITION

Object

To help the practical nurse develop an understanding of the basic principles of normal nutrition; the relationship of good nutrition to optimal health; the importance of the right kinds and amounts of foods in the daily diet; the application of basic nutrition principles to the nutritional and psychological needs of individuals at all ages (with special emphasis on the nurse's own personal well-being and needs); meal planning for individual and family needs; and programs in public health and community nutrition.

Introduction

Unit

1. FOOD, NUTRITION, AND HEALTH
2. NUTRIENTS IN FOOD AND NUTRITION
3. FOODS AND MEALS FOR GOOD NUTRITION
4. NUTRITION IN THE LIFE CYCLE
5. PUBLIC HEALTH AND COMMUNITY NUTRITION

Introduction

Object

To define basic terms and to point up to the practical nurse (1) the importance of a workable knowledge of nutrition for everyone, (2) the place of nutrition in the total nursing care of the patient, (3) the importance of the practical nurse's place on the nursing team of physician, professional nurse, dietitian, social worker, and other professional personnel, and (4) the part she will play in the nutritional care of her patients and in promoting better nutrition generally.

WHAT IS THE MEANING OF NUTRITION AND DIETETICS?

Nutrition is defined as "the combination of processes by which the living organism *receives* and *utilizes* the materials necessary for the maintenance of its functions and for the growth and renewal of its components."[1] In short, nutrition is the relationship of food to the nourishment of the body for optimal health, or, "nutrition is the food you eat and how the body uses it." The term nutrition is also used to indicate bodily condition or nutritional status (nutriture). Malnutrition is "a condition of the body resulting from an inadequate or excessive supply or impaired utilization of one or more essential food constituents."[2]

Dietetics is defined as "the combined science and art of feeding individuals or groups under different economic or health conditions according to the principles of nutrition and management"[3] (and with regard for sex, age, activity, and social and pyschologic factors).

Therapeutic nutrition (diet therapy or nutritive therapy), discussed in the second section of this book, deals with the use of food as a therapeutic (curative) measure in the treatment of disease.

HOW HAS INTEREST IN NUTRITION DEVELOPED?

From early times, humans have been interested in the food they consume, its passage through the body, and its effects. It has been said by some writers that the history of the world might be written in terms of food, as it has featured so largely in living, first with the use of wild native foods, then food cultivation, followed by specific health values ascribed to foods by early philosophical and Bible writers. With the development of chemistry in the late 1600's, some of man's questions regarding food began to find answers.

---

[1] D. F. Turner, *Handbook of Diet Therapy,* 5th edition. Chicago, University of Chicago Press, 1970, p.242.
[2] Ibid., p. 241.
[3] Ibid., p. 237.

When it was established that air was a life essential and that oxygen and carbon dioxide were gases of respiration, it was recognized that respiration was related in some way to the use of food by the human body. In the late 1700's a French nobleman, Antoine Lavoisier, observed that organic substances (those containing carbon) burned in the body in a manner similar to the burning of a fuel in a flame. Later experiments of Lavoisier marked the first era of true nutrition study and he became known as the Father of the Science of Nutrition. Detailed study of the energy or caloric value of carbohydrates, fats, and proteins (all carbon-bearing) followed.

At the beginning of this century interest in nutrition was primarily concerned with how much energy (calories) humans need and how carbohydrates, fats, and proteins compare in energy value, and proteins became the subject for special study. Minerals were subsequently discovered. Almost simultaneously with their discovery came that of another group of substances, the vitamins. Still later, amino acids of proteins, certain fatty acids of fats, trace mineral elements, enzymes and hormones, certain body regulators, and other substances and their relationships were to become subjects of detailed study.

The nutrition story is a never-ending one and discoveries, perhaps even more dramatic, are promised for the future, especially in regard to relationships among all known factors—an aspect of nutrition in which outstanding discoveries have been and continue to be made. The role of nutrition in the prevention and treatment of disease is also growing in importance.

IS NUTRITION A SCIENCE?

Nutrition stands as a science in its own right after many years of research. It is one of the newest of biological sciences. It is not an isolated subject, but has close relationships with other sciences. It is considered to stand at the crossroads of all medical sciences—bacteriology, biochemistry, endocrinology, physiology, and pathology.

"The science of nutrition is the study of food and its relationship to the well-being of the human body. It includes (1) the metabolism of foods, (2) the nutritive value of foods, (3) the qualitative and quantitative requirements of food at different ages and developmental levels to meet physiological changes and to meet activity needs, and (4) the selection and eating of foods at different economic, social and cultural levels and for psychological reasons. The science and practice of nutrition exists for and attempts to contribute to the advance of populations throughout the world toward longer and more secure living, relatively free of disease. The food we eat and do not eat has much to do with health."[4]

Nutrition research has progressed from the early chemical food analysis of the food chemist, through animal feeding experiments (bio-assay), the use of micro-organisms (micro-biologic assays) to observations on humans. Today the study of foods and their nutritional improvement, nutritional status studies on humans, and a better understanding of methods to prevent and treat certain metabolic disorders require combined team efforts of nutrition scientists, biochemists, physicists, laboratory technicians, food technologists, physicians, nurses, nutritionists, and even anthropologists and geneticists.

---

[4] M. V. Krause, *Food, Nutrition, and Diet Therapy*, 4th edition, Philadelphia, W. B. Saunders Company, 1966, page 3.

WHY STUDY NUTRITION?

"Food contributes to physical, mental, and emotional health. Food nourishes our bodies. When we eat in a favorable setting, we get another kind of well-being: A sense of belonging and other psychological and social values accrue from the pleasures of mealtime and from having our food with friendly companions.

"People devote much time and effort and thought to producing the assortments of food that they need and want and to processing, distributing, and serving food in the places, at the times, and in the forms it is wanted.

"People have always known that they must eat to live—children to grow normally and adults to keep strong. But food can do more than satisfy physiological hunger and carry psychological and social values. Modern science shows that all of us, regardless of purse, can add years to our life and life to our years if we apply knowledge about nutrition to our selection and use of food....Persons of every age and in every occupation require food of kinds and amounts that enable their bodies to maintain the best possible internal environment for all the cells and tissues."[5]

We are not instinctively able to make the right choices and select the right amounts of food for good nutrition. Plentiful food supplies and plenty of money in our purses do not insure desirable food habits. Even in our own country with its vast food supplies and a reasonable standard of living for almost everyone, it is estimated that a large percentage of the population is suffering from some degree of malnutrition. We need to learn what foods have functions far beyond the mere relief of hunger and the satisfaction of appetite in nourishing our bodies to their fullest potential for growth and life—to learn the difference between mere "hollow" hunger and "hidden" hunger.

Good nutrition is of utmost importance from both the personal and community standpoints. Nutrition education through every possible medium is being stressed both for better personal living and for community, national, and world betterment as well. Any educational program dealing with the health of society shares responsibility in this respect. Nutrition, now considered to be one of the important medical sciences, demands recognition in any nursing education program.

HOW IS NUTRITION AN ASPECT OF TOTAL NURSING CARE?

The total needs and care of the patient and the consideration of him as a person and community member, rather than in terms of his disorder or disease, are currently emphasized in nursing education programs. Nutrition is considered an integral part of nursing care along with the physical, social, psychiatric, economic, and other aspects. The patient, like the well person, requires an adequate nutritional intake to maintain an already good nutritional state or to improve a poor one. For many patients, food is the single factor or one of several factors used to restore him to good health.

Patient-centered educational activities are the accepted approach in choosing learning experiences for the nurse in training. Therefore, nurses require a better understanding of nutritive therapy in illness and recovery to health as well as in everyday living. Nutrition taught closely correlated with patient care and at the same time with some relation to the nurse's own nutritional needs can become a

---

[5] *Food, The Yearbook of Agriculture.* Washington, D. C., U. S. Department of Agriculture, 1959.

useful and vital field of knowledge for her. An understanding of its vital relationship to everyday living and to the total care of the patient is essential for effective nutrition learning and teaching. The nutritional well-being of a patient is, to a great degree, the responsibility of the nurse. While health may be restored without medicine, it cannot be maintained without proper nutrition.

WHAT IS THE ROLE OF THE PRACTICAL NURSE IN THE HEALTH OF SOCIETY?

Any nurse, professional or practical, bedside or public health, is in a favored position to promote better nutrition and the improvement of the health of society. Probably no other group, except dietitians and public health nutritionists (those professionally trained in the science of nutrition and its applications) and social workers, comes in contact with as wide a circle of persons as do nurses.

The responsibilities of nurses in the field of health have increased as new scientific discoveries have been made. The benefits of good nutrition to the general health of the individual, family, community, nation, and the world have proven greater than ever realized and nutritive therapy is more widely used than previously. The practical nurse cannot escape a share in these responsibilities since her acceptance on the nursing team of physician, professional nurse, dietitian, social worker, and others is so well established.

A nurse's contacts with patients provide unlimited teaching opportunities to promote better nutrition of many persons. Her own state of nutrition and attitudes toward food and nutrition, her own dietary habits, the manner in which she approaches the feeding of her patients, and her interest and ability in helping patients understand the importance of a basic normal diet and a therapeutic one will determine her success. The nurse can also, with good basic nutrition knowledge, do much to combat the misinformation forced on the public (by one or another method) by food faddists, quacks, and self-termed, untrained "health specialists." Food fads and fallacies are discussed in a later chapter (page 212).

WHAT ATTITUDES AND UNDERSTANDING WILL BE HELPFUL AS YOU STUDY NUTRITION?

1. An appreciation of the role of nutrition for optimal health, efficiency, longevity, and enjoyment of life for everyone, including yourself and family.
2. An appreciation of the importance of the right kinds and amounts of foods daily for good nutrition for yourself, your family, and your patients.
3. An appreciation of the role of nutrition in the total nursing care of the patient: to maintain good nutrition through an illness, to improve state of nutrition when necessary, or as a single or one of several therapeutic measures.
4. An appreciation of the social, racial, religious, economic, and psychological factors, as well as the physiologic factors, in feeding both well and ill persons.
5. An understanding of the patient's well-established patterns of eating.
6. An appreciation of the importance of *your* having the right attitude toward

food and nutrition habits for success in feeding patients and their willingness to accept diet modifications.

7. An appreciation of the importance of the normal basic diet as a foundation for any therapeutic modification.
8. An appreciation of your role and responsibility in educating patients, their families, and community members in good nutrition habits.

WHAT KNOWLEDGE AND SKILLS WILL BE OF VALUE IN MEETING PATIENTS' NEEDS?

Knowledge

1. Characteristics of good and poor nutritional status.
2. Nutrients for good nutrition and their functions in the body.
3. Nutritive values of foods in the various food groups.
4. Nutritional needs of individuals in different age groups and under varying activities.
5. Daily food guides for good nutrition.
6. Ways the normal diet is modified for therapeutic purposes.
7. Principles of meal planning for nutritional adequacy and palatability.
8. Food economics and selection.
9. Principles of food preparation for economy, retention of nutrients, and palatability.
10. Food fads and fallacies.
11. Agencies concerned with problems of nutrition and health.

Skills

1. Ability to recognize outward signs of good and poor nutrition.
2. Ability to apply basic principles of nutrition to the wise selection of your own daily foods and to those of your family.
3. Ability to plan adequate and palatable meals for yourself and family.
4. Ability to prepare simple, nutritious meals, as necessary.
5. Ability to serve food attractively and correctly to yourself, your family, and patients.
6. Ability to make simple modifications in the normal diet to conform to doctor's therapeutic diet orders; or to adapt a family meal for the family member requiring nutritive therapy.
7. Ability to answer questions of patients regarding food and nutrition and help them understand reasons for their nutritive therapy and the need for their cooperation.

WHAT IS YOUR NUTRITION I.Q. AS YOU BEGIN NUTRITION STUDY?

Some of the following statements are true; some are false. Read each question and then check your answer in the appropriate column, before you consult the list of correct answers at bottom of page 9.

	True	False
1. Toasted bread has the same number of calories as untoasted bread.	_____	_____
2. Rice, spaghetti, and macaroni have the same food value as potatoes.	_____	_____
3. Brown eggs have the same nutritive value as white eggs.	_____	_____
4. Gelatin is a "good" source of protein.	_____	_____
5. Fish and celery are brain foods.	_____	_____
6. Everyone should eat a good source of protein such as milk, or eggs, or meat, or fish, or poultry at every meal.	_____	_____
7. More food is needed when studying for examinations.	_____	_____
8. A diet for reducing should have fewer calories than a person needs but should have adequate amounts of protein, minerals, and vitamins.	_____	_____
9. Proteins and starches should not be eaten in the same meal.	_____	_____
10. Margarine and butter contain the same number of calories.	_____	_____
11. Vegetable juices have magic health-giving properties.	_____	_____
12. Frozen orange juice has the same food value as fresh orange juice.	_____	_____
13. All fruits and vegetables should be eaten raw.	_____	_____
14. Sour cream contains the same number of calories as sweet cream.	_____	_____
15. Milk and cheese are constipating foods.	_____	_____
16. One never outgrows the need for milk in the diet.	_____	_____
17. "Wonder foods" such as yogurt and blackstrap molasses help keep one young and fit.	_____	_____
18. Water is fattening.	_____	_____
19. There is no danger in eating fish or seafood and milk, or milk and cherries, or milk and tomatoes, in the same meal.	_____	_____
20. A well person who eats the right kinds and amounts of foods every day does not need to take vitamin pills.	_____	_____
21. Skipping meals is a good way to lose weight safely.	_____	_____
22. One must not drink water when trying to lose weight.	_____	_____
23. No food can be considered "fattening" or "slenderizing."	_____	_____
24. Natural sweets like honey have fewer calories than sugar.	_____	_____
25. Craving for a certain food does not mean that the body needs it.	_____	_____
26. Pasteurized milk has the same food value and is safer than unpasteurized milk.	_____	_____
27. Drinking water at meal time may aid digestion if it is not used to wash down food.	_____	_____
28. There is no danger in using aluminum cooking utensils in food preparation.	_____	_____
29. Vegetables eaten whole or simply cut up for preparation		

	True	False

are more nutritious than if put through a vegetable juicer.

30. People need calcium (milk) in their diets even after they are full grown adults and their bones are formed.

31. A teenager needs more milk every day than a pre-schooler.

32. A combination of honey and vinegar has special healthful properties.

33. Only a doctor can determine whether a person needs to take vitamin pills or concentrates.

34. "Fad diets" for reducing are not only ineffective for permanent weight reduction but they may be dangerous as well.

35. A daily diet containing the right amounts of milk, some meat or fish or poultry or eggs, fruits, vegetables, and enriched or whole grain breads and cereals will provide all the nutrients needed for good nutrition.

36. Most diseases are due to faulty diet.

37. At least one serving of a "good" protein should be eaten at every meal.

38. "Starve a fever and feed a cold."

39. Foods grown on poor soil or where chemical fertilizers are used have lower nutritional value than those grown in good soil.

40. True weight loss cannot be accomplished by reducing the amount of water in the diet.

41. "Enriched" foods are valuable in the diet because they contain added nutrients in kinds and amounts.

42. Brittle fingernails are improved by taking some gelatin in fruit juice several times daily.

43. Poor diets eaten by teenagers are deficient in several important nutrients.

44. Fruit juices cause an "acid reaction" in the body.

45. Some foods rich in vitamin C should be eaten daily as the body cannot store this vitamin.

Number correct answers _____
Number incorrect answers _____

How good do you think your Nutrition Score is?

Correct answers:

1. T	8. T	16. T	24. F	32. F	40. T
2. F	9. F	15. F	23. T	31. T	39. F
3. T	10. T	18. F	22. F	30. T	38. F
4. F	11. F	14. T	21. F	29. T	37. T	45. T
5. F	12. T	13. F	20. T	28. T	36. F	44. F
6. T	14. T	19. T	27. T	35. T	43. T
7. F		17. F	26. T	34. T	42. F
			25. T	33. T	41. T

MY "FOOD AND NUTRITION EXPERIENCE" DIARY

To help make you "food and nutrition-minded" as you study nutrition, jot down below any out-of-class food and nutrition comments, questions, or experiences you encounter in discussions with individuals and later as you give nursing care to patients (checking menus, setting up and/or observing and serving trays, feeding patients, etc.)

Date   *Food and Nutrition Experience*   *Comments*

Unit One

FOOD, NUTRITION, AND HEALTH

PART 1.   RELATION OF NUTRITION TO HEALTH

PART 2.   GUIDES FOR GOOD NUTRITION

Object

To discuss the meaning of health and the factors affecting health; ways food and nutrition contribute to health; the meaning, characteristics and evaluation of good nutrition; agencies interested in American and global nutrition; the development of food habits; recommended dietary allowances for nutrients; dietary guides; and also to record and evaluate one's own health and dietary habits.

PART 1.   RELATION OF NUTRITION TO HEALTH

HOW IS HEALTH DEFINED?

Health, as defined by the World Health Organization of the United Nations, is "a state of complete physical, mental, and social well-being, and not merely the absence of disease or infirmity."[1] While it is possible to have good nutrition without good health, the best or optimal health is impossible without good nutrition.

Great progress has occurred over the past 70 years in the improvement of the health of peoples. The increase in longevity is one example, average span of life now being 70 years as compared to 49 years in 1900. The control of preventable disease, particularly in the case of young folks, and also better nutrition for all are considered reasons for this increase in longevity. "Curative" medicine has been largely replaced by "preventive" medicine or, as termed by some, "productive health."

WHAT FACTORS AFFECT ONE'S STATE OF HEALTH?

Many factors affect one's state of health, such as proper functioning of all body organs, posture, good health and hygiene habits, a good mental attitude, and the correction of remediable defects. The figure on the following page indicates that the same factors which promote good nutrition also promote good health. It is

---

[1] *World Health Organization—What It Is, What It Does, How It Works.* Leaflet, Geneva, Switzerland. World Health Organization, 1956.

generally agreed that one of the most important environmental factors affecting health—of an individual, a community, or a nation—is good nutrition.

HOW ARE FOOD, NUTRITION, AND HEALTH RELATED?

Optimal (best or most favorable) health is founded on good nutrition. The right kinds and amounts of food and good dietary habits throughout the entire life cycle mean healthier bodies and minds, greater vitality and energy, greater resistance to disease, efficiency, happiness, and longevity. The role played by food in promoting and maintaining good health is, therefore, a major one. In other words, "food becomes our nutrition." Its role in fulfilling nonmetabolic needs of a social, socioeconomic, and emotional type needs to be recognized as well.

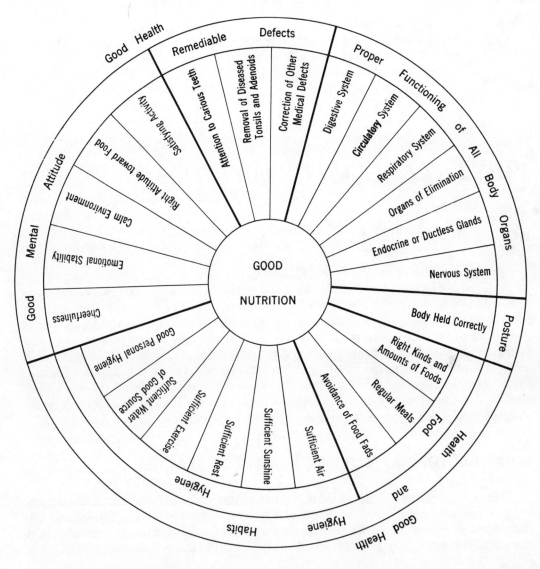

Factors in health and nutrition. (From M. T. Dowd and A. Dent, *Elements of Foods and Nutrition,* 2nd ed. New York, John Wiley and Sons, Inc., 1945.)

Personal aspects of good nutrition are far-reaching for the individual, since the assurance of one's own good health favors accomplishment and happiness. Good nutrition is likewise a community asset, paying valuable dividends. Continuing awareness of its importance has resulted in some improvements in dietary habits for many and lessened manifest nutritional deficiencies. However, there is still room for dietary improvement as a fairly large percentage of the population of every community exhibits partial dietary deficiencies. The international aspects of good nutrition are evidenced in the many world betterment programs under way.

Insufficient food (calories) and deficiencies of protein, minerals, and vitamins in the diet all affect physical fitness and work capacity. It has even been demonstrated that mental ability, associated with personality changes, as well as physical ability may be affected by a very poor diet.

WHAT STUDIES SHOW THAT FOOD REALLY MAKES A DIFFERENCE IN HEALTH?

1. Measurable improvement in growth, marked reduction of respiratory diseases, enlarged tonsils, minor illness and also unmeasurable changes in better school work and greater liveliness in work and play were noted by physicians in a large number of school children whose daily milk consumption was increased from one to three glasses over a period of two to three years.
2. Improvement in growth and bone development were noted in a group of children in a boarding school when one pint of milk was added daily to the usual meals served each child.
3. The blood of donors who ate an extra serving of meat daily after giving blood became normal at the end of two months instead of after the usual three months period.
4. A study of the physique and health of two African tribes showed that the tribe using meat and milk in daily meals had better health records, were taller by several inches, weighed more by several pounds, and were ill less often than the other tribe who lived chiefly on cereals, potatoes, and beans.
5. Several hundred Royal Air Force recruits who failed to pass army physical examinations were given extra fruit and milk in their diet for nearly a year and were allowed plenty of time for rest and exercise. Upon reexamination, 87 per cent passed the same physical examination they had previously failed.
6. Meat, milk, fruit, and vegetables added to the diets (rated poor) of pregnant women resulted in improved health of these pregnant mothers. They showed better general health, shorter labor period, and more success in nursing than pregnant women continuing on the poor diets. The babies of the mothers who received the additions to the diet were stronger, were ill less often, and none of them were premature.
7. A group of children in an Illinois school made slow gains in growth on diets which failed to meet daily requirements for all nutrients except vitamin A. After a year on the same diet plus additional milk and milk products, eggs, whole-grain cereals and fruit juice, their growth gains more than doubled previous gains.
8. In a breakfast study, schoolboys who omitted breakfast showed undesir-

able attitudes and poor scholastic work. Men and women who ate break-fasts supplying at least one-fourth of the daily needs could do more work and were more alert mentally than when they skipped breakfast or had only coffee.

9. Various observations on diets consumed by industrial workers demon-strated that those workers eating a nutritionally adequate diet showed less fatigue, greater efficiency, less absenteeism due to illness, and less prone-ness to accidents.

10. Medical examination of residents of Newfoundland, Canada, revealed symptoms of deficiencies in vitamins known to be low in their diet. Their flour was enriched with three B vitamins and their margarine was fortified with vitamins, A and D. Reexamined four years later, they showed im-provement—less mouth and face inflammation, fewer complaints of di-gestive disturbances and constipation, and greater alertness, especially in children; beriberi, previously widespread, was not in evidence.

11. Beriberi (due to a deficiency of thiamine, a B-complex vitamin) was reduced 90 per cent in an experimental zone in the Philippines when rice was en-riched. In a similar section where the people continued to eat unenriched rice, the number of deaths from beriberi increased.

WHAT ARE THE FUNCTIONS OF FOOD IN NUTRITION?

By definition, food is any material, solid or liquid, which after ingestion, diges-tion, and absorption from the intestinal tract is used to build and maintain body tissues, regulate body processes, and supply energy (calories). Any given food is a mixture of certain elements such as the minerals (calcium, phosphorus, sodium, iron, etc.) and certain compounds (carbohydrates, fats, proteins, some vitamins) and water, any of which is called a nutrient.

A nutrient is, therefore, any substance which performs one or more functions in the body. Nutrients include carbohydrates, fats, proteins, minerals, vitamins, and water. Some nutrients function in more than one way. Any single food might contain only one nutrient (carbohydrate in sugar) or several nutrients (protein, fat, calcium, vitamin A in milk). A variety of foods in the diet in the correct amounts will provide all the necessary nutrients (about 50 when the various amino acids, minerals, and vitamins are counted) in the correct amounts.

The chart on the following page shows the functions of food, the nutrients performing these functions, and the common food sources of the nutrients.

WHAT IS MEANT BY NORMAL OR GOOD NUTRITION?

Normal nutrition is defined as a "condition of the body resulting from the efficient utilization of sufficient amounts of the essential nutrients provided in the food intake."[2]

"Nutriture or nutritional status is the condition of physical health and well-being of the body as related to the consumption and utilization of food for growth, maintenance, and repair."[3] "Nutritional status may be good, fair, or poor, depending

---

[2] D. F. Turner, *Handbook of Diet Therapy*, 5th ed. Chicago, University of Chicago Press, 1970, p. 242.

[3] *Food, The Yearbook of Agriculture*, Washington, D. C., U. S. Department of Agriculture, 1959, p. 721.

FUNCTIONS OF FOOD IN NUTRITION

Function in Nutrition	*Nutrients*	*Foods*
1. Build and repair body tissue	Proteins	Meat, fish, poultry, eggs, milk, cheese, dried peas and beans, cereals, breads
	Minerals—Calcium	Milk, cheese, ice cream, collards, kale, mustard greens, turnip greens
	Iron	Lean meat, liver, eggs, green leafy vegetables, whole-grain and enriched cereals, dried peas and beans, dried fruits
	Water	See above.
2. Regulate body processes	Minerals	
	Vitamins—Vitamin A	Whole milk, butter, eggs, liver, dark green and yellow vegetables, fortified margarine, deep yellow or orange fruits
	Vitamin D	Vitamin D fortified milk, fish liver oils, sardines, salmon, tuna, small amounts in eggs
	Thiamine	Meat (pork high), fish, poultry, whole-grain and enriched bread and cereals
	Riboflavin	Milk, cheese, ice cream, meats, fish, poultry, eggs, liver, kidney
	Niacin	Lean meat, poultry, peanuts, beans, peas, whole-grain and enriched cereal products
	Ascorbic acid	Citrus fruits, strawberries, cantaloup, tomatoes, green peppers, broccoli, raw greens, cabbage, new potatoes
	Water	
	Proteins	See above.
3. Furnish energy	Carbohydrates	Sugars, sweets, molasses, flour, flour products, potatoes, starchy vegetables.
	Fats	Butter, margarine, shortenings, salad dressing, oils, meat fats, bacon, nuts, cream
	Also proteins to some extent; expensive source	See above.

not only on the intake of dietary essentials (nutrients) but on the relative need and the body's ability to utilize them."[4]

"Good nutritional status is noted when man benefits from the intake of a well-balanced diet. . . . Optimum nutrition means that the essential nutrients are supplied and utilized to maintain health and well-being at the highest possible level. It provides for a reserve. Good nutrition is essential for:

>   Normal organ development and function
>   Normal reproduction, growth, and maintenance
>   Optimum activity and working efficiency
>   Resistance to infection
>   Ability to repair bodily damage and injury.

"Poor nutritional status exists when man is deprived of an adequate amount of essential nutrients. This is relative. Demands may go up at times and the intake of food, being constant, may become inadequate."[5]

WHAT ARE THE CHARACTERISTICS OF GOOD NUTRITIONAL STATUS (NORMAL NUTRITION)?

Easily Observable Characteristics

Correct weight for height and age
Bones straight and without enlargements
Broad chest
Well-shaped head
Straight back with no protruding shoulder blades

Firm muscles
Smooth, clear, slightly moist skin of good color
Smooth glossy hair
Bright and alert eyes and expression
Well-formed jaws
Good posture
Unobstructed breathing

Less Easily Observable Characteristics

Sense of well-being
Absence of fatigue and tiredness
Good appetite
Restful sleep
Normal functioning of all processes: circulation, respiration, digestion, metabolism, elimination

Teeth well placed in jaws and free from caries
Cheerful disposition

Nutriture or nutritional status is appraised by
1. Determination of overweight and underweight
2. Clinical examination with special attention to the condition of the skin, eyes, mouth, tongue, gums, muscles
3. Blood pressure and pulse rate
4. Biochemical tests on the blood for various constituents associated with health
5. Tests of urine samples
6. Correlation of the above with a dietary history.

[4] Turner, op. cit., p. 242.
[5] M. V. Krause, *Food, Nutrition and Diet Therapy,* 4th edition. Philadelphia, W. B. Saunders Company, 1966 pp. 3–4.

HOW GOOD ARE AMERICAN DIETARY HABITS AND NUTRITION?[6]

The average American diet, as measured by the food available for consumption, is varied and sufficient to feed our population well. But, how well do Americans really eat and how good is their nutrition? Are we the best-fed nation in the world?

The first of several surveys (1940) of the food intake of men, women, and children in the United States made by the U.S. Department of Agriculture to evaluate food habits and their relation to nutritional status showed about one third of the diets to be nutritionally poor. These results gave impetus to the enrichment of flour and white bread with three of the B vitamins and iron, stimulated nutrition education programs, and indicated the need for a school lunch program.

In 1941 a nationwide program to promote better nutrition was launched at a National Nutrition Conference. Then the Food and Nutrition Board of the National Research Council established "Recommended Dietary Allowances" (RDA) of nutrients for different age and sex categories to provide a common goal for nutrition education. The 1968 revision of the RDA is shown on page 26.

A more intensive food intake study in 1955 showed fewer diets (about 10 per cent) to be poor nutritionally. Apparent improvement was thought to be due generally to better economic conditions, improved food marketing, flour and bread enrichment programs, and the broadening of nutrition programs in various agencies. However, many families were still not getting amounts of certain nutrients needed for good nutrition. The addition of synthetic nutrients to staple foods: vitamin D to milk; vitamin A to margarine; iron and certain vitamins to flour and white bread; and iodine to salt helped to improve American nutrition. This survey did provide data for new educational materials and the pilot stamp program and other food programs.

A nationwide dietary survey in 1965 showed that about half of U.S. households had "good diets" in which the Recommended Dietary Allowance for seven nutrients —protein, calcium, iron, vitamin A, thiamine, riboflavin, and ascorbic acid— was furnished. About a fifth had "poor diets" because they furnished less than two thirds of the Recommended Dietary allowance for one or more of the seven nutrients. The remainder of the households (about 30 percent) had diets between "good" and "poor."

Decreased use of milk and milk products (important calcium sources) and vegetables and fruits (most important sources of vitamins A and C) was chiefly responsible for the decline of "good diets" over the 10 year period. Agricultural Research Service food economists say that "if most U. S. households are to have good diets, *awareness* of foods to make up a good diet, a *desire* to choose these foods, and *sufficient money* to buy adequate food must become more universal." The following groups of persons are regarded as needing improved diets: adolescent girls and women age 9 through 64 years; older men and women; and infants and children under three years.

The 1965 survey emphasizes (1) intensified nutrition programs to guide all families, adapted to all age groups at all income levels (low *and* high), to meet nutritional needs in families' meals, snacks, and meals away from home and (2) increased consumption of milk and other good food sources of nutrients often found below

---

[6] Nutrition News, Sept.-Oct. 1969, and Press Releases 2/26/1968 and 2/19/1969, United States Department of Agriculture, adapted.

Recommended Dietary Allowances, and the use of enriched grain products and foods rich in iron, particularly for young children and for girls and women.

America is a land of plenty but the goal of the right kind and amount of food and optimum nutrition for every American has not yet been completely realized.

Even though overt clinical nutritional deficiencies are rare in this country, some of the numerous characteristics and symptoms associated with poor health may possibly be in the category of so-called sub-clinical deficiencies and be due to poor nutrition. The relation of nutrition to mental health, degenerative diseases, aging and dental caries provides a fertile field for study. The "National Nutrition Survey, begun in 1968 and being carried out by the U. S. Department of Health, Education and Welfare, the first comprehensive effort to assess nutritional status of the U. S. population, found an unexpectedly high prevalence of conditions associated with malnutrition".[7]

WHAT U. S. AGENCIES HELP TO IMPROVE NUTRITION?

"The basic tools to get food to people who are too poor, too young, too old, or too handicapped to provide fully for themselves are to be found in several food assistance programs of the Food and Nutrition Service of the United States Department of Agriculture." Operated through federal, state, and local governments, the tools (they must be activated locally, by public officials, private organizations, and volunteer citizens) can provide the following: FOOD FOR FAMILIES—(1) Donated Foods or (2) Food Stamps to low-income families at home, and (3) Supplemental Foods for health or selected highly nutritious foods to needy pregnant women, new mothers, and infants and young children; CHILD NUTRITION PROGRAMS—(1) School Breakfast, (2) School Lunch in elementary and secondary public and non-profit schools, and (3) Preschool Summer Food service and meals to preschool children in day-care centers and similar organized away-from-home activities.[8]

The Consumer and Food Economics Research Service and the Food and Nutrition Service of the U. S. Department of Agriculture are interested in the nutrition of the American family. Three branches of the U. S. Department of Health, Education and Welfare, namely the Children's Bureau, Food and Drug Administration, and Public Health Service, conduct nutrition research and/or provide services. Consult Unit Five, page 176, for a list of other federal, state, and local governmental agencies, non-governmental organizations, educational and industrial institutions, and private agencies interested in the nutritional welfare of the American family.

WHAT ARE WORLD PROBLEMS IN NUTRITION AND WHAT ARE THE INTERESTED AGENCIES?

Several World Food Surveys made from 1946 to 1963, the last one covering the largest number of countries and representing a very large percentage of the population, showed that the average total food intake (calories) as well as that of animal

[7] M. S. Read, "Malnutrition and Learning," Bethesda, Md., U.S. Department of Health, Education and Welfare, Public Health Service, National Institutes of Health, 1969.

[8] Tools to Fight Malnutrition, Leaflets, Food and Nutrition Service, U. S. Department of Agriculture, 1970, adapted.

protein of peoples in the less well developed countries is far below nutritional requirements. It was estimated that as much as one fifth of the population of these areas were undernourished and between one half to two thirds malnourished. The extent of calorie-protein malnutrition among children was extremely marked. Practically all nutritional deficiencies are still to found in many parts of the world, with lack of enough foods (calories) or the proper foods accounting for serious world nutrition problems.

The United States has developed various programs and campaigns over the years to assist developing countries in combating malnutrition by improving their food production through better agricultural practices and food technology and better and more complete use of their own food resources. The U. S. Foreign Aid and Food for Freedom programs and activities of AID (Agency for International Development) are coordinated with some or all of the following United Nations agencies which are interested in studying and improving nutritional standards all over the world.

FAO, the United Nations Food and Agriculture Organization studies various angles of world food problems, especially raising nutrition standards.

WHO, the World Health Organization concerns itself with health problems of the world.

UNESCO, the United Nations Educational, Scientific and Cultural Organization is interested in improving the standard of living of peoples all over the world.

UNICEF, the United Nations International Children's Emergency Fund has directed the distribution of milk to children all over the world through emergency relief, school feeding, and maternal and child health centers.

The activities of FAO, WHO, and UNESCO are coordinated by a joint Nutrition Advisory Committee of experts from different countries.

HOW DO FOOD AND DIETARY PATTERNS DEVELOP?

Our food selection patterns are habits which have been acquired in many different ways over the period of our lifetime. The cultural, religious, or regional groups in which we find ourselves are responsible for certain of our food patterns. Customs within individual family groups are influential in the development of likes and dislikes, "accepted" or "rejected" foods and certain eating habits. Many dietary habits in the individual can be traced to early association, pleasant or otherwise, of food with people, places, or events of one kind or another.

More recently recognized as powerful influences in our food choices and habits are emotional and psychological needs. Our physiological needs as a source of dietary habits are probably the least influential in the establishment of patterns. Unfortunately, lacks in our daily diet do not immediately show up in effects on the body, so we do not immediately become aware of the significance of food. Also, the food faddist and self-styled "nutrition specialist" (with very little or, more frequently, no knowledge of nutrition but with a product or idea to sell) influences food choice for far too many persons.

Improvement in food selection patterns (for bettering one's health) frequently means changing habits of long standing. This is a slow, step-by-step, almost never-ending process for which a real desire to change and a deep conviction that change is important (due to good teaching), and the willingness to substitute desirable food habits for undesirable ones are necessary. Persons dealing with nutrition improvement, while primarily concerned with the metabolic role of food in health, must also have some understanding of the circumstances under which diet habits are acquired and the various meanings food may have for different individuals (its nonmetabolic significance). This is especially true in dealing with patients whose disorder or disease imposes drastic changes in dietary habits if a cure is to be effected.

Since there appears to be no doubt that many nutritional deficiencies are due to poor dietary habits, the establishment of correct habits early in life and adherence to such throughout life is of extreme importance. A good diet insures good nutrition. The nurse has a unique opportunity in fostering good food habits.

TERMS TO UNDERSTAND

Nutrition	Normal nutrition	Optimal nutrition	Malnutrition
Health	Nutriture	Food functions	Nutritional deficiency
Food	Therapeutic nutrition	Science of nutrition	Dietetics
Nutrient	Nutritional status	Undernutrition	

STUDY QUESTIONS AND ACTIVITIES

1. Why should everyone have some knowledge of nutrition?

2. List five important factors which promote good nutrition and give an example of each.

3. List some characteristics of good nutritional status under the following headings: appearance, physical well-being, mental health.

4. What are the functions of food in nutrition? Which nutrients perform each function?

5. Be able to cite several instances which show that a change in diet improves nutrition.

6. Why are good food habits important? How are they formed? How can they be improved?

7. What is meant by the following statement: "Nutrition is an important aspect of nursing care"?

8. What are five good food habits for you to acquire and follow daily?

9. What does "food" mean to you? Write about 100 words on "What Food Means to Me."

10. List the foods you like; the foods you dislike; your good food habits; your poor food habits. How do you account for each item listed?

SUPPLEMENTARY READING[9]

Yearbook U.S.D.A., 1959, pages 1–22   Read: Malnutrition and Learning. 1969
Bogert: Chapters 1, 28   Mowry: Chapter 1   Robinson: Chapters 1, 2
Howe: Chapters 1, 2   Peyton: Chapter 1
    Leverton, R. M., *How Nutrition Relates to Learning*. Food and Nutrition, Food and Nutrition Service, U. S. Department of Agriculture, Washington. Vol. 1, No. 4, 1971, p. 12

---

[9] Sources of further reading are given at the end of each chapter, identified by the name of the author. Full references are given in the Appendix, page 291.

HOW GOOD IS YOUR HEALTH AND NUTRITION?

1. Does *your weight* meet the figure given by height-weight tables for persons of your height and age?[10]

    My height ___5'1½"___ inches (shoes with 1 inch heels).

    I weigh ___101___ pounds (indoor clothing).

    My desirable weight is _____ pounds

    I am _____ pounds over/under my desirable weight, which equals _____ per cent.

    Keep a record of your weight during your practical nurse training period, weighing yourself *weekly* on the same scales, at the same time of day, and with approximately the same amount of clothing.

    Date   *Wt.*   *Date*   *Wt.*   *Date*   *Wt.*   *Date*   *Wt.*

2. Using the graph paper on the following page, chart your weekly weight for the duration of your course. At left side of sheet, show pounds; along lower edge the weekly dates. Mark your weight *each week* and connect the marks with straight lines to show your weight curve.

3. What is your *Health Score*? Using the Health Score on page 23 check your state of health. Where a question applies, check the deduction score. Then add all deductions and subtract from 100 (the perfect score) to obtain your score.

HOW WELL DO YOU EAT?

1. Keep a record of your food intake, at meals and between meals, for one week on the chart on page 24.
2. Score your diet for each day and determine your average score for the week on the Food Selection Score Card on page 25.
3. What conclusions can you draw regarding your weight, health, and food and nutrition habits?

    What do you think may be possible causes for any low scores?

Check below.

Poor prenatal or early nutrition

Infection from teeth, tonsils, sinuses, etc.

Bad food habits:
  Overeating
  Eating too fast
  Irregular meals
  Lack of bulk
  Lack of water
  Lack of vitamins
  Lack of minerals

Constipation

Poor posture

Excessive use of tea or coffee

Cathartic habit

Lack of sleep and rest

Lack of exercise

Lack of fresh air—night or day

Glandular disorders

Overfatigue

Carelessness—neglect

Poorly fitting shoes

Incorrect seating

Disorders of stomach, heart, liver, kidneys

Can you do anything about any of the items you checked above? Explain.

---

[10] Consult Height–Weight Table on page 292.

WEIGHT CURVE CHART

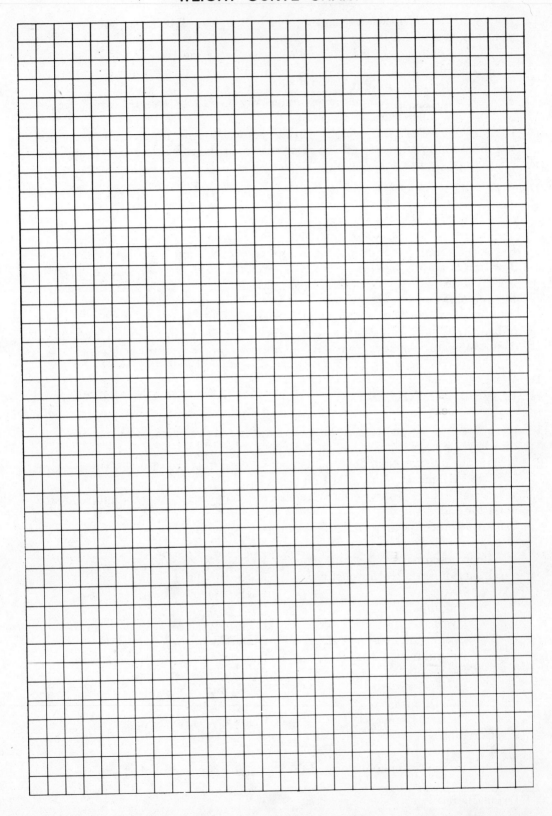

HEALTH SCORE

Deduct

1. Are you often tired? 2
2. Do you sleep less than 8 hours out of 24?................3
3. Do you ever sleep with windows closed? 2
4. Do you have more than one cold a year? 2
5. Are your nerves "jumpy"? Are you irritable? Do you lose your temper easily? 3
6. Do you worry needlessly?........1
7. Are you short of breath? 2
8. Do you have at least one hour's recreation or exercise in open air daily? 2
9. Do you have a good appetite for *all* foods? 4
10. Do you have indigestion? 2
11. Do you have sick headaches? 3
12. Do you have a coated tongue? ...1
13. Do you have bad breath? 1
14. Are you troubled with constipation? 5
15. Do you take less than two baths each week? 2
16. Do you ever handle food without washing your hands?....1
17. Do you have pains in your joints? 2
18. Do you have flat feet? 1
19. Do you have calluses on the bottoms of your feet? 1
20. Do you have corns? 1
21. Do you have a bent big toe with an enlarged joint? 1
22. Do you have weak ankles?.......1
23. Are you round shouldered? 2
24. Is your chest flat? 1
25. Have you a prominent abdomen? 1
26. Have you a sway back?..........1

Deduct

27. Have you winged shoulder blades? 1
28. Are you 10 to 20% underweight? 4
    Are you 10 to 20% overweight? .4
29. Are you 20% or more underweight? 5
    Are you 20% or more overweight?....................5
30. Are you deaf in one ear? 2
31. Are you deaf in both ears? 4
32. Do you have earache? 2
33. Do you have your teeth examined by a dentist less than once a year? 3
34. Do you brush your teeth less than twice a day? 4
35. Are your gums inflamed, soft, and bleeding? 3
36. Do you have decayed, uncared for teeth? 5
37. Do you have sore throat? 3
38. Do you breathe through your mouth? 4
39. Do you have pimples or other skin eruptions? 3
40. Is your skin sallow and colorless? 3
41. Do you have dark circles under your eyes? 1
42. Are your eyelids inflamed? 1
43. Have your eyes been tested in the last three years? 1
44. Do you neglect to wear glasses, if necessary? 2
45. Do you squint and scowl? 1
46. Is your hair thin? 2
47. Does your hair lack luster? 1
48. Do you have dandruff? 1

Total deductions ....

Subtract from 100 for total score _____

	BREAKFAST	BREAKFAST	BREAKFAST	BREAKFAST	BREAKFAST	BREAKFAST	BREAKFAST
	Orange juice, toast, bacon, egg 2, coffee	orange juice, cereal, coffee	orange juice, toast, coffee	orange juice, cereal, coffee			
	Orange juice, toast, cereal, milk, sugar, coffee						

	DINNER	DINNER	DINNER	DINNER	DINNER	DINNER	DINNER
	tossed salad, broiled fish, rice, lima beans	Roast beef, mashed potato, gravy, corn, celery + carrot sticks	hamburger, roll, french fries, pudding	Sausage, brown potatoes, green beans, rice pudding, baked apple, cake			
	Ham sandwich, potato chips, apple, cupcake, tea						

	SUPPER OR LUNCH	SUPPER OR LUNCH	SUPPER OR LUNCH	SUPPER OR LUNCH	SUPPER OR LUNCH	SUPPER OR LUNCH	SUPPER OR LUNCH
	tomato soup, grilled cheese sandwich, ice cream	noodle soup, bologna + cheese sand., ice cream	bologna + cheese sandwich, potato chips, banana, tea	tuna salad, rice pudding, fruit, tea			
	macaroni + cheese, stewed tomatoes, apple sauce						

	EXTRAS	EXTRAS	EXTRAS	EXTRAS	EXTRAS	EXTRAS	EXTRAS
	tangerine, popcorn	apple, potato chips	cookies	cake			
EXTRAS							

FOOD SELECTION SCORE CARD

Score your diet for each day and determine your average score for the week. If your final score is between 85 and 100, your food selection standard has been good. A score of from 75 to 85 indicates a fair standard. A score below 75 indicates a low standard.

MAXIMUM SCORE FOR EACH FOOD GROUP	CREDITS	COLUMNS FOR DAILY CHECK
20	Milk Group: Milk (including foods prepared with milk as cheese and ice cream) Adults: 1 glass, 10; 1½ glasses, 15; 2 glasses, 20 Children: 1 glass, 5; 1½ glasses, 10; 2 glasses, 15; 4 glasses, 20*	
25	Meat Group: Eggs, Meat, Cheese, Fish, Poultry, Dry Peas, Dry Beans, and Nuts 1 serving of any one of above, 10 1 serving of any two above, 20 If liver (beef, lamb, pork, or calf's) or kidney is used, extra credit, 5	
35	Vegetable—Fruit Group: Vegetables: 1 serving, 5; 2 servings, 10; 3 servings, 15 Potatoes may be included as one of the above servings If dark green or deep-yellow vegetable is included, extra credit, 5 Fruits: 1 serving, 5; 2 servings, 10 If citrus fruit, raw vegetable, or canned tomatoes are included, extra credit, 5†	
15	Bread—Cereal Group; Bread—dark whole grain, enriched or restored Cereals—dark whole grain, enriched or restored 2 servings of either, 10; 4 servings of either, 15	
5	Water (total liquid including milk, coffee, tea, or other beverage): Adults: 6 glasses, 2½; 8 glasses, 5 Children: 4 glasses, 2; 6 glasses, 5	
100	Final Score	

* Count 1/2 cup milk in soups, puddings, cream pies.

† Count 1/2 serving vegetables in soups or fruit in salad.

Deductions from final score: Each meal omitted, 10; Meals at irregular hours, 5; "Snacking" between meals, 5; Excessive soft drinks, 10.

From M. V. Krause, *Food, Nutrition and Diet Therapy,* 4th edition. Philadelphia, W. B. Saunders Co., 1966, adapted, p. 17.

FOOD AND NUTRITION BOARD, NATIONAL ACADEMY OF SCIENCES-NATIONAL RESEARCH COUNCIL

RECOMMENDED DAILY DIETARY ALLOWANCES,[a] Revised 1968

Designed for the maintenance of good nutrition of practically all healthy people in the U.S.A.

	Age[b] (years) From–Up to	Weight (kg)	Weight (lbs)	Height (cm)	Height (in.)	kcal	Protein (gm)	Vitamin A Activity (IU)	Vitamin D (IU)	Vitamin E Activity (IU)	Ascorbic Acid (mg)	Folacin[c] (mg)	Niacin (mg equiv)[d]	Riboflavin (mg)	Thiamin (mg)	Vitamin B6 (mg)	Vitamin B12 (μg)	Calcium (g)	Phosphorus (g)	Iodine (μg)	Iron (mg)	Magnesium (mg)
Infants	0–1/6	4	9	55	22	kg × 120	kg × 2.2[e]	1,500	400	5	35	0.05	5	0.4	0.2	0.2	1.0	0.4	0.2	25	6	40
	1/6–1/2	7	15	63	25	kg × 110	kg × 2.0[e]	1,500	400	5	35	0.05	7	0.5	0.4	0.3	1.5	0.5	0.4	40	10	60
	1/2–1	9	20	72	28	kg × 100	kg × 1.8[e]	1,500	400	5	35	0.1	8	0.6	0.5	0.4	2.0	0.6	0.5	45	15	70
Children	1–2	12	26	81	32	1,100	25	2,000	400	10	40	0.1	8	0.6	0.6	0.5	2.0	0.7	0.7	55	15	100
	2–3	14	31	91	36	1,250	25	2,000	400	10	40	0.2	8	0.7	0.6	0.6	2.5	0.8	0.8	60	15	150
	3–4	16	35	100	39	1,400	30	2,500	400	10	40	0.2	9	0.8	0.7	0.7	3	0.8	0.8	70	10	200
	4–6	19	42	110	43	1,600	30	2,500	400	10	40	0.2	11	0.9	0.8	0.9	4	0.8	0.8	80	10	200
	6–8	23	51	121	48	2,000	35	3,500	400	15	40	0.2	13	1.1	1.0	1.0	4	0.9	0.9	100	10	250
	8–10	28	62	131	52	2,200	40	3,500	400	15	40	0.3	15	1.2	1.1	1.2	5	1.0	1.0	110	10	250
Males	10–12	35	77	140	55	2,500	45	4,500	400	20	40	0.4	17	1.3	1.3	1.4	5	1.2	1.2	125	10	300
	12–14	43	95	151	59	2,700	50	5,000	400	20	45	0.4	18	1.4	1.4	1.6	5	1.4	1.4	135	18	350
	14–18	59	130	170	67	3,000	60	5,000	400	25	55	0.4	20	1.5	1.5	1.8	5	1.4	1.4	150	18	400
	18–22	67	147	175	69	2,800	60	5,000	400	30	60	0.4	18	1.6	1.4	2.0	5	0.8	0.8	140	10	400
	22–35	70	154	175	69	2,800	65	5,000	—	30	60	0.4	18	1.7	1.4	2.0	5	0.8	0.8	140	10	350
	35–55	70	154	173	68	2,600	65	5,000	—	30	60	0.4	17	1.7	1.3	2.0	5	0.8	0.8	125	10	350
	55–75+	70	154	171	67	2,400	65	5,000	—	30	60	0.4	14	1.7	1.2	2.0	6	0.8	0.8	110	10	350
Females	10–12	35	77	142	56	2,250	50	4,500	400	20	40	0.4	15	1.3	1.1	1.4	5	1.2	1.2	110	18	300
	12–14	44	97	154	61	2,300	50	5,000	400	20	45	0.4	15	1.4	1.2	1.6	5	1.3	1.3	115	18	350
	14–16	52	114	157	62	2,400	55	5,000	400	25	50	0.4	16	1.4	1.2	1.8	5	1.3	1.3	120	18	350
	16–18	54	119	160	63	2,300	55	5,000	400	25	50	0.4	15	1.5	1.2	2.0	5	1.3	1.3	115	18	350
	18–22	58	128	163	64	2,000	55	5,000	400	25	55	0.4	13	1.5	1.0	2.0	5	0.8	0.8	100	18	350
	22–35	58	128	163	64	2,000	55	5,000	—	25	55	0.4	13	1.5	1.0	2.0	5	0.8	0.8	100	18	300
	35–55	58	128	160	63	1,850	55	5,000	—	25	55	0.4	13	1.5	1.0	2.0	5	0.8	0.8	90	18	300
	55–75+	58	128	157	62	1,700	55	5,000	—	25	55	0.4	13	1.5	1.0	2.0	6	0.8	0.8	80	10	300
Pregnancy						+200	65	6,000	400	30	60	0.8	15	1.8	+0.1	2.5	8	+0.4	+0.4	125	18	450
Lactation						+1,000	75	8,000	400	30	60	0.5	20	2.0	+0.5	2.5	6	+0.5	+0.5	150	18	450

[a] The allowance levels are intended to cover individual variations among most normal persons as they live in the United States under usual environmental stresses. The recommended allowances can be attained with a variety of common foods, providing other nutrients for which human requirements have been less well defined. See text for more-detailed discussion of allowances and of nutrients not tabulated.

[b] Entries on lines for age range 22–35 years represent the reference man and woman at age 22. All other entries represent allowances for the midpoint of the specified age range.

[c] The folacin allowances refer to dietary sources as determined by *Lactobacillus casei* assay. Pure forms of folacin may be effective in doses less than 1/4 of the RDA.

[d] Niacin equivalents include dietary sources of the vitamin itself plus 1 mg equivalent for each 60 mg of dietary tryptophan.

[e] Assumes protein equivalent to human milk. For proteins not 100 percent utilized factors should be increased proportionately.

PART 2. GUIDES FOR GOOD NUTRITION

HOW ARE STANDARDS FOR NUTRIENT REQUIREMENTS SET UP?

"Nutrition is a science of the quantity, as well as the nature, of the substances we need from food for good health. Supplying some of any essential nutrient does not insure good nutrition: The body must have a large enough supply of each nutrient to meet all of its needs all of the time. A reserve supply in the body for use during emergencies is most desirable also.

"Good judgement must go into interpreting the results of investigations into the quantitative requirements for a nutrient and the application of the results to develop dietary standards or guides. . . . The Food and Nutrition Board of the National Academy of Sciences–National Research Council (appointed in 1940 to advise our government on matters of food and nutrition) is the scientific group in the United States that is assembled to interpret the results of research and to set up dietary standards. . . . One of the first responsibilities of this board was to develop a dietary guide for the United States—a guide that would state the amounts of calories and certain nutrients needed to keep the population of the country well nourished and that would be of help in planning adequate diets for healthy individuals and population groups."[11]

WHAT ARE RECOMMENDED DIETARY ALLOWANCES?

Formulations of daily nutrient intakes, designated as "Recommended Dietary Allowances" (RDA) and judged to be adequate for the maintenance of good nutrition in essentially all healthy persons in the United States under current conditions of living, have been developed by the Food and Nutrition Board. The first edition of RDA was published in 1943, and has been updated periodically as new nutritional research findings have become available. The 1968 revision appears on the preceding page. It includes the addition of nutrient amounts for a new age category, that of 18 to 22 year olds; tabular data on several nutrients not included in previous revisions: phosphorus, iodine, magnesium, vitamin B_6, vitamin E, vitamin B_{12} and folacin and separate tabulation of allowances for infants under 1 year of age in relation to energy needs.

Except for calorie requirements the RDA provide a margin of safety above the average physiological requirements to cover variations among individuals in the general population and to act as a buffer against increased needs during common stresses. They are not considered adequate to meet additional nutritional requirements imposed by disease or injury.

"The primary objective of the RDA is to permit and encourage the development

---

[11] *Food, The Yearbook of Agriculture.* Washington, D. C., U. S. Department of Agriculture 1959, p. 227.

of food practices by the population in the United States that will allow for the greatest dividends and disease prevention. With the exception of iron, patterns of food consumption and food supplies permit ready adaptation and compliance with the RDA."[12] Iron supplementation may be required.

HOW ARE RECOMMENDED ALLOWANCES TRANSLATED INTO FOODS FOR THE DAY?

The technical information supplied by "Recommended Dietary Allowances," sometimes referred to as "The Nutrition Yardstick," must be interpreted in terms of a selection of foods to be eaten daily if it is to be valuable from the practical standpoint. Various basic diet patterns may be devised to serve as guides in food selection. The "Basic Seven Food Groups" plan was early used for this purpose.

"A Daily Food Guide," (shown on the opposite page) by the Consumer and Food Economics Research Division, Agricultural Research Service, U. S. Department of Agriculture shows one way to choose daily foods wisely. Most foods contain more than one nutrient but no single food provides all the necessary nutrients in the correct amounts for good health. With the help of this guide, it is possible to obtain all the nutrients needed daily from a variety of common foods. Directions for using the guide are given below.

HOW IS THE DAILY FOOD GUIDE USED?[13]

The main part of your daily diet is selected from the four broad food groups shown on the chart on the opposite page and listed more fully on page 30.

In using the plan:

1. Choose at least the minimum number of servings from each of the broad food groups. Serving sizes will differ—small for young children, extra large (or seconds) for very active adults and teenagers. Pregnant and nursing women also require more food from these groups.
2. Make choices within each group according to suggestion under each food group. Foods within each group are similar, but not identical, in food value.
3. Choose the additional foods to round out your meals both from foods in the four food groups and from foods not listed in these groups. These additional foods should add enough calories to complete your food energy needs for the day. Children need enough food energy to support normal growth; adults need enough to maintain body weight at a level most favorable to health and well-being.
4. Try to have some meat, poultry, fish, eggs or milk at each meal.

---

[12] *Recommended Dietary Allowances,* 7th edition. Publication No. 1694. Washington, D. C., National Academy of Sciences—National Research Council, 1968, adapted.

[13] *Food for Fitness, A Daily Food Guide,* Leaflet No. 424. Washington, D. C., U. S. Department of Agriculture, Revised 1967, adapted.

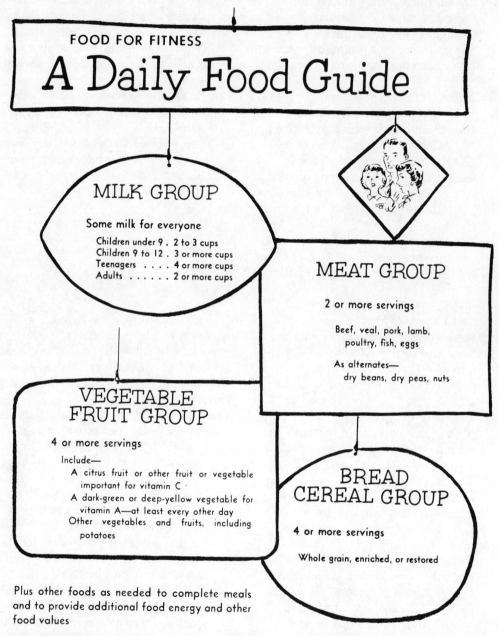

FOOD FOR FITNESS

A Daily Food Guide

MILK GROUP

Some milk for everyone

Children under 9 . 2 to 3 cups
Children 9 to 12 . 3 or more cups
Teenagers . . . . 4 or more cups
Adults . . . . . . 2 or more cups

MEAT GROUP

2 or more servings

Beef, veal, pork, lamb,
poultry, fish, eggs

As alternates—
dry beans, dry peas, nuts

VEGETABLE FRUIT GROUP

4 or more servings
Include—
A citrus fruit or other fruit or vegetable
important for vitamin C
A dark-green or deep-yellow vegetable for
vitamin A—at least every other day
Other vegetables and fruits, including
potatoes

BREAD CEREAL GROUP

4 or more servings

Whole grain, enriched, or restored

Plus other foods as needed to complete meals
and to provide additional food energy and other
food values

Food for Fitness, A Daily Food Guide. Leaflet No. 424. Washington, D. C., U. S. Department
of Agriculture, Revised 1967.

Milk Group

Some milk every day for everyone:

2 to 3 cups for children under 9

3 or more cups for children 9 to 12

4 or more cups for teenagers

2 or more cups for adults

3 or more cups for pregnant women

4 or more cups for nursing women

Use *Milk:*   fluid whole, evaporated, skim, dry, buttermilk

Cheese and ice cream may replace part of milk on basis of calcium content as follows:

1-inch cube cheddar-type cheese = 1/2 cup milk

1/2 cup cottage cheese = 1/3 cup milk

2 tablespoons cream cheese = 1 tablespoon milk

1/2 cup ice cream = 1/4 cup milk

Meat Group

2 or more servings every day

Use beef, veal, lamb, variety meats such as liver, heart, kidneys

Poultry and eggs; fish and shellfish

Alternates — dry beans, dry peas, lentils, nuts, peanuts, peanut butter

Count as one serving: 2 to 3 ounces of lean cooked meat, poultry, or fish — all without bone; 2 eggs; 1 cup cooked dry beans, dry peas, or lentils; 4 tablespoons peanut butter

Vegetable-Fruit Group

4 or more servings every day including:

(1) **1** *serving* of a *good* source of vitamin C *OR*

2 *servings* of a fair source of vitamin C

(2) **1** *serving at least every other day,* of a *good* source of vitamin A, such as dark green or deep yellow vegetables

(3) The remaining 1 to 3 servings may be any vegetable or fruit including those that are valuable for vitamin C and vitamin A.

Count as one serving: 1/2 cup vegetable or fruit or a portion as ordinarily served, such as 1 medium apple, banana, orange, or potato, or half a medium cantaloup or grapefruit, or juice of 1 lemon.

Bread-Cereal Group

4 servings or more daily. Or, if no cereals are chosen, have an extra serving of bread or baked goods which will make at least 5 servings from this group daily.

Use: all breads and cereals that are whole-grain, enriched, or restored (check label to be sure); breads, cooked cereals, ready-to-eat cereals, cornmeal, crackers, flour, grits, macaroni, spaghetti, rice, noodles, rolled oats, quick breads, and other baked goods if made with whole-grain or enriched flour. Parboiled rice and wheat may also be included in this group. Count as one serving: 1 slice bread, 1 oz. ready-to-eat cereal, 1/2 to 3/4 cup cooked cereal, cornmeal, grits, macaroni, noodles, rice or spaghetti.

Other Foods

To round out meals and to satisfy the appetite other foods not specified will be used by everyone, in amounts to maintain weight at the desired

Use: butter, margarine, and other fats, oils, sugars, unenriched refined grain products (often ingredients in baked goods and

level and to add to total nutrients of meals; also meet energy needs.

mixed dishes). Fats, oils, and sugars are also added to foods during preparation or at the table. Try to include some vegetable oil among the fats used.

HOW DO THE FOUR FOOD GROUPS SUPPLY NEEDED NUTRIENTS?

The Food Value Wheel is a handy visual reminder of nine of the 17 nutrients for which allowances have been recommended, and the food group which is the major source of each nutrient. The outside rim shows the four food groups. The inner rim of the wheel lists the name of nine key nutrients for which complete analytical data

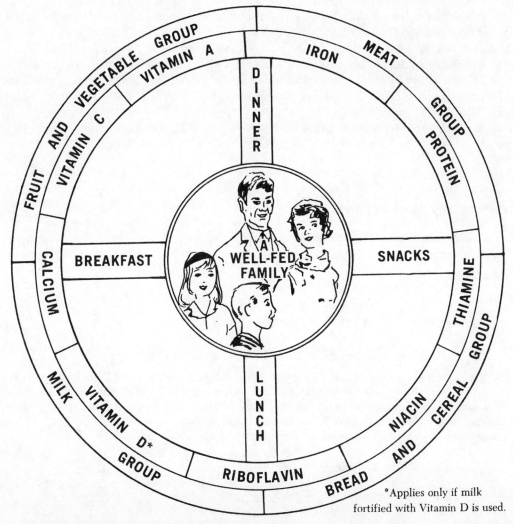

A Food Value Wheel. (From Home Economics Extension Leaflet 25. Ithaca, New York, New York State College of Home Economics. Revised 1965.)

regarding food supply and human needs are available. (See page 26 for RDA.) These recommendations are standards of plenty. They represent the amount of a nutrient required by the body plus extra amounts to provide for times of increased need and the wide differences between individual needs. At present, it is probable that diets furnishing adequate amounts of the nutrients on the Food Value Wheel will also supply sufficient quantities of all other nutrients needed by normally healthy individuals.

The selection, preparation for cooking, and the principles underlying correct food preparation will be discussed more fully in Unit Three, Part 1.

HOW CAN ONE LEARN THE NUTRITIVE VALUE OF A FOOD?

Information on the composition and nutritive value of over 2,000 food items is available in a publication by the U. S. Department of Agriculture: *Composition of Foods—Raw, Processed, Prepared.* (Agriculture Handbook No. 8. Washington, D. C., Agricultural Research Service, U. S. Department of Agriculture, 1963.)

A shorter table of nutritive values for common household measures of foods, based on a revised form of the above is: *Nutritive Value of Foods.* (Home and Garden Bulletin No. 72. Washington, D. C., U. S. Department of Agriculture, 1970.)

In the Appendix of this book you will find a still shorter food composition table: *Food Composition Table for Short Method of Dietary Analysis,* 3rd revision, Principles of Nutrition, by E. D. Wilson, K. H. Fisher and M. E. Fuqua, New York, John Wiley and Sons, 1965, pp. 528–533.

An additional food value table is: *Food Values of Portions Commonly Used,* 11th ed., by C. E. Church and H. N. Church. (Philadelphia, J. B. Lippincott Company, 1970.)

TERMS TO UNDERSTAND

RDA	Food composition	UNESCO
Daily Food Guide	WHO	UNICEF
Four Food Groups	FAO	

STUDY QUESTIONS AND ACTIVITIES

1. What is meant by Recommended Dietary Allowances?

2. Underline in *red pencil* the figures on the table of Recommended Dietary Allowances on page 26, which indicate the requirements for calories and each of the nutrients listed for a person of your age (in other words, *your* daily requirements for calories, protein, calcium, iron, vitamin A, thiamine, riboflavin, niacin, ascorbic acid, vitamin D) and jot them down below. You will be referring to these figures throughout the course.

My RDA:	Calories	2,000		Thiamine	1.0	mg.
	Protein	55	gm.	Riboflavin	1.5	mg.
	Calcium	0.8	gm.	Niacin	13	mg.
	Iron	18	mg.	Ascorbic acid	55	mg.
	Vitamin A	5000	I.U.	Vitamin D		I.U.

To call to your attention the additional seven nutrients which appear for the first time on the 1968 RDA, underline *in green your* daily requirements for vitamin E activity, folacin, vitamin B_6, vitamin B_{12}, phosphorus, iodine, and magnesium.

3. Why is breakfast such an important meal of the day? What constitutes a good breakfast? What are some of the dangers of skipping breakfast or eating an inadequate breakfast?

4. Review your week's diet record and score in Part 1 of this unit in the light of the more detailed daily food guide discussed on pages 28–32.

Can you see further improvements which it might be desirable for you to make in your daily food selection?

5. This menu was eaten by a teenager:

Breakfast:	Banana	Lunch:	Hot dog on roll	Dinner:	Broiled hamburger
	Cornflakes		Relish		Baked potato and
	Cream and sugar		Chocolate cake		margarine
	Toast, butter and		Coke		Harvard beets
	jelly				Cherry pie

Judge the meals according to the Four Food Group Diet Plan.
List the foods and amounts lacking for a teenager.

SUPPLEMENTARY READING:

Howe: Chapter 1   Mowry: Chapter 1   Peyton: Chapter 2
                                                      Bogert: Chapter 1
                                                      Robinson: Chapter 4
                                                      Yearbook; 1959: p. 267
                                                                  1965: p. 393

Note: Canadian Dietary Standards for adults and for boys and girls have been developed and published by the Canadian Council on Nutrition, an advisory group to the Canadian Department of National Health and Welfare. The latest revisions of these tables appear on pages 296 and 297 in the Appendix.

Unit Two

NUTRIENTS IN
FOOD AND NUTRITION

PART 1. CARBOHYDRATES

PART 2. FATS

PART 3. PROTEINS

PART 4. ENERGY REQUIREMENTS

PART 5. MINERALS AND WATER

PART 6. VITAMINS

PART 7. HOW THE BODY USES FOOD
(DIGESTION, ABSORPTION, METABOLISM)

Object

To study the characteristics, functions, daily requirements, best food sources, and the use by the body of the nutrients required for good nutrition; and evaluation of one's own diet for weight control and adequacy of essential nutrients.

PART 1. CARBOHYDRATES

WHAT ARE CARBOHYDRATES?

Carbohydrates, mostly plant products in origin, include sugars, starches, and cellulose and are composed of the elements carbon, hydrogen, and oxygen. Carbohydrates are formed by all green plants by a complex process known as photosynthesis. In this process sugar is first formed from carbon dioxide and water in a series of reactions, one or more of which are dependent upon the aid of sunlight and the green plant pigment known as chlorophyll. Some of the sugar remains in the plant sap; the rest of the sugar units can be converted into starch and other carbohydrates, even of very complex form. The dry matter of most plants is largely carbohydrate and provides energy directly when eaten as food by man and animals.

HOW DO CARBOHYDRATES FEATURE IN DIETS?

Cereals and cereal products, fruits, vegetables, sugars, and syrups are the chief sources of carbohydrates in the average diet. For a very large part of the world, grains of one sort or another and root vegetables constitute a major food source, ranging from the approximate 50 per cent in the American diet to a much higher proportion — as much as 80 per cent — in other countries. Wheat in the form of breads, cereals, and pastes (macaroni, noodles, spaghetti) feature in the Western world; corn in the diet of the Indians in America as well as in the diet of the Negro in the South; wheat and rye in Europe; wheat and rice in the Near East; and rice in the diet of Orientals.

Carbohydrates are the most readily available and easily digested of the energy foods and, in the case of breads, cereals, and potatoes, inexpensive. For this reason, they feature largely in diets at lower economic levels. They are also generally popular and palatable. Cereals can be grown almost every place and can be transported and stored easily. Refined sugar and cornstarch are the only pure carbohydrate foods.

From the early 1900's to the present time both the amount and types of carbohydrates have decreased in the American diet by almost 25 per cent. The consumption of flour, cereals, breads, and potatoes has decreased markedly; because of this a larger proportion of calories have been consumed as fat. A 25 per cent increase has occurred in the consumption of sugar and syrups. This increased consumption of sugar is thought by some nutritionists to be a factor in dental caries and obesity.[1]

WHAT ARE DIFFERENT KINDS AND SOURCES OF CARBOHYDRATES?

Carbohydrates are either small single units (molecules) or larger units, consisting of two units or several, or still larger and more complex ones consisting of many small units linked together. Those which have special significance in nutrition are the simple sugars—glucose, fructose, and galactose; the double sugars—sucrose, lactose, and maltose; and the more complex forms—starch, glycogen, and cellulose.

Simple Sugars
(monosaccharides)

Glucose   (grape sugar, corn sugar, dextrose): fruits, certain roots, corn, honey; less sweet than ordinary sugar; cheap; form of sugar in the blood; end product of all carbohydrate digestion; and form in which all carbohydrates are absorbed; only fuel central nervous system can use; form given for immediate energy (by mouth or intravenous) as it is ready for utilization; stored as glycogen in liver.

Fructose (fruit sugar):   honey; many fruits and vegetables; combined with glucose in ordinary sugar; gives characteristic flavor to honey.

Galactose: produced from lactose in milk; does not occur free in nature.

Double Sugars
(disaccharides; changed to simple sugars in digestion)

Sucrose (cane sugar, beet sugar, table sugar):   maple and other syrups; molasses; maple sugar; many fruits and vegetables

---

[1] Recommended Dietary Allowances, 7th edition, Publication No. 1694, Washington, D. C., National Academy of Sciences–National Research Council. 1968, pp. 9–10.

Lactose (milk sugar):   produced only by mammals; less soluble and less sweet than cane sugar and more slowly digested

Maltose (malt sugar):   malt and malt products; made from starch in sprouting grains; not free in nature; formed in change of starch to sugar during digestion; appears with dextrin (a polysaccharide) in a carbohydrate source for infant feeding.

Complex Compounds

(polysaccharides; many simple sugar units)

Starch: reserve store of carbohydrate in plants (grains, seeds, roots, potatoes, green bananas, other plants); changed to glucose in digestion through intermediate steps of dextrin and maltose.

Glycogen ("animal starch"):   body stores carbohydrate as glycogen in liver; constitutes reserve form of carbohydrate; quickly changed in body to and from glucose as necessary.

Cellulose (fiber):   pulp and skins of fruits and vegetables; structural parts of plants; coverings of seeds and outer covering of nuts; indigestible so it provides bulk and stimulation for intestinal tract; agar-agar and pectin (hemicelluloses related to cellulose) absorb water and add bulk to intestines; pectins in fruits and seeds give jellying properties; agar-agar gives thickening properties.

Dextrin: formed from starch breakdown by heat or in digestion (starch is converted to dextrin with toasting).

HOW DO CARBOHYDRATES FUNCTION IN NUTRITION?

Primary function: specific need for carbohydrate as energy source for brain and other specialized purposes; after these needs met, interchangeable with fat for energy and comparable in protein sparing; readily converted to fat. 1 gram carbohydrate yields 4 calories. Carbohydrates provide 40 to 50 per cent of calories in American diet.[2] (1 gram carbohydrate yields 4 calories).

Spare the burning of protein for energy (protein has more important functions).

Aid in the more efficient and complete oxidation (burning) of fats for energy.

As *sugar,* a quick energy producer.

As *starch,* provides most economical and abundant source of energy after change to glucose.

As *lactose*, has certain laxative properties (remains in intestine longer and encourages desirable bacterial growth).

As *cellulose* (insoluble and indigestible), aids in normal intestinal functioning.

WHAT ARE COMMON FOOD SOURCES OF CARBOHYDRATES?

Plant Sources

Cereal grains.   Rice, wheat, corn, oats, rye, barley, buckwheat, millet. Cereal grains also contain some protein, minerals and vitamins. Whole-grain and enriched sources contain iron and B complex vitamins.

---

[2] Ibid., p. 10.

Vegetables. Green leafy vegetables lowest in carbohydrates; roots, tubers, and seeds contain more carbohydrate; starchy vegetables—corn, dried peas and beans, and potatoes—contain the most. Sugar in fresh green peas changes to starch after harvesting. Vegetables also contain cellulose.

Fruits. Fruits contain a large proportion of water. Their carbohydrate content is mostly sugar and, except in dried fruits, it is low. Starch in immature bananas changes to sugar in ripening. They contain some cellulose. Nuts contain 10 to 20 per cent carbohydrate (also high in protein and fat).

Sweets. Ordinary table sugar, molasses, maple syrup and sugar, corn syrup, honey, sorghum syrup; concentrated with "empty" calories.

Animal Sources

None of importance except possibly lactose in milk; traces of glycogen in meat, poultry, fish, eggs, and small amounts in liver and scallops.

WHAT IS THE DAILY CARBOHYDRATE REQUIREMENT?

"Adaptation to diets very low in carbohydrate is possible but, in individuals accustomed to normal diets, at least 100 grams of carbohydrate per day appear to be needed. Since diets compatible with good health contain a widely varying proportion of carbohydrate, there is no basis for a recommended allowance."[3]

DIGESTION AND METABOLISM

In the mouth	In the stomach	In the small intestine		Absorption, small intestine	Metabolism
Starch	No action	Starch	Sucrose	In the form	Oxidized for
↓	except con-	↓	Lactose	of	energy to carbon
Dextrin	tinued action	Dextrin	Maltose	glucose	dioxide and water
	of ptyalin	↓	↓		
↓	until destroyed	Maltose	Glucose		Changed to
Maltose	by HCI	by action	by action of		glycogen and
by action of		of amylopsin	sucrase		stored in liver
ptyalin		(enzyme)	lactase		
(enzyme)			maltase		Changed to fat
			(enzymes)		and stored as
					fatty tissue

WHAT HAPPENS TO CARBOHYDRATES IN THE BODY?

Carbohydrates are easily digested and the degree of absorption is high. Digestion of starch starts in the mouth and is completed in the small intestine. Double sugars are digested in the small intestine.

Simple sugars like glucose and fructose are ready for absorption in the digestive tract. Double sugars like sucrose must be changed to simple sugars for absorption.

---

[3] Ibid., p. 10.

Complex carbohydrates like starch require two steps in digestion for their change to simple sugar (glucose) for absorption in the intestinal tract. Cooking starch facilitates digestion as it breaks down the cell walls, making easier the action of digestive enzymes. Cellulose (fiber) is indigestible and passes through the intestinal tract unchanged.

Glucose, formed from all carbohydrate in food eaten, is absorbed into the blood stream through the walls of the small intestine and metabolized as shown below.

WHAT IS MEANT BY "ENRICHMENT"?

Whole grain products contribute not only considerable amounts of carbohydrate to the diet but also some protein and appreciable amounts of some minerals and vitamins. When milled, to produce the popular white product with better keeping quality (with removal of bran layers and germ), most of the B vitamins—thiamine, riboflavin, and niacin—and iron are lost. The addition of these nutrients in synthetic form to cereals and their products or "enrichment" to replace those removed in the milling process is now approved. It is estimated that about 80 to 90 percent of the flour and bread on the market are enriched. Enrichment of other foods is mentioned on page 112.

WHAT ARE THE FUNCTIONS, REQUIREMENTS, AND SOURCES OF FIBER (CELLULOSE)?

Functions	*Requirements*	*Sources*
Indigestible carbohydrates: cellulose or fiber (roughage, bulk) acts as regulator.	Daily requirements vary among different individuals.	Vegetables and fresh fruits: 1 gram per serving.
Fiber facilitates good elimination by absorbing water.	Average requirement: 5–6 grams daily	Dried fruits: 1.5 grams per serving.
Body has no enzymes to digest cellulose or fiber.		Whole grain breads and cereals: 0.5 gram per serving.
Digestive juices and bacterial action soften tough fibers.		Nuts: 0.5 gram per ounce.
Intestinal muscular contractions reduce cellulose to smaller portions.		Average requiremnet of 5–6 grams provided by the average mixed diet including: 1 serving raw vegetable, 1 serving cooked vegetable; 2 servings fruit, one with skin; 1 serving whole grain cereal; several slices of whole grain bread.

TERMS TO UNDERSTAND

Carbohydrate	Hormone	Enzymes
Cellulose	Insulin	Enrichment
Pectin	Glycogen	Fiber
Agar-agar	Digestion	Roughage

STUDY QUESTIONS AND ACTIVITIES

1. What are the important food sources of carbohydrates?

2. What are the different kinds of carbohydrates?

3. In what ways, other than providing energy, are carbohydrates important in the diet?

4. What happens to carbohydrates in the body?

5. What is meant by the "fiber" or "bulk" or "roughage" content of food?

6. What happens to fiber in the body? Why can it not be digested even though it is a carbohydrate? What is its important function? What are food sources?

7. Is your fiber intake adequate for your needs? Do you require bran or other additional bulk in your diet for the proper functioning of your intestinal tract? If so, do you think you could choose your foods more carefully so as to include more fruits, vegetables, and whole wheat products and rely on the use of bran or other bulk only occasionally, if at all?

8. What might be the dangers of eating *excessive* bran or other rough substances?

9. What changes would you make in the following meals to increase the fiber or cellulose content?

(1)	(2)	(3)
Applesauce	Tomato juice	Mixed fruit juice
Cornflakes	Meat loaf	Creamed chicken on
Cream and sugar	Mashed potatoes	steamed rice
Enriched toast	Buttered carrots	Hubbard squash
Butter and jelly	Roll and butter	Muffin and butter
Milk or coffee	Lemon meringue pudding	Baked caramel custard
	Tea	Coffee

10. Why is an excess of sugars and sweets in the diet undesirable?

11. Using your week's diet record (page 24), list below the foods you ate under the following headings:

Predominantly sugar   *Predominantly starch*   *Contain considerable fiber*

SUPPLEMENTARY READING:

Bogert: Chapter 2   Mowry: Chapter 2   Robinson: Chapter 7
Howe: Chapter 3   Peyton: Chapter 3   Yearbook, 1959: pages. 88–100

PART 2. FATS

WHAT ARE FATS?

Fats and oils constitute a second group of nutrients which provide energy in the diet. They and certain fat-like substances are classified as lipids. Fats are compounds of fatty acids—three molecules of fatty acids and one molecule of glycerol (triglycerides)—which, like carbohydrates, contain carbon, hydrogen and oyxgen but in different proportions. When oxidized, they give about $2\frac{1}{4}$ times more energy than carbohydrates.

The kinds and types of fatty acids present in a fat determine whether it is liquid or solid at room temperature, its flavor and other properties. Common fats found in foods include stearin (stearic acid) in beef suet and other animal fats, palmitin (palmitic acid) in both animal and vegetable fats, olein (oleic acid) in almost all fats and oils, and butyrin (butyric acid) in butter.

Fat-like substances having important roles in the body include phospholipins (fat plus the mineral phosphorus) and sterols (ergosterol in plants and cholesterol in animal tissues).

HOW DO FATS FEATURE IN DIETS?

Approximately one-third to one-half of the total calories in the American diet come from fat, a figure which is high compared with that in other countries. Only about 10 to 20 percent of the calorie intake comes from fat in diets in European and Asian countries. The consumption of fats, both in kind and amount, has increased in our country during the past 50 years. More oils and margarines, but less butter, are now used; the greater consumption of meat, poultry, fish, and milk has increased fat intake from these sources.

WHAT ARE THE DIFFERENT KINDS OF FAT?

Any fats that remain fluid at ordinary room temperatures are called oils; those that remain solid are called fats. For convenience, food fats are classed as "visible" fats or those purchased and used as fats and "invisible" fats or those which are parts of natural foods.

"Visible" fats		*"Invisible" fats in*	
Bacon	Salt pork	Meat	Eggs
Lard	Salad dressings	Fish	Baked goods
Oils	Other shortenings	Poultry	Cream
Margarine	such as cooking fats	Whole milk	Cheese
Butter		Ice cream	Nuts

Hydrogenated fats are made by treating liquid fats—vegetable oils such as cotton, corn, soybean, etc.—with hydrogen to produce a plastic fat for cooking purposes or a table fat for a butter substitute. Cooking fats and margarines found on the market, each under a different trade name, are examples of this type of fat.

Margarines may be further treated for use as table fats by churning with cultured milk to improve flavor and fortifying with the vitamin A equivalent of butter.

WHAT DO "SATURATED" AND "UNSATURATED" FATS MEAN?

Fatty acids, a variety of which are present in different food fats, are classified as "saturated" and "unsaturated" depending on the absence or presence of double bonds between the carbon atoms in the molecule. No hydrogen can be added to saturated fatty acids as they have no double bonds; their predominance makes a solid fat. Hydrogen atoms can be added to unsaturated oleic acid with its one double bond (*mono*saturated) or to linoleic acid and linolenic acid with 2 and 3 double bonds, respectively (*poly*unsaturated); this makes possible the conversion of oils into plastic fats (margarines) by hydrogenation mentioned on the previous age.

Food fats contain a mixture of both kinds of fatty acids. If saturated acids predominate, the fat is solid and called a saturated fat; if unsaturated acids predominate, the fat is called a polyunsaturated fat. Several of these unsaturated fatty acids are essential in nutrition, especially linoleic acid, and must be furnished in the diet.

Fat-rich foods "high in *saturated fatty acids* include whole milk, cream, ice cream, cheeses made from whole milk, egg yolk; medium fat or fatty meats; beef, lamb, pork, ham; bacon, beef tallow, butter, coconut oil, lamb fat, lard, regular margarine, salt pork, hydrogenated shortenings; chocolate, chocolate candy, cakes, cookies, pies, rich puddings."[4]

Fat-rich foods "high in *polyunsaturated fatty acids* include vegetable oils: safflower, corn, cottonseed, soybean, sesame, sunflower; salad dressings made from the above oils: mayonnaise, French and others; special margarines: liquid oil listed first on label; fatty fish: salmon, tuna, herring."[5]

The relative amounts of fatty acids in foods and diets is referred to as a P/S Ratio (P = polyunsaturated/S = saturated fatty acids).

Certain of the newer margarines ("special") on the market are made by combining vegetable oils containing unsaturated fatty acids with just enough hydrogenated fat to get the right plastic state. These margarines will have more of the free unsaturated fatty acids than the older types. The labels on such margarines will list the liquid oil first, may be marked "high in polyunsaturates," and may also state the amount and type of fatty acids present.

WHAT SHOULD ONE KNOW ABOUT CHOLESTEROL?

Cholesterol, one of the "fat-like" sterols is found in various concentrations in all animal tissue and the blood and has important functions in the body, food intake or synthesis within the body being responsible for its presence. A fatty deposit containing cholesterol (which interferes with the flow of blood) is characteristic of a cardiovascular disease known as atherosclerosis, the exact cause of which is unknown. "The relationship of dietary fat to coronary heart disease and other mani-

---

[4] C. H. Robinson, Basic Nutrition and Diet Therapy, 2nd edition, New York, The Macmillan Company, 1970, p. 52

[5] Ibid., p. 53

festations of atherosclerosis has received special attention from the Food and Nutrition Board."[6]

Studies in various parts of the world show an association in many populations between a high intake of "saturated" fats and the prevalence of coronary heart disease while populations subsisting on diets low in fats appear to be relatively free of coronary disease. The former so-called "high-risk" populations show a higher plasma concentration of cholesterol (and also trigylcerides) while the latter "low-risk" populations tend to lower amounts of lipids in the blood.[6]

It has been observed that the substitution in the diet of polyunsaturated fats for the more saturated fats lowers significantly the amount of cholesterol in the blood and further reductions occur when the diet cholesterol is also reduced. The exact mechanism for these results is not as yet well understood. For this reason, the Food and Nutrition Board states that "evidence warrants only tentative decisions as to desirable amounts of fats and fatty acid patterns for the general population; for many Americans, dietary modifications designed to lower levels of cholesterol (and also triglycerides) appear to be indicated on an individual basis with due regard for consideration of the possible role of other known risk factors."[6]

HOW DO FATS FUNCTION IN NUTRITION?

Primary function—to serve as concentrated source of heat and energy (1 gram of fat yields 9 calories, 2-1/4 times that of carbohydrate); "with the exception of the central nervous system, virtually all tissues of the body utilize fatty acids directly as a source of energy."[6] About one-third to one-half of calories in the American diet comes from fat.

Spare burning of protein for energy.

Add flavor and palatability to diet.

Give satiety value to diet; fats slow digestion and retard development of hunger.

Animal fats and fortified margarines carry certain fat soluble vitamins (A, D, E, K) and aid in their absorption and also essential fatty acids.

Excess fat in diet is stored as adipose tissue reserve and insulates and protects organs and nerves.

Phospholipids have an important role in metabolism.

Lubricate the intestinal tract.

WHAT ARE REQUIREMENTS FOR FATS?

No recommended allowances have been set for fats by the Food and Nutrition Board. Good health appears to be possible with widely different variations in fat content. Some peoples remain healthy on fat intakes of 10 to 20 percent of total calories while in the United States the fat intake is as high as 40 percent. Some authorities recommend that fat should provide about 25 per cent (1/4) of the total calories needed. See 2nd paragraph top of page for Food and Nutrition Board statement.

---

[6] Recommended Dietary Allowances, 7th edition, Publication No. 1694, Washington, D. C., National Academy of Sciences–National Research Council, 1968, pp. 11–12

WHAT ARE COMMON FOOD SOURCES OF FAT?

Animal sources		*Plant sources*	
Whole milk	Bacon	Vegetable oils—corn, cotton, peanut etc.	
Butter	Cheese	Margarines	Salad dressings
Lard	Cream	Chocolate	Nuts, Olives
Meat fats	Egg yolk	Peanut butter	Avocadoes

Note: Mineral oil, frequently used in salad dressings, is not a food fat as it can not be digested and utilized by the body. Its use as a substitute for salad oils should be avoided as it interferes with the absorption of fat-soluble vitamins in the intestine. When used as a laxative, if at all, it should never be taken near meal time.

WHAT HAPPENS TO FATS IN THE BODY?

Fats, being insoluble in water, require special treatment in the gastrointestinal tract so that their end products can be absorbed through the intestinal wall. No digestion of fat takes place in the mouth. Only finely emulsified fats such as found in butter, cream, and egg yolk can be digested in the stomach. For the most part, fats are digested in the small intestine by enzymes from the pancreatic juice after the fats have been emulsified by bile and bile salts. Fats are changed to glycerol and fatty acids during digestion.

Fatty foods are digested without difficulty but they require a longer time for digestion than do carbohydrates. Softer fats are more completely digested and absorbed than harder fats. Fried foods are not necessarily indigestible but more slowly digested.

The presence of carbohydrates in the diet is necessary for the complete oxidation of fats in the tissues; otherwise, acetone bodies accumulate, resulting in ketosis.

DIGESTION AND METABOLISM

In the mouth	*In the stomach*	*In the small intestine*	*Absorption small intestine*	*Metabolism*
No action	Emulsified fats ↓ Fatty acids and glycerol by action of gastric lipase	Fats After emulsification by bile ↓ Fatty acids and glycerol by action of pancreatic and intestinal lipase	In the form of fatty acids and glycerol which are recombined into a new fat during absorption	New fat ↓ oxidized for energy to carbon dioxide and water or stored as fatty tissue Some fat combines with phosphorus to form phospholipids

TERMS TO UNDERSTAND

"Visible fat"   Hydrogenated fat   Saturated fat

"Invisible fat"   Cholesterol   Unsaturated fat

                                                        Polyunsaturated fat

STUDY QUESTIONS AND ACTIVITIES

1. What important functions, in addition to energy, are performed by fats?

2. How do fats and carbohydrates compare in energy value?

3. Name several plant sources of fats; several animal sources.

4. Using your week's diet record (page 24), list the fat-containing foods you ate under the following headings:

        Visible fats   Invisible fats

5. What is the calorie value of a food which contains 12 grams of fat and 25 grams of carbohydrate?

6. How do butter and margarine compare in food value?

7. If you require 2000 calories and 25 percent or one-quarter of the calories should come from fat, how many *grams* of fat will be in your diet?

8. Collect several labels of "special" margarines and compare information on the labels.

SUPPLEMENTARY READING

Bogert: Chapter 3   Mowry: Chapter 4   Robinson: Chapter 6
Howe: Chapter 4   Peyton: Chapter 4   Yearbook, 1959: pages 74–87

PART 3. PROTEINS

WHAT ARE PROTEINS?

Proteins are complex food substances (nutrients) made up of amino acids composed of carbon, hydrogen, and oxygen, the same elements found in carbohydrates and, *in addition, nitrogen*. The presence of nitrogen makes them different from carbohydrates and fats: proteins are capable of building body tissues in addition to furnishing heat or energy. Sulphur, phosphorus, and iron may also be present.

Twenty-two amino acids—called "building stones" or units—are known to be physiologically important and are found in different amounts and combinations in food proteins. Eight of these amino acids are called "essential" and must be supplied adequately in the daily food of the adult. At least one additional one, and possibly a second, are needed for growth in children. These "essential" or "indispensable" amino acids can not be synthesized by the body in adequate amounts.

Plants are able to build their own protein from the nitrogen in certain substances in the soil, carbon dioxide from the air and with water, the energy needed for this process being supplied by the sun. Animals and humans must get their protein preformed from plants and other animals. These preformed proteins are then digested and the end products used to build special types of body proteins as necessary.

HOW DO PROTEINS FEATURE IN DIETS?

In the United States there are adequate sources of good quality protein and, on the whole, the average person probably eats sufficient protein. Some studies show, however, that the amount of protein may be inadequate in the diet of some persons, for economic or other reasons. In many parts of the world, protein may be adequate but of poor quality; in still other parts there is a definite shortage of protein foods and this constitutes a health hazard. Also, many countries lack sufficient information about their protein food supply and how to use it. Superstition and poor sanitary conditions may also account for inadequate consumption of protein. In some instances, limited available sources may be too expensive for low-income groups.

Short stature is a characteristic of peoples in areas where protein is derived largely from plant sources; in other parts, meat featured in diets means better stature and stronger, heavier physiques. A protein nutrition problem due to a very restricted intake in many of the newly emerged and emerging nations is the deficiency seen in children—kwashiorkor—resulting in retarded growth and development, lowered resistance to disease, loss of appetite, changes in skin and hair, and severe edema. Treatment of this condition with reconstituted nonfat dry milk brings improvement as does a product—INCAPARINA—developed in some areas from a combination of inexpensive local grain and vegetable protein sources by the Institute of Nutrition of Central America and Panama (INCAP).

Various divisions of the United Nations are interested in developing locally produced vegetables as sources of protein in underdeveloped areas, with financial support arranged for by various national and international organizations. The right combination of vegetable protein sources can provide a protein of better quality than that present in any single vegetable.

WHAT ARE THE DIFFERENT KINDS OF PROTEINS?

The nutritional quality of a protein depends on the assortment of amino acids in the protein. On this basis, a protein is referred to as being a "complete" or an "incomplete" one.

A "complete" protein will contain the amino acids necessary both for growth and for maintenance and repair of body tissues and is said to have a high "biologic" value. Generally speaking, animal sources of protein—meat, fish, poultry, eggs, milk and its products—contain complete proteins.

An "incomplete" protein will maintain life (repair worn out tissue) but it will not support growth because it lacks the amino acids required for building (growth). Vegetable and other plant sources contain incomplete proteins of poor "biologic" value. Incomplete proteins can be supplemented by complete proteins from animal sources as in cereal and milk, toast and eggs, macaroni and cheese. The protein quality of bread can be improved by making it with milk instead of water.

If one knew exactly how to combine cereals and vegetables in the right mixtures and amounts, he could provide himself with the right assortment of amino acids to meet his protein needs. This is not practical, of course, and so the daily diet should contain both animal sources of protein (about 1/3 of the total requirement) and some plant sources. It is desirable to have some animal protein in every meal, the total daily amount being divided about equally among the three meals of the day.

HOW DO PROTEINS FUNCTION IN NUTRITION?

Protein is a part of all protoplasm in every living cell in muscles, organs, and glands and is found in all body fluids except bile and urine. Protein in the diet provides nitrogen to be utilized in the synthesis of body proteins and other nitrogen-containing substances and is involved in a variety of important metabolic functions:

It is essential for life: supplies material to repair or replace worn out tissues.

It is essential for growth: supplies material for tissue building.

It supplies some energy (four calories per gram) but it is an expensive source.

It supplies certain essential substances necessary for the construction and proper functioning of important body compounds: enzymes, hormones, hemoglobin, antibodies, other blood proteins, glandular secretions.

Certain amino acids play very special and vital roles in nutrition.

To carry out tissue building functions efficiently and adequately, it is essential that all the necessary amino acids for the building at hand be present simultaneously. This is another reason why it is important to have the day's supply of protein about equally divided among the three meals. Sufficient amounts of carbohydrates and fats to provide for energy needs will prevent some of the protein needed for building and repair from being diverted for energy.

WHAT ARE RECOMMENDED DIETARY ALLOWANCES FOR PROTEIN?

The recommended allowance for protein for adults is about one gram per kilogram of body weight amounting to 65 grams daily for a man; 55 grams daily for a woman. An additional 10 grams of protein per day or a total of 65 grams is recommended during pregnancy to meet the needs of the growing fetus and accessory tissues; an additional 20 grams per day or a total of 75 grams during lactation is recommended to cover milk secretion.

The protein requirement during growth is relatively higher than that of the adult since nitrogen must be provided for the formation of new tissue.

Protein requirement is increased in any condition where the body protein is broken down: hemorrhage, burns, poor protein nutrition previous to surgery, wounds, long convalescence. Deficiency of protein over a long period of time results in loss of weight, reduced resistance to disease, skin and blood changes, slow healing of wounds, and a condition known as nutritional edema.

Exercise in itself does not increase the need for protein, if the diet contains sufficient carbohydrates and fats to meet increased energy needs. As energy foods are added to the diet to meet energy requirements, some increase in protein foods will occur naturally.

WHAT ARE COMMON FOOD SOURCES OF PROTEIN?

Animal sources		*Plant sources*
(complete: more expensive)		(incomplete: less expensive)
Milk	Meat	Vegetables—generally poor sources
Cheese	Fish	except dry peas, beans, lentils,
Eggs	Poultry	peanuts (legumes)
Variety meats		Cereals Breads Nuts
Supply nutritionally essential amino acids.		Lack one or more nutritionally essential amino acids.
Should provide about 1/3 of the daily dietary protein.		Inadequate for building purposes.
Called "high quality" protein.		Need to be supplemented in the diet with complete proteins
(Gelatin, although an animal source, lacks several essential amino acids so is *incomplete*).		May supplement each other with a careful choice among the different sources.
		Soybeans, although of plant origin, contain high quantity and quality protein

Foods with Same Amount of Protein

Meat	Poultry	Fish*	Eggs
Small Serv.	Small Serv.	Small Serv.	2 jumbo
2 oz. cooked, boneless	2 oz. cooked, boneless	2 oz. boneless	
Cottage Cheese*	**Cheese***	**Baked Beans****	**Peanut Butter****
1/2 cup creamed	2 slices Cheddar 2 oz.	1 cup	4 rounded tbsp. 4 oz.

Also 2 Glasses or 1 Pint of Milk

*Advise iron-rich foods with these, such as greens, eggs, prunes.

**Advise milk, cheese or another food from animals with these to improve the quality of their protein.

Nutrition Source Book, Chicago, National Dairy Council, 1970, p. 12.

The following chart shows the daily recommendations and food sources of protein in average servings.

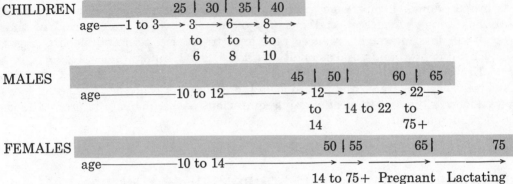

PROTEIN*
DAILY RECOMMENDATIONS

GRAMS

CHILDREN   25 | 30 | 35 | 40
age——1 to 3——→ 3——→ 6——→ 8——→
                     to   to   to
                     6   8   10

MALES   45 | 50 | 60 | 65
age————————10 to 12————————→ 12——→ ————→ 22——→
                                 to   14 to 22   to
                                 14   75+

FEMALES   50 | 55   65 | 75
age————————10 to 14————————————→ ——→ ————————→ ————————→
                              14 to 75+ Pregnant Lactating

GOOD SOURCES OF PROTEIN†

GRAMS

Veal   3½ oz.   33
Liver   3½ oz.   30
Beef   3½ oz.   30
Pork   3½ oz.   28
Lamb   3½ oz.   27
Frankfurters   13
    2 med.
Luncheon Meat   10
    2 oz.

Turkey   3½ oz.   32
Chicken   3½ oz.   30
Fish   3½ oz.   26
Canned Fish   12
    1¾ oz.
Egg   1 med.   6

Milk   1 cup   9
Cottage Cheese   8
    ¼ cup
Cheese   1 oz.   7

Dried Beans   13
and Peas ¾ cup
Peanut Butter   8
    2 tblsp.
Nuts   ¼ cup   5

Cereal   ½ cup   2
Bread   1 slice   2

*Lesson on Meat, Chicago, National Livestock and Meat Board, 1970, page 14.
†Average nutrient content as food is served. *(Note: 3½ ounces equals approximately 100 grams.)*

WHAT HAPPENS TO PROTEINS IN THE BODY?

The proteins in the daily diet must be broken down into their component parts, the amino acids, by digestion before the body can absorb them into the blood from the small intestine and use them. Digestion of protein is started in the stomach by enzymes in the gastric juice and is continued (and completed) in the small intestine by enzymes from the pancreatic and intestinal juices.

DIGESTION AND METABOLISM

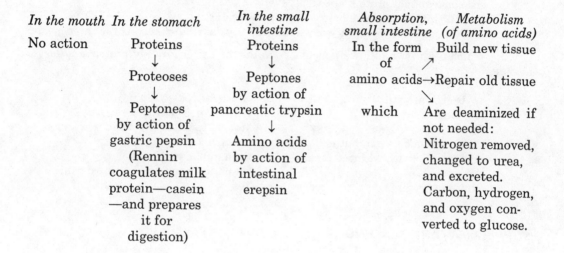

In the mouth	*In the stomach*	*In the small intestine*	*Absorption, small intestine*	*Metabolism (of amino acids)*
No action	Proteins ↓ Proteoses ↓ Peptones by action of gastric pepsin (Rennin coagulates milk protein—casein —and prepares it for digestion)	Proteins ↓ Peptones by action of pancreatic trypsin ↓ Amino acids by action of intestinal erepsin	In the form of amino acids→ which	Build new tissue ↗ Repair old tissue ↘ Are deaminized if not needed: Nitrogen removed, changed to urea, and excreted. Carbon, hydrogen, and oxygen con- verted to glucose.

TERMS TO UNDERSTAND

Protein
Amino acid
"Essential" amino acid

Complete protein
Incomplete protein
Legumes
Enzyme

Hormone
Hemoglobin
Antibodies
Kwashiorkor
Marasmus

STUDY QUESTIONS AND ACTIVITIES

1. How do proteins differ from carbohydrates and fats?

2. What is a complete protein? Where are they found?

3. What is an incomplete protein? Where are they found?

4. Why is it possible for proteins to build and repair tissues in addition to furnishing energy?

5. Why is it uneconomical to use protein foods for energy?

6. When does an adult need more than the RDA for protein?

7. Why is the protein requirement about the same for an athlete and a non-athlete?

8. Why are amino acids called building stones?

9. Why should a complete protein be included in every meal?

10. How much protein do you require every day? See RDA on page 26.

11. Using your week's dietary record (page 24), list all the protein foods you ate under the following headings:

Complete proteins	*Incomplete proteins*
(animal sources)	(plant sources)

Did some animal protein appear at every meal?
Do you think you ate sufficient protein every day?
Was the protein eaten every day about equally distributed among the three meals?

12. Which of the two following menus contains the better kinds of protein *and* larger amounts? Why?

(1)	(2)
Soybean loaf with tomato sauce	Cream of pea soup
Buttered green beans	Whole wheat crackers
Cornmeal muffins and butter	Molded tomato jelly salad with tuna fish and mayonnaise
Fruited jello with whipped cream	Bran muffins and butter
Cookies	Prune whip with soft custard sauce
Fruit punch	Tea

SUPPLEMENTARY READING

Bogert: Chapter 4	Mowry: Chapter 3	Robinson: Chapter 5
Howe: Chapter 5	Peyton: Chapter 5	Yearbook, 1959: Pages 57–73

PART 4. ENERGY REQUIREMENTS

WHAT IS THE MEANING OF "ENERGY," "CALORIE," AND "METABOLISM"?

Energy is defined as the power to do work. Some energy (calories, fuel, heat) is needed for even the slightest movements of the body. It is provided by the oxidation (burning) of the carbon-containing nutrients—carbohydrates, fats, and proteins. Without sufficient calories in the food intake, the body burns its own tissues for needed energy.

A "calorie" is simply a unit of measure to express the fuel value of these nutrients just as an inch measures length, an ounce weight, etc. The large calorie (or Kilo-Calorie, abbreviated as C. or Cal.) used in nutrition represents the amount of heat necessary to raise the temperature of one kilogram of water one degree centigrade.

Metabolism is a general term covering all changes food nutrients undergo after their absorption from the gastrointestinal tract and their utilization by the body cells. If the change is of a constructive nature building up new substances, it is called anabolism; if of a destructive or oxidative nature, it is called catabolism. Energy metabolism refers to the oxidation of nutrients within the body, with the release of heat and energy; protein metabolism refers to protein changes in the body.

WHAT ARE THE DAILY ENERGY NEEDS?

"The body requires food energy for resting metabolism, synthesis of body tissues (growth, maintenance, pregnancy, lactation), physical activity, excretory processes, and to maintain thermal balance (also for physiological and psychological stress."[7]

1. Internal (involuntary) activities or work—known as basal metabolism or the amount of energy needed when the body is lying at rest, in repose in a comfortable environment, several hours after any heavy exercise, and without food for 12 to 15 hours. It covers activities of organs and tissues and oxidation within the tissues, circulation, respiration, digestion, elimination, maintenance of muscle tone, heart beat, etc. All internal activities continue 24 hours each day, during sleeping and nonsleeping hours.

The basal metabolic rate varies from person to person for various reasons but, on the average, it amounts to approximately 1/2 Cal. per pound per hour, or 1200–1400 Cal. per day for women; 1600–1800 Cal. per day for men. This minimum calorie need usually accounts for more than half the total daily calorie need of a moderately active adult; even more for less active adults.

A basal metabolism test, formerly used extensively for diagnostic purposes in disturbances affecting the metabolic rate, is taken in the morning before rising, usually, and before eating. It measures the minimum amount of energy which will "keep life in process." More recently, a diagnostic blood test to measure the protein-bound iodine (PBI)—combination of iodine and thyroxine with certain blood proteins—is employed for this purpose. Thyroid hormone (Thyroxine) affects notably the metabolic rate.

---

[7] Recommended Dietary Allowances, 7th edition, Publication No. 1694, Washington, D. C., National Academy of Sciences, National Research Council, 1968, p. 1.

2. Effect of food eaten: The stimulating effect (specific dynamic action or SDA) each food exerts on basal metabolism after digestion and absorption amounts to a rise of about 10 percent of the total energy needs of a person eating a mixed diet.

3. External (voluntary) activities: Muscular movements and other activities in moving about and carrying on daily activities and work raise the energy requirement 30–100 percent above basal needs depending on severity and extent of activity:

30 % above: very light activity   75 % above: moderate activity

50% above: light activity   100% above: strenuous activity

Sufficient calories to cover the above three needs will permit an adult to maintain his desirable weight. Additional energy is needed by an adult to help in building new tissue following a wasting disease or malnutrition, or during pregnancy and lactation. Energy needs decrease as one grows older.

4. Growth needs: children need sufficient calories to provide for the above three conditions plus additional calories to permit growth of new tissues and increase of body weight. This need continues throughout the teens.

WHAT ARE CALORIE ALLOWANCES FOR ADULTS?

CALORIE ALLOWANCES FOR ADULT INDIVIDUALS OF VARIOUS BODY WEIGHTS AND AGES

(At a mean environmental temperature of 20° C. [68° F.] assuming light physical activity)

Body Weight	Calorie Allowance		
pounds	22 years	45 years	65 years
MEN			
110	2,200	2,000	1,850
121	2,350	2,150	1,950
132	2,500	2,300	2,100
143	2,650	2,400	2,200
154	2,800	2,600	2,400
165	2,950	2,700	2,500
176	3,050	2,800	2,600
187	3,200	2,950	2,700
198	3,350	3,100	3,800
209	3,500	3,200	2,900
220	3,700	3,400	3,100
WOMEN			
88	1,550	1,450	1,300
99	1,700	1,550	1,450
110	1,800	1,650	1,500
121	1,950	1,800	1,650
128	2,000	1,850	1,700
132	2,050	1,900	1,700
143	2,220	2,000	1,850
154	2,300	2,100	1,950

Age Adjustments
(% of Calorie Allowance at age 22)

Age	Adjustment	Age	Adjustment	Age	Adjustment
22–35	100–95	45–55	92–89	65–75	84–79
35–45	95–92	55–65	89–84	75–85	72

From *Recommended Dietary Allowances,* 7th edition. Publication No. 1964. Washington, D. C., National Academy of Sciences—National Research Council, 1968, page 5.

HOW DOES THE BODY GET ENERGY FROM FOOD?

In some ways the body is like an engine. An engine needs fuel which can be burned for work. The body needs food (carbon-containing) which, after digestion and absorption into the blood stream, can be oxidized (burned) to do work. The body differs from a machine in several ways. First, an engine uses but one kind of fuel; the body can use three kinds interchangeably—carbohydrates, fats, and proteins. When an engine stops working, it requires no fuel. The body never stops working as internal or involuntary activities continue even during sleep, so there is a 24 hour need for upkeep and repair.

HOW CAN ONE DETERMINE ONE'S ENERGY REQUIREMENT?

1. Simplest method: Multiply your desirable weight (see page 54) in pounds by 18 (for a woman, 21 for a man) for the approximate number of calories needed by a moderately active adult. Add 1/4 more calories if very active; subtract 1/4 if sedentary.

2. Keep a record of your different activities during a representative 24 hour period, listing the time spent in each activity. With the help of the table on page 61, the energy expenditure and food calories needed may be quickly determined for the period of time spent in each activity and total figure obtained for the 24 hours. You will be doing this problem for yourself on page 60.

3. Consult RDA Table on page 26. You have already underlined in red the figure which represents your daily calorie requirement.

HOW DOES ONE KNOW IF ONE IS IN ENERGY BALANCE?

One's weight is a good index of one's energy balance; that is, if one is at the desirable weight for height and age. If no weight gain or loss occurs over a period of time, it may be assumed that the number of calories eaten daily is sufficient or about equal to one's energy expenditure or needs. If fewer calories are eaten than the energy expended, some of the body tissues will be burned and there will be a weight loss. If more calories are eaten than calories expended, there will be a storage of fatty tissue and weight gain. "Energy balance" means that the calories in the diet equal the calories expended by the body. Or, if one eats the same number of calories as expended and increases physical activity, there will be a weight loss; weight gain will occur with decreased physical activity.

WHY IS OVERWEIGHT CONSIDERED A HEALTH PROBLEM?

Medical scientists consider overweight a major health problem in the United States because of its relation to degenerative diseases. Early guides to desirable weights for adult men and women were based on average weights at different ages, compiled from insurance company records which indicated advantages, in terms of health and longevity, of slight overweight under 30 years and underweight over 30 years. Recent tables of desirable weights for adults recognize differences in frame (small, medium, and large) but do not allow for increases with age. They are published by the Metropolitan Life Insurance Company. People who are well below the average weights of the population have lower mortality rates (longer life) than heavier people; and also less illness. It is now considered that, in the interest of good health and longevity, one should weigh no more in the years after 25 than the indicated normal weight for height and body build at 25. A weight 15 to 20 percent more than this figure indicates overweight; 25 percent more indicates one as very fat or obese. See page 293 for height-weight tables.

Underweight and undernutrition are also considered health hazards. Some causes and disadvantages of overeating and undereating as to calories are listed below.

WHAT ARE CAUSES AND DISADVANTAGES OF OVERWEIGHT AND UNDERWEIGHT?

Overweight	Underweight
Causes	
1. Calorie intake in excess of needs	1. Calorie intake inadequate for needs
2. Insufficient exercise	2. Overactivity and tenseness
3. Good appetite with special fondness for rich foods	3. Poor appetite: satisfied with less than required amount of foods or with low calorie foods
4. Frequent snacking due to irregular meals or skipping meals	4. Skipping meals—hard to fulfill day's needs
5. Food may serve as compensation for emotional problems	5. Emotional problems affect appetite
6. Failure of older persons to reduce food intake with lowering metabolism	6. Various illnesses lower food intake
7. More generous family meal patterns	7. Limited family meal patterns for economic or other reasons
Disadvantages	
1. Inconvenience	1. Physical fatigue—less energy
2. Unattractive appearance	2. Poor appearance
3. Inefficiency	3. Nervousness and irritability
4. Predisposition to functional diseases of heart, circulatory system, and others	4. Lack of vitality and endurance
5. Lessened life expectancy	5. Susceptibility to infections—tuberculosis in young

Overweight	Underweight
6. Slower recovery following serious illness and surgery	6. Lessened life expectancy
7. Children handicapped in athletics and socially	7. Anemia

WHAT ARE ENERGY FOODS?

The energy value of a food depends on its chemical composition: how much carbohydrate, fat, and protein is present.

1 gram carbohydrate	yields 4 calories
1 gram fat	yields 9 calories
1 gram protein	yields 4 calories

Example: 1 cup whole milk (8 oz.) contains

12 gm. carbohydrate	× 4	48 calories
9 gm. fat	× 9	81 calories
8.5 gm. protein	× 4	34 calories
		163 calories

Refer to Food Composition Table in Appendix for the carbohydrate, fat, and protein content and calorie value of different foods.

In general, foods high in calories are rich in fat or low in water: fatty foods, cheese, nuts, dried legumes, dried fruits. Foods moderate in calories are lean meats, cereals, starchy vegetables. Calories in the Four Food Groups are shown below and on the following page. Bar graphs illustrating the approximate number of calories in average servings of some common foods follow on page 59.

CALORIES IN FOUR FOOD GROUPS

Adapted from a Cornell extension bulletin.

Milk Group

Milk, whole, 1 cup	165
Milk, skim 1 cup	90
Buttermilk, 1 cup	90
Cheese, Am. Cheddar, 1 oz.	115
Cheese, Cottage, 1/2 cup	100
Ice cream, vanilla, 2/3 cup	200
Cream, coffee, 1/4 cup	125
Cream, whipping, 1/4 cup	200

Cereals—Bread

Bread, whole wheat or enriched	
Bakery, 1 slice	65
Homemade, 1 slice	100
Breakfast cereals, whole-grain, 3/4 cup cooked	100

Meat Group

Meat, cooked, 4 oz. ser.	
Beef, veal	250–425
Lamb	300–475
Pork	375–450
Note: variation depends on fat content	
Poultry, cooked 4 oz. ser. (without added fat)	
Broiler-fryer	175
Roaster	225
Hens	350
Liver—1 tsp. fat	235
Heart	150
Tongue	300

Cereals-Bread

Breakfast cereals, whole-grain, dry, 1 oz.	100
Cornmeal, farina, spaghetti, macaroni, noodles, rice, 3/4 cup cooked	100
Crackers, graham, 2 med.	55
saltines, 3	50
Flour, whole wheat or enriched, 1 cup	400
1 Tbsp.	25

Meat Group

Fish

Lean—broiled, baked, haddock, cod	125
Fat—broiled, baked, halibut, salmon, tuna	225
Shrimp	150
Oysters, 1/2 cup	100
Eggs, one	75
Dry beans, peas, 1/2 cup cooked	100
Nuts, 1 Tbsp.	50
Peanut butter, 1 Tbsp.	100

Vegetables-Fruits
1/2 cup servings

15 calories:
Asparagus, green
Peppers, green
Snap beans, green
Salad greens
Cabbage, raw
Peppers, raw
Cantaloup
Celery
Cucumbers
Eggplant
Lettuce, head
Radishes
Squash, summer

25 calories:
Broccoli
Carrots
Greens, cooked
Pumpkin
Squash, winter
Tomato, 1 med.

25 calories:
Tomato, canned or fresh cooked
Tomato juice
Beets
Brussels sprouts
Cabbage, cooked
Cauliflower
Rutabagas
Turnips
Apricots, canned with water
Peaches, canned with water

50 calories:
Grape fruit juice
Orange juice
Lemon juice

50 calories:
Strawberries
Peach, 1 med.
Pears, canned with water
Pineapple, raw
Onions
Parsnips
Applesauce
Blackberries
Blueberries
Grapes
Pineapple juice
Plums
Raspberries

75 calories:
Peas
Lima beans
Sweet corn
Apple, 1 med.
Apple juice

75 calories:
Sweet potato, 1/2 med.
Potato, 1 med.
Banana, 1 med.
Pear, 1 med.
Apricots, dried
Watermelon, 4″ wedge
Pineapple, canned or frozen

Miscellaneous

Fats

Butter, 1 Tbsp.	100
Margarine, fortified, 1 Tbsp.	100
Cooking fats, salad oils, 1 Tbsp.	125
Mayonnaise, 1 Tbsp.	100
Bacon, broiled, 2 strips	100

Sweets

Sugar, 1 Tbsp.	50
Molasses, 1 Tbsp.	50
Candy, 1 oz.	100–150
Jam or jelly, 1 Tbsp.	50
Pies, homemade	
Fruit, 2 crust	500
Single-crust pies	365
Cakes	
Angel or sponge, no icing, 2″ piece	100
With fat, iced	400

CALORIES IN THE FOUR FOOD GROUPS

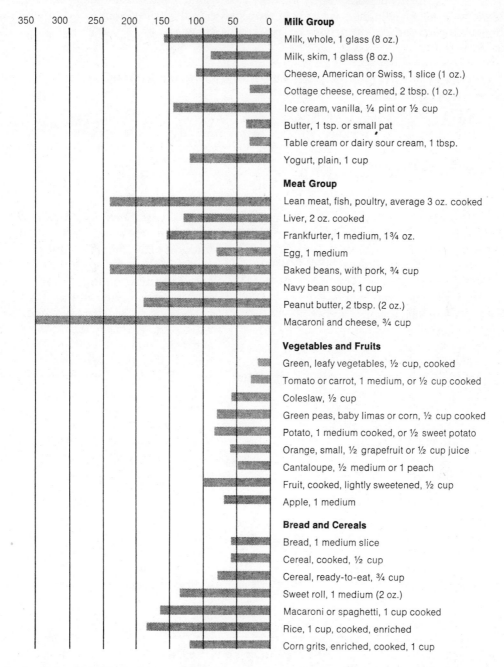

| 350 | 300 | 250 | 200 | 150 | 100 | 50 | 0 |

Milk Group

Milk, whole, 1 glass (8 oz.)

Milk, skim, 1 glass (8 oz.)

Cheese, American or Swiss, 1 slice (1 oz.)

Cottage cheese, creamed, 2 tbsp. (1 oz.)

Ice cream, vanilla, ¼ pint or ½ cup

Butter, 1 tsp. or small pat

Table cream or dairy sour cream, 1 tbsp.

Yogurt, plain, 1 cup

Meat Group

Lean meat, fish, poultry, average 3 oz. cooked

Liver, 2 oz. cooked

Frankfurter, 1 medium, 1¾ oz.

Egg, 1 medium

Baked beans, with pork, ¾ cup

Navy bean soup, 1 cup

Peanut butter, 2 tbsp. (2 oz.)

Macaroni and cheese, ¾ cup

Vegetables and Fruits

Green, leafy vegetables, ½ cup, cooked

Tomato or carrot, 1 medium, or ½ cup cooked

Coleslaw, ½ cup

Green peas, baby limas or corn, ½ cup cooked

Potato, 1 medium cooked, or ½ sweet potato

Orange, small, ½ grapefruit or ½ cup juice

Cantaloupe, ½ medium or 1 peach

Fruit, cooked, lightly sweetened, ½ cup

Apple, 1 medium

Bread and Cereals

Bread, 1 medium slice

Cereal, cooked, ½ cup

Cereal, ready-to-eat, ¾ cup

Sweet roll, 1 medium (2 oz.)

Macaroni or spaghetti, 1 cup cooked

Rice, 1 cup, cooked, enriched

Corn grits, enriched, cooked, 1 cup

These bar graphs illustrate the approximate number of calories in average servings of some common foods. The calorie values are averaged, rounded figures and are practical for everyday use. From *Nutrition Source Book*. Chicago, Ill., National Dairy Council, page 31.

Even though calories are essential in the diet and we can not live without an adequate number for our needs (undernutrition in many parts of the world is due to insufficient calories), they are not the only dietary essential. They must be accompanied by "leader" nutrients—proteins (amino acids), fats (fatty acids)—and many different minerals and vitamins. Calories in food unaccompanied by these other dietary essentials are frequently referred to as "empty calories" or "lone-wolf calories." "Choose Your Calories by the Company They Keep," a slogan of the National

Dairy Council, emphasizes the importance of "choosing calories which keep company with a wealth of nutrients until all our nutritional needs . . . except energy . . . have been supplied. Then we can choose calories from any source . . . including 'lonewolf calories' . . . until our energy requirement is met."[8]

HOW MANY CALORIES ARE EXPENDED IN VARIOUS ACTIVITIES?[9]

The approximate number of calories per hour it takes to perform each of the five different types of activity is given in the tabulation below; these figures include the basal calorie need.

Type of activity	Cal./hour	Type of activity	Cal./hour
Sedentary activities:	80–100	*Moderate activities:*	170–240
Reading, writing, eating, watching TV or movies, listening to radio, sewing, playing cards; typing, miscellaneous office work, and other activities done while sitting that require little or no arm movement.		Making beds; mopping and scrubbing; sweeping; light polishing and waxing; laundering by machine; light gardening and carpentry work; walking moderately fast; other activities done while standing that require moderate arm movement; and activities done while sitting that require more vigorous arm movement.	
Light activities:	110–160		
Preparing and cooking food; doing dishes; dusting; hand washing small articles of clothing; ironing; walking slowly; personal care; miscellaneous office work and other activities done while standing that require some arm movement; and rapid typing and other activities done while sitting that are more strenuous.		*Vigorous activities:*	250–350
		Heavy scrubbing and waxing; hand washing large articles of clothing; hanging out clothes; stripping beds; other heavy work; walking fast; bowling; golfing; gardening.	
		Strenuous activities:	350 and more
		Swimming; playing tennis; running; bicycling; dancing; skiing; and playing football.	

"A range of calorie values is given for each type to allow for differences in activities and in persons. Of the sedentary activities, for example, typing uses more calories than watching TV. And some persons will use more calories in carrying out either activity than others; some persons are more efficient in their body actions than others. Values closer to the upper limit of a range will give a better picture of calorie expenditures for men and those near the lower limit a better picture for women."[9]

---

[8] *Choose Your Calories by the Company They Keep.* Chicago, Ill., National Dairy Council, 1970.

[9] *Food and Your Weight,* Home and Garden Bulletin no. 74, Washington, D. C., U. S. Department of Agriculture, 1969, p. 4.

TERMS TO UNDERSTAND

Energy	Basal metabolism	Overweight
Calorie	Energy metabolism	Underweight
Metabolism	Obesity	"Empty" calories
		"Lone-wolf" calories

STUDY QUESTIONS AND ACTIVITIES

1. What factors affect the total number of calories one needs daily? Which have the greatest effect?

2. Why does a child need more energy in proportion to size than an adult?

3. What is meant by "empty" or "lone-wolf" calories?

4. Why is overweight undesirable? When is a person overweight? Obese?

5. Why is underweight undesirable? When is a person underweight? Mildly? Seriously?

6. What is the effect of eating too many calories? Too few?

7. Why is it incorrect to say that any food is "fattening" or "slimming"?

8. Two slices of whole wheat bread contain 22 grams carbohydrate, 2 grams fat, and 4 grams protein. How many calories do the two slices contain?

9. How many calories are needed daily by a woman weighing 125 pounds who is employed in a sedentary occupation? A man weighing 180 pounds who is engaged in very active employment?

10. Comment on the following: "Choose Your Calories by the Company They Keep."

SUPPLEMENTARY READING

Bogert: Chapters 5, 6, 7   Mowry: Chapter 5   Peyton: Chapter 6
Robinson: Chapters 8, 21
Yearbook 1959: Pages 304–314

The Healthy Way to Weigh Less. Chicago, Council on Foods and Nutrition, American Medical Association, 1966.

Food and Your Weight, Home and Garden Bulletin no. 74, Washington, D. C., U. S. Department of Agriculture, 1969.

Metropolitan Life's Four Steps to Weight Control. New York, Metropolitan Life Insurance Company, 1969.

Calories and Weight. The U. S. D. A. Pocket Guide. Washington, D. C. Home and Garden Bulletin No. 153, U. S. Department of Agriculture, 1968.

The Brand Name Calorie Counter. C. Retzer, New York, Dell Publishing Company, 1969.

HOW MANY CALORIES DO YOU EXPEND DAILY?

Keep a record below of the number of hours or part of hours you spend in each of the activities or similar ones for an average 24 hour period and complete the table to obtain an approximate figure for your day's energy expenditures.

ENERGY EXPENDITURE FOR EVERYDAY ACTIVITIES[10]

Activity	No. hrs. (or fraction of hr. engaged in activity)	Cal. per lb. per hr.	Total for period
Asleep		0.4	
Bicycling, moderate speed		1.7	
Cello playing		1.1	
Dancing, foxtrot		2.4	
Dancing, waltz		2.0	
Dishwashing		1.0	
Dressing and undressing		0.9	
Driving an automobile		1.0	
Eating a meal		.7	
Horseback riding, trot		2.6	
Ironing		1.0	
Laundry, light		1.1	
Lying still and awake		0.5	
Painting furniture		1.3	
Playing ping-pong		2.7	
Piano playing, moderate		1.2	
Reading aloud		0.7	
Running		4.0	
Sewing by hand		0.7	
Sewing, electric machine		0.7	
Sitting quietly, watching TV		0.6	
Skating		2.2	
Standing relaxed		0.8	
Sweeping, vacuum sweeper		1.9	
Swimming, 2 m.p.h.		4.5	
Tailoring		1.0	
Typing rapidly		1.0	
Walking, 3 m.p.h.		1.5	
Walking, 4 m.p.h.		2.2	
Writing		0.7	
	24	Total per lb.	x

Desirable wt. in lb. _____

Total number of calories expended per day _____

Note: For any one of your daily activities for which no figure is given above, use the figure for a similar activity.

HOW MANY CALORIES DO YOU CONSUME?

Keep a record below of all the food you eat for one day: at breakfast, during morning, at noon meal, during afternoon, at evening meal, at night. You will be referring to this food record as you progress with your study of nutrition so keep it

[10] C. M. Taylor, G. MacLeod, and M. S. Rose, *Foundations of Nutrition,* 5th edition. New York, Macmillan Company, 1956, adapted.

as accurately as possible. Determine the calorie and protein content of the foods on the food record. (Refer to Food Composition Table, Appendix, p. 298.)

Date: _____

Meal	Foods	Size of Serving	Calories	Protein Gm.

How does the calorie content of the above food record compare with your calculated requirement on page 62.

How does the protein content compare with your protein requirement? See page 26.

PART 5. MINERALS AND WATER

WHAT ARE MINERALS?

Minerals belong to a group of chemical elements in plant and animal tissues which include:

Group 1	Group 2		
Non-metallic elements (96 % body weight)	"Inorganic" elements or "ash" constituents remaining after organic portions of food and body tissues are burned (4% body weight)		
Carbon (C)			
Hydrogen (H)	Calcium (Ca)	Iron (Fe)	Selenium (Se)
Oxygen (O)	Cobalt (Co)	Magnesium (Mg)	Silicon (Si)
Nitrogen (N)	Chlorine (Cl)	Manganese (Mn)	Sodium (Na)
	Fluorine (Fl)	Molybdenum (Mo)	Sulfur (S)
	Iodine (I)	Phosphorus (P)	Zinc (Zn)
		Potassium (K)	

Calcium and phosphorus are present in the body in the largest amounts. Certain minerals, present in very small amounts but having important functions, are sometimes referred to as micronutrients or trace elements.

Minerals are found in all body tissues and fluids. They exist in the form of inorganic salts as sodium and chlorine in sodium chloride, calcium salt, phosphates, and sulfates or in organic combination as iodine in thyroxine, iron in hemoglobin, phospholipids, and phosphoproteins. Some are in soluble form, giving certain properties to body fluids (lymph, blood plasma, fluids around cells and soft tissues); some in insoluble form as found in hard tissues of bones and teeth.

Minerals occur in different forms in natural foods along with carbohydrates, fats, and protein, remaining in the ash after foods are burned. Figures are available for 10 or more minerals in many foods but the figures for calcium and iron are the ones chiefly used in planning normal diets. For certain therapeutic diets, adjustments (increase or decrease) in one or more minerals may be necessary.

HOW DO MINERALS FUNCTION IN NUTRITION?

Minerals have both building functions, taking part in the structure of all body tissues, hard and soft, and also body regulating functions. The trace elements are also thought to help enzymes, hormones, and vitamins play their roles in the body. Although each mineral has a specific function, minerals are interrelated in their functioning, with each mineral affecting the performance of one or more of the other minerals. For example, the correct amounts and ratios of five different minerals in body fluids are necessary for muscle contraction and relaxation; three for bone formation; and three (along with other substances) for hemoglobin formation.

As *builders,* minerals enter into the formation of
    Bony tissues: Ca and P in

As *regulators,* mineral salts in solution in body fluids (lymph, blood plasma, and around cells)

bones and teeth; Fl in teeth

Soft body tissues (muscles, nerves, and glands), all salts, especially P, K, S, Cl

Hair, nails, skin: S

Nerve tissue: all salts, especially P

Blood: all salts, especially Fe for hemoglobin and Cu for red blood cells

Glandular secretions: Cl in gastric juice; Na in intestinal juice: I in thyroxine; Mn in endocrine secretions; Zn in enzymes

Assist in muscle contraction and relaxation: Ca, K, Na, P, Cl

Assist nerves in irritability functions: all salts with a balance between Ca and Na

Aid in water balance in body: all salts, especially Na and K

Help in blood clotting: Ca

Aid in oxidation processes in tissues and blood: Fe and I

Regulate acid-base balance in blood and tissues: balance between acidic and basic compounds

Perform important functions in muscle physiology: phosphates

WHAT ARE FUNCTIONS AND FOOD SOURCES OF CALCIUM AND PHOSPHORUS?

Calcium

Functions

1. Major mineral constituent of body: as calcium phosphate 99% in bones (giving rigidity) and teeth with remainder in blood, other body fluids, and soft tissues
2. With other minerals helps muscles contract and relax normally; helps nervous system to function properly; helps passage of materials into and out of cells.
3. Aids in blood coagulation
4. Helps certain enzymes function
5. Needed daily throughout life. Vitamin D required for proper absorption and utilization.

Inadequate Ca:
   Poor bone and tooth development
   Stunted growth
   Rickets in children
   Osteomalacia and osteoporosis in adults

Food Sources

Best sources:
   Milk and milk products
   Cheese—cheddar type (less Ca in cottage)
   Ice cream
   (Difficult to meet daily requirement without some milk or cheese in diet)

Other sources
   Green leafy vegetables: turnip and mustard greens, kale, collard, broccoli (Ca in chard, beet greens, spinach, and rhubarb is not available to the body as it forms an insoluble salt with the oxalic acid present).

American diet apt to be lacking in Ca. Good supply of dairy products in the United States should insure adequate intake for every one.

Thin fragile bones
Poor blood clotting
RDA for Ca usually stated in grams; sometimes in milligrams. See RDA, page 26.

Phosphorus

Functions

1. Second to Ca in amount in body. Largest amount with Ca in bones, remainder in soft tissues and fluids
2. Performs many functions in body: in bone and tooth structure; present in nuclei of all cells; helps in oxidation of carbohydrates and fats; helps enzymes act in energy metabolism; aids in maintaining body's acid-base balance.

Food Sources

A diet adequate in protein and calcium will provide sufficient phosphorus for body needs. Rich sources include milk, meat, eggs, cheese, dry beans, nuts, and whole-grain cereals.

RDA for phosphorus equal to that for calcium for all age groups except young infant.

Each of the following lists of foods supply the RDA for Ca for the adult (0.8 gm. or 800 mg.). As the amount of milk is decreased in each list, more of less-rich calcium foods must be added. These lists show how difficult it is to get adequate calcium without milk or milk products in the diet.

(1)	mg. Ca*
3 glasses milk (1–1/2 pints)	864

(2)	mg. Ca*
2 glasses milk (1 pint)	576
1 inch cube cheese	129
1/6 qt. ice cream	130
2/3 cup green beans	42
2 slices bread	44
	921

(3)	mg. Ca
1 glass milk (1/2 pint)	288
1/2 cup creamed cottage cheese	115
2/3 cup broccoli	91
1 cup orange juice (frozen; reconstituted)	25
2 slices whole wheat bread	50
2/3 cup mustard greens	128
1 tablespoon molasses	33
6 medium oysters	113
	843

(4)	mg. Ca*
4 Tbsp. nonfat instant dry milk	220
3 oz. pink salmon with bones	167
1 cup baked beans	95
2/3 cup turnip greens	168
2 eggs	54
4 dried prunes	14
2 large lettuce leaves	34
3 Tbsp. light cream	45
3 dried figs	78
	875

Equivalent quantities of various milk products in calcium will be found on page 100.

The chart on page 68 shows the daily recommendations and food sources for calcium in average servings.

---

* Calculated from *Nutritive Value of Foods,* Home and Garden Bulletin no. 72, Washington, D. C., U. S. Department of Agriculture, 1970.

MILK IS OUR MAIN SOURCE OF CALCIUM
FOR BONES, TEETH, MUSCLES, NERVES, BLOOD

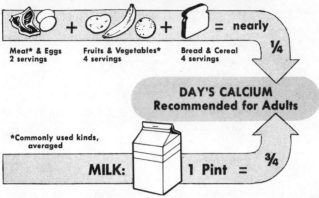

Meat* & Eggs
2 servings

Fruits & Vegetables*
4 servings

Bread & Cereal
4 servings

= nearly ¼

DAY'S CALCIUM
Recommended for Adults

*Commonly used kinds, averaged

MILK: 1 Pint = ¾

From *Nutrition Source Book*. Chicago, National Dairy Council, 1970, p. 11.

WHAT ARE FUNCTIONS AND FOOD SOURCES OF IRON?

Functions

1. Very small amounts of iron in body perform many very important functions in all cells.
2. More than half of the four to five grams of iron in the body is in hemoglobin; about 1/3 in liver, spleen and bone marrow; small amounts in muscle, blood serum and oxidative enzymes in cells.
3. Hemoglobin in blood cell carries oxygen from lungs to tissue cells and the carbon dioxide formed in oxidation away from cells, facilitating tissue respiration.
4. Copper, adequate protein and other substances are necessary for hemoglobin synthesis.

Food Sources

Excellent:
    Liver, heart, kidney
Good:
    Meat (lean), oysters
    Eggs (yolk)
    Dark green leafy vegetables
    Potatoes
    Dried fruits
    Whole-grain and enriched cereals and bread
    Dried peas and beans
    Molasses and raisins, if eaten generously

Inadequate iron: "Iron-deficiency" anemia (also occurs from poor iron absorption); weakness.

Reserve supply of iron in infant's body at birth depleted after 3 months.

RDA for iron stated in milligrams. See RDA, page 26.

"The allowance of 18 milligrams of iron recommended for girls and women is almost impossible to obtain through ordinary foods; iron supplementation is often required. Many foods, as breakfast cereals, are being fortified with iron at increasingly higher levels to meet this allowance for girls and women."[11]

The chart on page 69 shows the daily recommendations and food sources for iron in average servings.

---

[11] Nutritive Value of Foods. Home and Garden Bulletin No. 72, Washington, D. C., U. S. Department of Agriculture, 1970, p. 3.

CALCIUM*

DAILY RECOMMENDATIONS

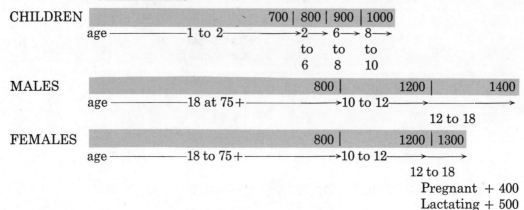

MILLIGRAMS

CHILDREN 700 | 800 | 900 | 1000
age ————— 1 to 2 —————→ 2 → 6 → 8 →
to   to   to
6   8   10

MALES 800 | 1200 | 1400
age ————— 18 at 75 + ————→ 10 to 12 ——→
12 to 18

FEMALES 800 | 1200 | 1300
age ————— 18 to 75 + ————→ 10 to 12 ——→
12 to 18
Pregnant + 400
Lactating + 500

GOOD SOURCES OF CALCIUM†

MILLIGRAMS

Food	Serving	Milligrams
Milk	1 cup	288
Cheese	1 oz.	219
Cottage Cheese		53
Sardines	3½ oz.	205
Canned Fish	1¾ oz.	80
Fish	3½ oz.	33
Egg	1 med.	27
Dark Green Leafy Vegetables	½ cup	99
Broccoli	½ cup	66
Sweet Potato	1 med.	43
Cabbage	½ cup	31
Potato	1 med.	10
Orange	1 med.	58
Canned Figs	3	40
Cantaloup	½ med.	27
Dried Fruit	½ cup	27
Grapefruit	½ med.	22
Molasses	1 tblsp.	46
Bread	1 slice	21
Cereal	½ cup	6

* Lessons on Meat, Chicago, National Livestock and Meat Board, 1970, p. 24.
† Average nutrient content as food is served. *(Note: 3½ ounces equals approximately 100 grams.)*

IRON*

DAILY RECOMMENDATIONS

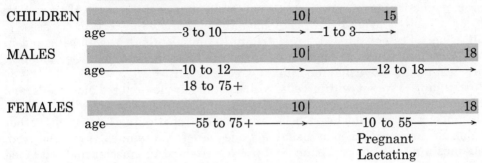

MILLIGRAMS

CHILDREN	10	15
age	3 to 10 →	─1 to 3─→
MALES	10	18
age	10 to 12 →	12 to 18 ─→
	18 to 75+	
FEMALES	10	18
age	55 to 75+ →	10 to 55 ─→
		Pregnant Lactating

GOOD SOURCES OF IRON†

MILLIGRAMS

Liver	3½ oz.	8
Heart	3½ oz.	5.4
Beef	3½ oz.	3.7
Pork	3½ oz.	3.5
Veal	3½ oz.	3.3
Lamb	3½ oz.	2.0
Luncheon Meat	2. oz.	2.0
Oysters	6-9 med.	6.6
Chicken	3½ oz.	1.5
Egg	1 med.	1.1
Fish	3½ oz.	1.1
Canned Fish	1 3/4 oz.	1.0
Dried Beans and Peas	¾ cup	3.6
Dried Fruit	½ cup	2.5
Dark Green Leafy Vegetables	½ cup	1.0
Potato	1 med.	8
Molasses	1 tblsp.	1.1
Nuts	½ cup	1.1
Cereal	½ cup	.6
Bread	1 slice	.6

* Lessons on Meat, Chicago, National Livestock and Meat Board, 1970, page 25.
† Average nutrient content as food is served. *(Note: 3½ ounces equals approximately 100grams.)*

WHAT FUNCTIONS DO OTHER MINERALS PERFORM IN NUTRITION?

Sodium.   Present for the most part in extracellular fluids (blood plasma and around tissues). Aids in water balance of body, osmotic pressure, acid-base balance, and proper functioning of muscles and nerves. Requirement is more than met by usual nutritionally adequate diet—may have to be restricted in certain diseases.

Chlorine.   Present as HCL in gastric juice and also both within cells and in extracellular fluids. Aids in maintaining osmotic pressure and acid-base balance. Requirement met by the usual food intake and table salt.

Potassium.   Present within cells, with most in muscles and red blood cells, and small amounts in extracellular fluids. Aids in functioning of muscles and nerves, fluid balance, regularity of heart beat, and enzyme functioning (along with other minerals). Requirements met by usual diet adequate in protein, calcium, and iron.

Magnesium.   Present in bones in form of salts and in muscles and red blood cells. Functions with other minerals in the functioning of various tissues—cardiac, muscle, nervous, skeletal—and aids enzymes. Recommended allowances have been set at 350 mg. per day for adult males and 300 mg. per day for adult females. See RDA, page 26. Requirement met by usual diet including whole-grain cereals, dark green vegetables, nuts, and legumes.

Sulfur.   Present in all cells as part of protein. Functions in formation of hair, nails, and skin and as part of several important body compounds. Requirement met by a diet adequate in protein.

Iodine.   Present as an integral part of the hormones of the thyroid gland and also in other tissues. Functions as part of thyroxine in regulating energy metabolism. Requirement met by supplementing diet with iodized salt. Need increased during adolescence and pregnancy. Lack causes simple goiter. Recommended dietary allowances have been established. See RDA on page 26.

Fluorine.   Present in bones and teeth. In the *proper amounts,* it helps reduce incidence of dental caries. Some evidence that it is related to use of Ca in bone formation. "The Food and Nutrition Board recommends fluoridation of public water supplies where it is needed because of low fluoride concentration."

Copper.   Aids in the absorption of iron from intestinal tract and also in production and survival of red blood cells. Requirement met by ordinary diet which supplies two to five milligrams. Copper deficiency is extremely rare in man.

Microelements. Certain trace- or microelements are thought to be essential nutritionally. These include *chromium,* concerned with carbohydrate metabolism, *cobalt,* an integral part of vitamin B_{12}, *manganese,* needed for normal bone structure, *molybdenum, selenium,* and *zinc.* A mixed diet may be expected to supply adequate amounts of these microelements and the risk of a deficiency in the United States is slight. Green leafy foods, fruit, whole grains, organ meats, and lean meats usually serve as generous sources of these elements.[12]

HOW ARE MINERALS RELATED TO ACID-BASE BALANCE IN BODY?

A very important regulating function performed by minerals in the body is the

---

[12] Recommended Dietary Allowances, 7th edition, Publication No. 1694. Washington, D. C., National Academy of Sciences–National Research Council, 1968, pp. 61–62.

role they play in helping to maintain the neutrality of the body. The blood of a person in normal health is almost at the neutral point expressed by the term pH 7.0 (actually just slightly on the alkaline side—7.3 to 7.5). Should the blood become too alkaline, a condition of alkalosis would result; if too acid, a condition of acidosis, either of which would be undesirable. To maintain the blood at this almost neutral point, the body calls upon proteins which can combine with either excess acid or excess base elements, certain neutralizing systems, including *minerals,* and the kidneys which can adapt to an acid or alkaline urine.

Mineral elements in the food intake which are left in the blood and tissues after the foods are digested, absorbed, and burned for energy possess acid-forming properties if Cl, S, and P predominate, or base-forming properties if Ca, Na, K, and Mg predominate. In an ordinary, well selected diet, a good balance probably exists between acid and base elements.

Fruits, especially citrus fruits, even though acid to taste, are not acid-forming after reaching the tissues. The acids giving the sour taste to these foods are actually organic in nature and can be burned in the body just like any other carbon-containing nutrient, leaving a basic residue, like the other base-forming foods. Even plums, prunes, and cranberries, listed below with the acid-forming foods, actually have an excess of basic over acidic elements and should leave a basic residue in the tissue. However, these fruits contain, in addition, an inorganic acid which the body can not burn and which offsets the base present.

The use of diets predominating in either acidic or basic elements may be prescribed for certain therapeutic purposes.

Base-forming foods (alkaline-ash)	*Acid-forming foods* (acid-ash)	*Neutral foods*
Milk	Meat, fish, shellfish, eggs, poultry	Butter
Vegetables (except corn and lentils)	Cheese (all types)	Margarine
Fruits (except prunes, plums, cranberries, and some nuts) coconut, almonds, chestnuts	Cereals, crackers, cookies, cakes, breadstuffs	Lard, oils
	Prunes, plums, cranberries	Cornstarch
	Filberts, peanuts, walnuts, Brazil nuts	Tapioca, arrowroot
Sweets—jams, jellies, honey	Corn and lentils	Refined sugar
Molasses	Pastes—macaroni, noodles, spaghetti	Cooking fats
		Syrups
		Candy (plain)

WHAT ARE FUNCTIONS, REQUIREMENTS, AND SOURCES OF WATER?

Functions	*Requirements*	*Sources*
Principal constituent of body — 1/2 to 3/4 of body weight.	Fluid balance is important —intake must balance output.	Water as such. Water in foods — foods contain 10–98% water.

Functions	Requirements	Sources
Important for life — a few days' deprivation causes death.	Requirements closely related to salt requirement and intake	Water formed in body in metabolic processes
Most of water in cells (intracellular), remainder in blood, lymph, various secretions and excretions, and around cells (extracellular).	Increased amounts needed under conditions of extreme heat or excessive sweating.	—end products of oxidation.
Helps every organ function.	Absorbed in small intestine with digested food and also in colon.	Average diet with milk (87% water) contains about 1000 ml water.
Aids digestion, absorption, circulation, excretion.	Not stored so daily intake is necessary — 6 to 8 glasses total including that in food, and beverages.	
Solvent for body constituents. Medium for all chemical changes.	Water lost in urine, in expired air, in feces and from skin.	
As part of blood, carries nutrients to and waste products from cells.	Water requirements increased for infants on high protein formulas, comatose patients, and those with fever, polyuria, diarrhea, or receiving high protein diets.	
Regulates body temperature.		
Lubricates moving parts of body.		
Necessary for building and repair processes.		

TERMS TO UNDERSTAND

Mineral	Base-forming foods	Anemia	Edema
Water balance	Rickets	Osteomalacia	Inorganic
Dehydration	Intracellular	Acid-forming foods	Osteoporosis
Ash	Fluoridation	Extracellular	

STUDY QUESTIONS AND ACTIVITIES

1. Why must minerals be supplied daily in the diet?

2. Where are minerals found in the body? In what different forms?

3. List several ways minerals build or enter into the structure of certain parts of the body.

4. List several ways in which minerals play a role in regulating vital life processes.

5. What are important calcium functions in nutrition?

6. What vitamin helps in the utilization of calcium by the body?

7. Explain why milk and milk products are the best calcium foods.

8. What do you think of the following statement "One never outgrows the need for milk in the diet"?

9. What are important iron functions in nutrition?

10. Why is an anemic person usually tired and listless?

11. If your doctor tells you your hemoglobin is low, what foods will you stress in your daily diet?

12. Why might a person with leg cramps be told to check on the adequacy of milk in his diet?

13. Is the taste of food always an indication whether it will produce an acid or alkaline reaction in the body tissues and blood? Why?

14. Why is it difficult to get the right amount of calcium in the diet if milk or milk products are not used?

15. What suggestions could you give a person about getting sufficient calcium if he or she can not drink milk for some reason?

16. How does water function in the body? Why must there be a balance between intake and output?

17. Is it desirable to drink water with meals?

18. Will water make one fat?

19. Is your fluid intake adequate? For a couple of days jot down below the amounts of fluids consumed each day and compare the amount with your requirements.

20. Which of the following menus is better for hemoglobin building? Why?

(1)	(2)
Broiled hamburger	Broiled liver
Mashed potatoes	Baked potato
Buttered green beans	Buttered swiss chard
Cabbage and carrot salad	Tossed salad
Enriched bread and butter	Whole wheat bread and butter
Baked apple and milk	Prune whip with custard sauce

21. Why are requirements for calcium and iron increased during pregnancy and lactation?

SUPPLEMENTARY READING

Bogert: Chapter 9
Howe: Chapters 6, 8

Mowry: Chapter 6
Peyton: Chapters 8, 9

Robinson: Chapter 9
Yearbook, 1959: Pages 112–129

HOW ADEQUATE IS YOUR MINERAL INTAKE?

Determine the calcium and iron content of your day's food record on page 24.[13]
The calcium content of the foods on my food record totals_____ grams.
My recommended allowance for calcium is_____ grams.
The iron content of the foods on my food record totals_____ milligrams.
My recommended allowance for iron is _____ milligrams.
What suggestions can you make regarding your mineral intake?

NOTE: This activity may be omitted and students asked to list all foods on
their week's diet record (page 24) which are good sources of calcium and
also those which are good sources of iron and judge their intake for
adequacy for both these minerals.

Jot down below your RDA for the additional three minerals which appear for the
first time on the 1968 RDA revision. [14] See page 26.
My RDA for phosphorus is _____ milligrams.
iodine is _____ milligrams.
magnesium is _____ milligrams.

---

[13] Use Food Composition Table, **Appendix,** page 299.
[14] See RDA page 26.

PART 6. VITAMINS

WHAT ARE VITAMINS?

Long before the beginnings of nutrition science, it was a common observation that certain foods cured certain diseases. Lemons and limes added to the diet of sailors in the British navy on long voyages with limited rations prevented the scurvy so frequently encountered. Beriberi, the scourge of the Japanese navy, was prevented when the limited diet of polished rice and fish was supplemented. It is now thought that the potatoes and fruits eaten by early New England and Pilgrim settlers curbed deaths from scurvy during those early days. The incidence of pellagra in the United States has decreased with dietary changes.

Only at the beginning of this century did it become evident that something was needed for good health in addition to carbohydrates, fats, proteins, and minerals. The term "vitamine," later changed to "vitamin," was coined to cover these new substances, occurring in minute amounts in food and needed only in minute amounts. As each new vitamin, with specific functions, was discovered, an alphabetical designation was given. Five letters were originally used. The number of letters was extended as new vitamins were discovered. Some of the original letters were given subnumerical designations where a vitamin was found to be made up of several parts. A name indicating a "curative" property was frequently attached to each vitamin, as "antiscorbutic" for vitamin C, "antineuritic" for vitamin B_1, etc.

When a vitamin could be isolated from a food, its chemical formula determined, and, in some instances, its synthesis accomplished, it was learned that each of these vitamins was a distinct chemical substance organic in nature, with a chemical formula all its own and with specific nutritional functions. Names indicating chemical nature or coined names have now replaced the alphabetical designations for most of the vitamins. Some vitamins are groups of factors and are called complexes. Some vitamins are simple, some complex, and others have not yet been identified.

Solubility of vitamins in either fat or water provided an early basis for classification into fat-soluble and water-soluble groups. This classification continues in use for convenience in study, even though the vitamins in each group differ from one another in characteristics, functions, and sources.

WHAT IS THE ROLE OF VITAMINS IN NUTRITION?

Vitamins are present in foods and needed by the body only in minute amounts but proper growth and development and optimal health are impossible without them. Some may be synthesized in the body but, for the most part, they must be supplied in the daily diet of normal healthy persons. Vitamin supplements may be prescribed by a physician for therapeutic purposes. Vitamins, although organic in nature, do not provide energy but they do help carbohydrates, fats, and proteins to be metabolized more efficiently. It is thought that vitamins act as catalysts. Early attention to the clear-cut manifest diseases caused by vitamin deficiencies (avitaminoses), seldom seen now, obscured for a time the very important function of vitamins in the promotion of optimal health. They are not, as advertising might lead us to believe, a cure-all for every ill. Nor do they lessen the importance in the diet of the other essential nutrients such as proteins and minerals. Unlike minerals, vitamins are not a part of various body structures.

Vitamins are classed as *body regulators* because they:

Promote normal growth and development, reproduction, and lactation.

Are essential for optimal health at all ages by promoting better tissue structure and function, strength, endurance, stability, normal function of the digestive tract and other parts of the body, the utilization of all nutrients, resistance to infection, and good appetite.

Prevent certain nutritional deficiency diseases.

WHAT ARE FUNCTIONS AND SOURCES OF FAT-SOLUBLE VITAMINS?

Each of the four fat-soluble vitamins—A, D, E, K—is a distinct chemical entity and performs a specific function in the body. All are absorbed along with dietary fats, requiring the same favorable conditions for intestinal absorption; mineral oil interferes with absorption. These vitamins can be stored in the body to a certain degree but are not normally eliminated in the urine. Excessive amounts (hypervitaminosis) may be harmful. Some vitamins can be synthesized—vitamin A from chlorophyll and carotene (precursors), the green and yellow coloring substances in plants.

Vitamin	Functions	Sources
Vitamin A and Provitamin A (carotene)	Influences growth, development, pregnancy and lactation.	*Animal* (preformed Vitamin A)
First vitamin recognized.	Influences normal bone, tooth, and skin development.	Liver (animal and fish)
Allowances stated in International Units (I.U.)	Necessary for normal vision and eye health (prevents night blindness).	Whole milk, butter, cream
With prolonged excessive intake may be toxic (hypervitaminosis).	Maintains healthy epithelial tissues throughout the body.	Whole milk cheese, cream cheese
		Egg yolk
		Plant (provitamin A—carotene)
	Increases resistance to disease ("anti-infective")	Dark green leafy and stem vegetables
		Deep yellow or orange fruits
	Prevents eye disease (xerophthalmia).	Fortified margarines
		Food supplements
		Concentrates: fish liver oils

Deficiency: night blindness (nyctalopia), dry and rough scaly skin (keratinized), infections (mucous membranes), xerophthalmia. Dietary fat needed for absorption. Protein malnutrition results in decreased absorption and blood transport of vitamin. Normal functioning of G. I. tract (especially bile secretion) necessary for absorption. Laxatives, biotics, mineral oil, and disease decrease absorption.[15]

---

[15] Recommended Dietary Allowances, 7th edition, Publication 1694, Washington, D. C., National Academy of Sciences–National Research Council, 1968, p. 23.

The following chart shows daily recommended allowances and food sources for vitamin A in average servings.

VITAMIN A Value*
DAILY RECOMMENDATIONS

INTERNATIONAL UNITS

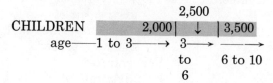

	2,500	
CHILDREN	2,000 ↓ 3,500	
age——1 to 3—— →	3—— →	—— →
	to	6 to 10
	6	

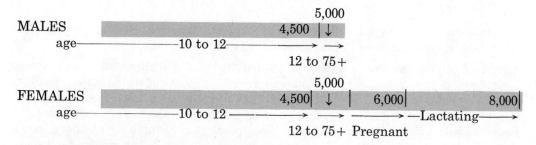

	5,000
MALES	4,500 ↓
age——————————10 to 12—————— → —→	
	12 to 75+

	5,000		
FEMALES	4,500 ↓ 6,000		8,000
age——————10 to 12 ——————→ —→ ———→ —Lactating—→			
	12 to 75+ Pregnant		

GOOD SOURCES OF VITAMIN A†

INTERNATIONAL UNITS

Food	Serving	I.U.
Liver	3½ oz.	43,875
Sweet Potato	1 med.	9,600
Spinach	½ cup	7,245
Carrots	½ cup	6,830
Dark Green Leafy Vegetables	½ cup	5,137
Winter Squash	½ cup	4,305
Broccoli	½ cup	1,875
Tomato	½ cup	1,136
Asparagus	½ cup	747
Peas	½ cup	491
Cantaloup	½ med.	6,540
Dried Fruit	½ cup	2,283
Peach	1 med.	935
Orange	1 med.	275
Banana	1 med.	190
Egg	1 med.	590
Cheese	1 oz.	350
Milk	1 cup	350
Butter or Margarine	1 pat	230

* Lessons on Meat, Chicago, National Livestock and Meat Board, 1970, p. 21.
† Average nutrient content as food is served. (*Note: 3½ ounces equals approximately 100 grams.*)

Vitamin	*Functions*	*Sources*
Vitamin D Requirement for vitamin D in adult life not known; usual mixed diet and exposure to sunlight will meet need. Precursors: ergosterol in plants; a form of cholesterol in body. Calciferol a crystalline form.	Needed throughout growth period. Essential at all ages for utilization of Ca and P and for soundness of teeth and skeleton.	Very small amounts in a few foods — butter, egg yolk, liver, tuna, salmon, sardines Fresh and evaporated milk fortified to 400 I.U. per quart Fortified margarines and some cereal foods. Concentrates Fish liver oils

Deficiency: rickets in children, with skeletal deformities, soft bones, poor teeth, bowed legs, enlarged joints; osteomalacia in adults.

Vitamin	*Functions*	*Sources*
Vitamin E (alpha tocopherol) Allowances stated in I. U. (vitamin E activity), Requirement related to fat intake (especially unsaturated fatty acids).	Essential nutrient for man. Protects red blood cells from rupture (hemolysis) by oxidizing agents. Protects oxidative destruction of vitamin A in intestine.	Wide distribution in foods. Vegetable oils, shortenings, margarines. Dark leafy vegetables. Stable to ordinary cooking processes except deep fat frying.
Vitamin K No RDA established.	Related to formation of prothrombin and other clotting factors. Complex relationship exists between vitamin K and other nutrients and hormones. Coumarin products (anticoagulants) act as antagonists.	Average diet probably contains adequate amounts. Green leaves excellent sources. Pork liver. Heat, light, and air stable Some body synthesis — lessened with antibiotics.

Deficiency: hemorrhage, lack of synthesis, poor absorption, disturbance in bile flow in newborn, biliary tract disease.

WHAT ARE FUNCTIONS AND SOURCES OF WATER-SOLUBLE VITAMINS?

The Vitamin B Complex

This term includes all water-soluble vitamins except ascorbic acid (vitamin C). Vitamin B was the first of this group to be discovered and was known as the "antiberiberi" or "antineuritic" vitamin or simply as vitamin B. Thiamine was the first to be obtained in pure form and is known as vitamin B_1. With further study, vitamin B proved to be not a single substance but a combination of a number of factors, each one of which was given a letter or a descriptive term, or, later, a chemical designation as its chemical nature became known.

Twelve factors in the vitamin B complex are recognized today. RDA have been established for six: thiamine (B_1), riboflavin (B_2—formerly G), niacin (nicotinic acid), B_6, B_{12}, and folacin. See page 26 for RDA. Important functions in the body have been assigned to biotin, choline and pantothenic acid in the 1968 RDA revision but no definite daily allowances are established. It is thought that the amount needed daily in each case will be met by the average daily diet.

All of the 12 substances now recognized to be included in the vitamin B complex are essential to nutrition in one or more ways and must be supplied in the daily diet. Some are available in pure form. Several are components of one or more coenzyme systems which function as "catalysts" in the use of nutrients for energy and building and repair processes. All are closely interrelated. A lack of vitamins of the B complex is one of the widespread forms of malnutrition. Because of the similar distribution of the B vitamins in foods, a deficiency of several factors is observed oftener than a deficiency of a single factor. The interrelationship of many of these vitamins in life processes means that signs of a deficiency are often similar when the diet lacks any one of several factors. Many physiological and pathological stresses influence the need for the B vitamins. Needs are increased during pregnancy and lactation, growth, fevers, hyperthyroidism, injury, and before and after surgery.

Thiamine and ascorbic acid are most easily destroyed because of water solubility, dehydration and cooking; their destruction is speeded by the presence of alkali, copper, and iron and release of enzymes by cutting raw foods. Foods cooked properly for thiamine and ascorbic acid retention retain other water-soluble vitamins. Riboflavin is light sensitive. Amounts of riboflavin eaten in excess of needs are eliminated in urine; there is very little body storage.

Vitamin	Functions	Sources
Thiamine (B_1). Need is small but important, based on calorie requirement. Regular daily supply needed as body stores little. Amounts eaten in excess of needs eliminated in urine. RDA stated in mg. The following chart shows recommended daily allowances and food sources of thiamine in average servings	Functions in carbohydrate metabolism. Promotes good appetite and good functioning of digestive tract. Helps nervous system, heart and muscles function properly. Prevents beriberi. Needed throughout life for tissue functioning. Increased need during pregnancy and lactation.	Many foods contain small amounts. Whole-grain enriched flour and bread. Meats, fish, poultry; especially organ meats Pork contains three times as much as other meats Dry beans and peas, peanuts Small amounts in milk and eggs Dry yeast, wheat germ Lost in cooking unless cooking water is used. Alkali (baking soda), high temperature and long cooking destroy thiamine.

Deficiency: Polyneuritis, beriberi, fatigue, depression, poor appetite, and poor functioning of intestinal tract, and nervous instability.

THIAMINE*
DAILY RECOMMENDATIONS
MILLIGRAMS

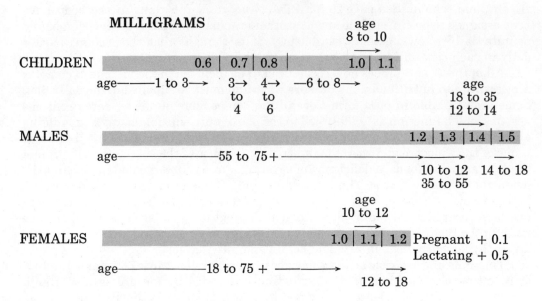

GOOD SOURCES OF THIAMINE†
MILLIGRAMS

Pork	3½ oz.	1.03
Pork Sausage	2 oz.	.46
Liver	3½ oz.	.33
Lamb	3½ oz.	.22
Veal	3⅓ oz.	.18
Luncheon Meat	2 oz.	.17
Beef	3 oz.	.10

Dried Beans and Peas	¾ cup	.19
Peas	½ cup	.15
Orange	1 med.	.14
Potato	1 med.	.12
Dark Green Leafy Vegetables	½ cup	.07

Oysters	6–9 med.	.17
Nuts	¼ cup	.17
Fish	3½ oz.	.09
Poultry	3½ oz.	.08
Egg	1 med.	.05

Cereal	½ cup	.09
Bread	1 slice	.06

Milk	1 cup	.08

* Lessons on Meat, Chicago, National Livestock and Meat Board, 1970, p. 17.
† Average nutrient content as food is served. *(Note: 3½ ounces equals approximately 100 grams.)*

Vitamin	Functions	Sources
Riboflavin (B₂) Requirement stated in mg. is related to calorie need. Excess intake over needs eliminated in urine.	Essential for certain enzyme systems which aid in metabolism of carbohydrates, proteins and fats. Promotes general well-being. Important for eye, skin, lip and tongue health.	Milk, cheese, eggs, Green leafy vegetables, Organ meats, liver, kidney, heart Dry yeast Peanuts, peanut butter. Adequate milk consumption important for adequacy. Heat, acid, and oxidation resistant

Deficiency: cheilosis, tongue inflammation, scaling and burning skin, sensitive eyes, ariboflavinosis.

The following chart shows daily recommended allowances and food sources of riboflavin in average servings.

RIBOFLAVIN*

DAILY RECOMMENDATIONS

MILLIGRAMS

CHILDREN   0.6 | 0.7 | 0.8 | 0.9 | 1.1 | 1.2
age   1 to 2→ → → → –6→ →
                 2   3   4   to   8
                to   to   to   8   to
                 3   4   6   10

MALES   1.3 | 1.4 | 1.5 | 1.6 | 1.7
age————————10 to 12————————→ 12→ 14→ 18→ 22
                                        to   to   to   to
                                        14   18   22   75 +

FEMALES   1.3 | 1.4 | 1.5 | 1.8 | 2.0
age————————10 to 12——————→ → →———————→———————→
                                        12   16 Pregnant Lactating
                                        to   to
                                        16   75 +

---

* Lessons on Meat, Chicago, National Livestock and Meat Board, 1970, p. 18.

GOOD SOURCES OF RIBOFLAVIN†

MILLIGRAMS

Food		mg
Liver	3½ oz.	4.46
Beef	3½ oz.	.39
Veal	3½ oz.	.35
Lamb	3½ oz.	.32
Pork	3½ oz.	.29
Luncheon Meat	2 oz.	.27
Tongue	2 oz.	.17
Pork Sausage	2 oz.	.12
Oysters	6–9 med.	.22
Poultry	3½ oz.	.17
Fish	3½ oz.	.17
Egg	1 med.	.15
Milk	1 cup	.42
Cottage Cheese	¼ cup	.14
Cheese	1 oz.	.12
Asparagus	½ cup	.13
Spinach	½ cup	.12
Squash	½ cup	.11
Bread	1 slice	.04
Cereal	½ cup	.03

Vitamin	Functions	Sources
Niacin (nicotinic acid) Requirement stated in mg. is related to calorie intake. Excess intake over needs eliminated in urine. Chart on following page shows recommended allowances and food sources of niacin in average servings.	Functions as part of two important enzymes which regulate energy metabolism Promotes good physical and mental health. Helps maintain health of skin, tongue, and digestive system. Helps prevent pellagra.	Organ meat—liver, kidney, heart Meat, poultry, fish Whole grain and enriched cereal products Meat drippings, yeast Niacin can be synthesized in body from an amino acid, tryptophan, in protein. Precursor of niacin in milk and eggs. Heat, oxidation, light, acid, alkali stable.

Deficiency: Pellagra with skin and mouth affections, gastro-intestinal disturbances, and mental disturbances.

---

† Average nutrient content as food is served. *(Note: 3½ ounces equals approximately 100 grams.)*

NIACIN*
DAILY RECOMMENDATIONS

MILLIGRAMS

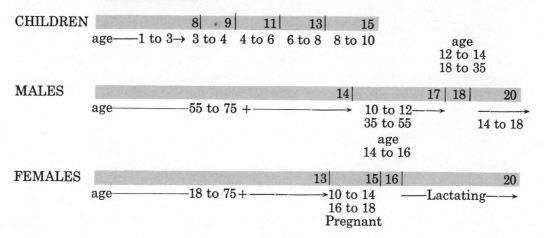

CHILDREN

8| · 9| 11| 13| 15

age——1 to 3→ 3 to 4   4 to 6   6 to 8   8 to 10

age
12 to 14
18 to 35

MALES

14| 17| 18| 20

age————————55 to 75 + ——————→   10 to 12——→   ———————→
35 to 55   14 to 18
age
14 to 16

FEMALES

13| 15| 16| 20

age————————18 to 75+ ————→10 to 14   ——Lactating——→
16 to 18
Pregnant

GOOD SOURCES OF NIACIN†

Food	Amount	mg
Liver	3½ oz.	20.1
Lamb	3½ oz.	7.6
Veal	3½ oz.	7.2
Beef	3½ oz.	4.5
Pork	3½ oz.	4.4
Luncheon Meat	2 oz.	2.4
Pork Sausage	2 oz.	2.4
Tuna Fish	3 oz.	10.1
Poultry	3½ oz.	8.1
Fish	3½ oz.	5.5
Peanut Butter	2 tblsp.	4.8
Potato	1 med.	1.8
Dried Fruit	½ cup	1.5
Peas	½ cup	1.3
Dried Beans and Peas	¾ cup	1.3
Corn	½ cup	1.3
Sweet Potato	1 med.	0.8
Banana	1 med.	0.7
Cereal	½ cup	0.7
Bread	1 slice	0.7

* Lessons on Meat, Chicago, National Livestock and Meat Board, 1970, p. 19.
† Average nutrient content as food is served. (*Note: 3½ ounces equals approximately 100 grams.*)

Vitamins	*Functions*	*Sources*
Other B Complex vitamins:	Functions in energy metabolism but more related to protein and amino acid metabolism.	Three forms present in varying amounts in different foods.
Vitamin B6—collective term for 3 substances; pyridoxine (plants), pyridoxal and pyridodoxamine (animal products).	Possibly of importance in red blood cell regeneration and normal nervous system functioning.	Recommended amounts of food in the Four Food Groups will meet requirements.
Allowances stated in mg. Increased need with high protein diets, pregnancy, and certain tuberculosis therapy.		Heat, light and oxidation stable; high heat detrimental.
Vitamin B12 (cobalamin) RDA stated in micrograms (μg.)	Essential for normal function of all cells, particularly cells of bone marrow, nervous system, G. I. tract.	Present mostly in foods of animal origin, bound to protein. Little in vegetables. High in kidney and liver; moderate amount in meat.
Cobalt essential part of B_{12}.	Important in energy metabolism but especially folic acid metabolism	Milk; most cheeses. Shellfish; most fish. Whole egg and egg yolk.
Deficiency: pernicious anemia, caused by lack of "intrinsic factor" of aid in B_{12} absorption.	Deficiency: certain types of anemia with muscle, nerve, skin and G. I. disturbances.	Severe heating of meat and products detrimental.
Folacin Active form is folinic acid formed from folacin by vitamin C.	Functions in formation of red blood cells. Aids in metabolism of protein.	Wide variety of foods of animal and plant origin, particularly glandular meats, yeast, dark green vegetables, dry beans, peanuts, walnuts, lentils, filberts.
RDA stated in mg. Some body synthesis.	Readily absorbed by G. I. tract and stored primarily in liver.	

Requirements increased by pregnancy and other stressful conditions, including various diseases and alcohol consumption. "Folacin allowance refers to dietary sources."

Deficiency: certain types of anemia with sore mouth and G.I. disturbances; causes—inadequate food intake, impaired absorption, excessive body demands, metabolism abnormalities.

Biotin	***Choline***	***Pantothenic Acid***
No RDA established. Essential for activity of many enzyme systems.	Constituent of several compounds necessary in certain aspects of	Essential constituent of complex enzymes concerned with fatty

Biotin

Found in great many foods: richest liver, kidney, milk, egg yolk, yeast.

Diet deficiency only when diet contains large amounts of raw egg white. Protein avidin (inactivated by heating) in egg white binds biotin and prevents its absorption.

Adequate diet provides any need of 150–300 mg.

Pregnancy and lactation increase need.

Choline

nerve function and lipid metabolism.

Deficiency not demonstrated in man.

Average mixed diet consumed in U. S. (500–900 mg.), including its precursor, betaine, adequate when compared with animal needs.

No RDA established.

Pantothenic Acid

acid metabolism and synthesis of certain products.

Presence assured in diets otherwise adequate in B complex vitamins.

Widely distributed, occurring abundantly in animal tissues, whole grain cereals, and legumes, and lesser amounts in milk, vegetables, and fruit.

No RDA established; daily intake of 5–10 mg. considered adequate for children and adults. Usual diet contains 10–15 mg. daily.

Vitamin

Ascorbic acid (vitamin C)
Requirement stated in mg.

Daily intake necessary as this vitamin is not stored.

Excessive intake excreted in urine; body has saturation point.

The chart on page 86 shows RDA and food sources of ascorbic acid in average servings.

Deficiency: Scurvy with sore mouth, cutaneous hemorrhages, bleeding gums, loose teeth, weak-walled capillaries.

Vegetable-Fruit Group on the Daily Food Guide (see page 28) only group furnishing vitamin C in appreciable amounts.

Functions

Performs multiple functions.

Aids in formation and maintenance of intercellular cement substance of body tissue: important for tooth dentine, bones, cartilage, connective tissue, blood vessels.

Protects body against infections.

Helps in wound healing and recovery following operations.

Helps in formation of red blood cells in bone marrow.

Helps change folacin to folinic acid.

Helps absorption of iron in intestine.

Sources

Fruits and vegetables the main source; contain more of vitamin when fresh.

Citrus fruits, strawberries, cantaloup, some green leafy vegetables.

Potatoes, if cooked properly.

Tomatoes, green peppers, broccoli, raw greens, cabbage, newly harvested potatoes.

Ascorbic acid most sensitive of vitamins to cooking procedures—heat, oxygen, alkalis, high temperature, long cooking.

See pages 108–109 for correct procedures for vegetable cookery to conserve this vitamin.

ASCORBIC ACID   Vitamin C*
DAILY RECOMMENDATIONS
MILLIGRAMS

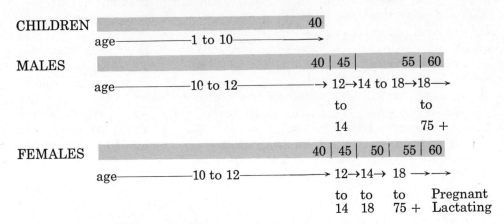

CHILDREN — 40
age————1 to 10————→

MALES — 40 | 45 | 55 | 60
age————10 to 12————→ 12→14 to 18→18—→
                        to   to
                        14   75 +

FEMALES — 40 | 45 | 50 | 55 | 60
age————10 to 12————→ 12→14→ 18 —→—→
                      to to to   Pregnant
                      14 18 75 + Lactating

GOOD SOURCES OF ASCORBIC ACID†
MILLIGRAMS

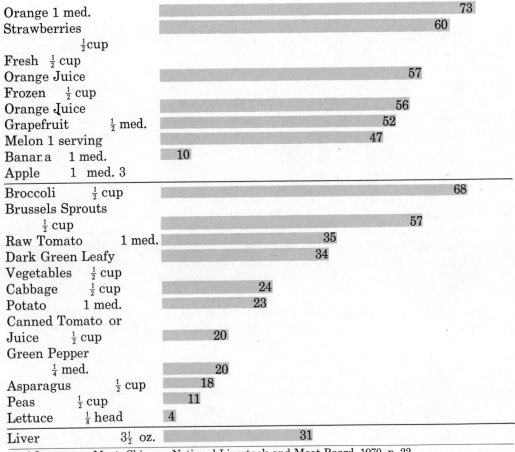

Food	mg
Orange 1 med.	73
Strawberries ½ cup	60
Fresh ½ cup Orange Juice	57
Frozen ½ cup Orange Juice	56
Grapefruit ½ med.	52
Melon 1 serving	47
Banana 1 med.	10
Apple 1 med.	3
Broccoli ½ cup	68
Brussels Sprouts ½ cup	57
Raw Tomato 1 med.	35
Dark Green Leafy Vegetables ½ cup	34
Cabbage ½ cup	24
Potato 1 med.	23
Canned Tomato or Juice ½ cup	20
Green Pepper ¼ med.	20
Asparagus ½ cup	18
Peas ½ cup	11
Lettuce ⅛ head	4
Liver 3½ oz.	31

* Lessons on Meat, Chicago, National Livestock and Meat Board, 1970, p. 22.
† Average nutrient as food is served. *(Note: 3½ ounces equals approximately 100 grams.)*

WHAT FACTORS AFFECT VITAMIN VALUE OF FOODS?

Variety of food: some varieties have more or less of a certain vitamin.

Soil variations and climate: same food grown in one area may have more or less than same food grown elsewhere.

Degree of maturity: some foods have more of a vitamin when underripe; others when ripe.

Type of diet fed animal used as food.

Storage after harvesting or production: may have destructive effect.

Freezing: some vitamins lost in preliminary blanching.

Drying: certain losses occur.

Canning: less loss in acid food than in non-acid food.

Cooking of food affects vitamins in various ways.

Antivitamin factors: certain substances may inactivate the vitamins, be antagonistic to them, interfere with their absorption and metabolism or synthesis in the body. Antibiotics and other drugs may kill intestinal bacteria which help in the synthesis; oxidation may be destructive.

Favorable food handling practices for vitamin retention:

Store vegetables properly to avoid wilting and drying out which cause loss of vitamin A.

Cook vegetables whole as often as possible: cutting releases oxidative enzymes and increases cut surfaces where water-soluble vitamins leach out.

Use cooking water and canned food juices to conserve soluble nutrients.

Avoid use of baking soda in cooking vegetables as it is destructive to thiamine and ascorbic acid; also avoid long cooking for the same reason.

Store fats properly to prevent rancidity, a destructive factor for vitamin A.

Keep milk in glass bottles away from light which is destructive to riboflavin.

Use drippings when cooking meat to conserve thiamine and niacin.

Keep fruit juices covered and cold to prevent oxygen from destroying ascorbic acid.

Don't stir while cooking foods with ascorbic acid as oxygen destroys vitamin.

Cook vegetables covered, quickly, and just until fork-tender. Store leftovers covered and cold: reheating causes further loss of vitamins.

IS IT NECESSARY TO USE VITAMIN SUPPLEMENTS?

Nutrition scientists agree that if a healthy person chooses his daily diet from the Four Food Groups on the Daily Diet Plan (pages 28–31), he will obtain not only an adequate supply of essential vitamins but also the right amounts of the other essential nutrients. Therefore, it should not be necessary for him to supplement the vitamins in his food intake with pill, liquid, or capsule forms of vitamins. Not only is it nutritionally advantageous to purchase one's vitamins in foods from the supermarket rather than the drug store, it is much more economical, as well.

Vitamins are not a cure-all for the many ailments for which they are advertised; neither are they a substitute for good eating habits. Also, some evidence exists which shows that excessive intakes of certain vitamins may prove deleterious. Moderate amounts of vitamin A and other fat-soluble vitamins may be stored. It is important that concentrates of fat-soluble vitamins be taken only in the exact a-mounts prescribed. Amounts of water-soluble vitamins consumed in excess of needs are excreted, constituting a waste of money for something not usable.

If for some reason—physical or psychological—the amount or quality of a food must be restricted in the diet or if absorption from the intestinal tract is impaired, vitamin supplements may be indicated. This is a medical problem and should be in the hands of a physician. Vitamin D supplements are usually ordered by the physician for infants and young children and pregnant and lactating women. Only the exact dosage prescribed should be used.

It is estimated that about 300 million dollars are spent yearly for vitamin products, most of which are purchased on the basis of self-diagnosis. Some of these products contain larger amounts of vitamins than are needed by the body even in extreme cases of depletion; excesses of certain vitamins that the body can not store, which are quickly eliminated; some vitamins and minerals not yet found to be required by humans; and excessive amounts of some vitamins which might be definitely harmful to the body. Amounts of vitamins may also be found in therapeutic doses which no person should be taking "on his own" and which should not be available without prescription. In one case "sale without prescription of vitamin preparations recommending doses of more than 0.1 milligram folic acid per day is prohibited (Federal Register July 20, 1963)."[16]

TERMS TO UNDERSTAND

Vitamin	Avitaminosis	Vitamin deficiency
Provitamin	Hypervitaminosis	Vitamin precursor
Precursor	Epithelial	Antivitamin

STUDY QUESTIONS AND ACTIVITIES

1. Vitamins are sometimes called "accessory food factors" or "coordinators." Can you suggest some reasons?

2. Name several reasons why vitamins are body "regulators."

3. Why must foods containing vitamins be eaten daily? What vitamins can be stored? Which ones can not be stored?

4. What important function of vitamin A accounts for its being called "anti-infective"?

5. Why is vitamin D sometimes called the "sunshine" vitamin? How is it related to rickets?

6. What is meant by the vitamin B complex? What foods will you be sure to have in your daily diet to insure adequate amounts of the vitamin B complex vitamins?

7. How can you be sure to have the required amount of ascorbic acid in your daily diet?

8. Will milk in paper containers possibly have more or less riboflavin than milk in glass bottles? Why? What special care is needed for milk in clear glass bottles?

9. Ascorbic acid is the vitamin most easily destroyed in preparation of foods for cooking, actual cooking, and serving of foods. Name several procedures in food care, preparation, and cooking which will help retain the vitamin.

---

[16] *Recommended Dietary Allowances,* 6th edition. Publication No. 1694. Washington, D. C., National Academy of Sciences—National Research Council, 1968, p. 37.

10. List the foods in the Four Food Groups with correct servings which will help meet your requirements for vitamins. Why is special emphasis placed on whole milk, meat, dark green or yellow vegetables, citrus fruits, and whole grain or enriched cereals and bread?

SUPPLEMENTARY READING

Bogert: Chapters 12, 13, 14, 15   Mowry: Chapter 7   Robinson: Chapters 10–11
Howe: Chapter 9   Peyton: Chapter 7   Yearbook, 1959: pages 130–161
Vitamin Supplements and their Correct Use. Chicago, American Medical Association, 1970.

The summary chart of key nutrients, their functions and sources, on page 90 will be helpful to you in reviewing parts 1 to 6 of Unit Three.

HOW ADEQUATE IS YOUR VITAMIN INTAKE?

Determine the vitamin A, thiamine, riboflavin, niacin, and ascorbic acid content of your day's food record on page 24.[17]

Vitamin content of my food record

My recommended allowances for vitamins[18]

Vitamin content of my food record			My recommended allowances for vitamins[18]		
Vitamin A	_____	Int. Units	Vitamin A	_____	Int. Units
Thiamine	_____	mg.	Thiamine	_____	mg.
Riboflavin	_____	mg.	Riboflavin	_____	mg.
Niacin	_____	mg.	Niacin	_____	mg.
Ascorbic acid	_____	mg.	Ascorbic acid	_____	mg.

What suggestions can you make regarding your vitamin intake?

Jot down below your RDA for the additional four vitamins which appear for the first time in the 1968 RDA revision. See page 26.

My RDA for vitamin	E activity is	_____	Int. Units
	Folacin is	_____	mg.
	Vitamin B_6 is	_____	mg.
	Vitamin B_{12} is	_____	mg.

NOTE: This activity may be omitted and students asked to list all foods on their week's diet record (page 24) which are good sources of vitamin A, thiamine, riboflavin, niacin, and ascorbic acid and judge the adequacy of their intake of these vitamins.

---

[17] Use Food Composition Table, Appendix, pages 298.
[18] RDA, p. 26.

Key Nutrients	Important Functions	Important Sources
Protein	Builds and repairs all tissues Helps build blood and form antibodies to fight infection Supplies energy	Meat, fish, poultry, eggs Milk and all kinds of cheese Dried beans and peas Peanut butter, nuts Bread and cereals
Fat	Supplies large amount of energy in a small amount of food. Helps keep infant's skin healthy by supplying essential fatty acids Carries vitamins A, D, E and K	Butter and cream Salad oils and dressings Cooking and table fats Fat in meat
Carbohydrate (Sugars and Starch)	Supplies energy	Bread and cereals Potatoes, lima beans, corn Dried beans and peas Dried fruits, sweetened fruits; smaller amounts in fresh fruits Sugar, syrup, jelly, jam, honey
Minerals Calcium	Helps build bones and teeth Helps blood clot Helps muscles and nerves to work Helps regulate the use of other minerals in the body	Milk Cheese, but less in cottage cheese, ice cream Sardines, other whole canned fish Turnip and mustard greens Collards, kale, broccoli
Iron	Combines with protein to make hemoglobin, the red substance in the blood that carries oxygen to the cells	Liver, other meat and eggs Dried beans and peas Green leafy vegetables Prunes, raisins, dried apricots Enriched or whole grain bread and cereals
Iodine	A constituent of thyroxine, a hormone that controls metabolic rate	Seafoods, iodized salt
Vitamins Vitamin A	Helps keep skin clear and smooth Helps keep mucous membranes firm and resistant to infection Helps prevent night blindness and promote healthy eyes Helps control bone growth	Liver, eggs Dark green and deep yellow vegetables Deep yellow fruits, such as peaches or cantaloup Butter, whole milk, fortified skim milk, cream Cheddar-type cheese, ice cream

Key Nutrients	Important Functions	Important Sources
Thiamine or Vitamin B₁	Helps promote normal appetite and digestion Helps keep nervous system healthy and prevent irritability Helps body release energy from food	Meat, fish, poultry—pork supplies about 3 times as much as other meats Eggs Enriched or whole grain bread and cereals Dried beans and peas Potatoes, broccoli, collards
Riboflavin	Helps cells use oxygen Helps keep eyes, skin, tongue and lips healthy Helps prevent scaly, greasy skin around mouth and nose	Milk All kinds of cheese, ice cream and cereals Meat, especially liver Fish, poultry, eggs
Niacin or Its Equivalent	Helps keep nervous system healthy Helps keep skin, mouth, tongue, digestive tract in healthy condition Helps cells use other nutrients	Peanut butter Meat, fish, poultry Milk (high in tryptophan) Enriched or whole grain bread and cereals
Ascorbic Acid or Vitamin C	Helps make cementing materials that hold body cells together Helps make walls of blood vessels firm Helps in healing wounds and broken bones Helps resist infection	Citrus fruits—orange, grapefruit, lemon, lime Strawberries and cantaloup Tomatoes Green peppers, broccoli Raw or lightly cooked greens, cabbage White potatoes
Vitamin D, The Sunshine Vitamin	Helps absorb calcium from the digestive tract and build calcium and phosphorus into bones.	Vitamin D milk Fish liver oils Sunshine on skin (not a food)

From Nutrition Source Book. Chicago, National Dairy Council, 1970, p. 5.

Thiamine

or

Vitamin B₁

Water is also an essential, although people do not usually think of it as a food. Water helps in carrying nutrients to cells and waste products away, in building tissue, regulating temperature, aiding digestion, replacing daily water loss.

Other B-Vitamins are essential human nutrients: vitamin B_6, B_{12} and folacin. Folacin and vitamin B_{12} have antianemic properties, while vitamin B_6 helps enzyme and other biochemical systems to function normally. The three vitamins are widely distributed in foods—from meat, fish, poultry, whole grain and enriched bread and cereals, dark green and leafy vegetables. Milk provides vitamin B_{12} and folacin.

Although the exact biochemical mechanism whereby vitamin E functions in the body is still unknown, it plays an important role as an intracellular antioxidant, thus inhibiting the oxidation of unsaturated fatty acids and vitamin A. It is found in a variety of foods such as wheat germ oil, vegetable oil, egg yolk, milk fat, meats, butter, cereal germs and leafy vegetables.

PART 7. HOW THE BODY USES FOOD (DIGESTION, ABSORPTION, METABOLISM)

HOW ARE FOODS PREPARED FOR BODY USE?

1. Digestion. Change of food from complex to simpler forms and from insoluble to soluble state in the digestive tract to facilitate absorption through intestinal walls into the circulation for eventual use by the body.

Processes (occur simultaneously)

Physical (mechanical). Breaks up food into small particles (chewing in mouth), mixes it with digestive juices, (churning in the stomach action) and propels it through the digestive tract (peristaltic action)

Chemical. Enzymes in digestive juices change food nutrients—carbohydrates, fats, and proteins—into simple soluble forms which can be absorbed. Each enzyme has a specific action and optimum conditions under which it acts. The name of each group of enzymes ends in *ase:* amylases act on starch; lipases on fat; proteases on protein. Other chemical substances such as hydrochloric acid (HCl) and mucin in the gastric secretion, bile from the liver excreted into the duodenum, and certain hormones assist in the physical and chemical processes.

Results. Carbohydrates are changed to simple sugars; fats to fatty acids and glycerol; proteins to amino acids. Water, simple sugars, salts, and vitamins require no digestion.

2. Absorption. Passage of soluble digested food materials through the intestinal walls into the blood, either directly or by way of the lymph, by means of osmosis.

Alimentary Canal and Digestive Juices

Part	Juice
Mouth	Saliva
Stomach	Gastric
	HCl
Intestine (small)	Intestinal
Liver	Bile
	(no enzymes)
Pancreas	Pancreatic

Pancreatic and intestinal juices and bile combine in intestinal tract.

Labels: Salivary glands, Esophagus, Liver, Gallbladder, (Pylorus), Duodenum, Large intestine (colon), Jejunum, Ileum, Rectum, (Fundus), Stomach, Pancreas, Small intestine

Absorbed materials are carried by blood to various organs and tissues to be used as needed. Greater part of absorption takes place in small intestine, lower duodenum, and upper jejunum. Tiny fingerlike projections called villi, containing small capillaries and lacteals (part of the lymph circulation), line the intestinal wall. Simple sugars, amino acids, a few fatty acids, minerals, and water soluble vitamins reach the general circulation through the capillaries; the rest of the fatty acids, certain fat molecules, and fat soluble vitamins reach the lymph circulation through the lacteals. Absorbed materials are carried by blood to various organs and tissues to be used as needed. Water is also absorbed from large intestine. Body is able to digest and absorb about 90 to 98% of an average mixed diet.

3. Metabolism. The use that organs and tissues make of the absorbed food materials. Comprises all the chemical changes that the products of digestion (simple sugars from carbohydrates, fatty acids and glycerol from fats, amino acids from proteins) undergo from the time of absorption into the blood stream until they are utilized in one way or another and waste products are excreted through lungs, kidney, and skin. Metabolic processes are dependent upon the proper functioning of the endocrine glands and are assisted by systems of enzyme reactions. Metabolism includes (1) anabolism or building up of new tissue (constructive) and (2) catabolism or the breaking down of substances with energy release (destructive).

WHAT ROLE IS PLAYED BY EACH PART OF THE DIGESTIVE TRACT?

Parts of Digestive Tract	Mechanical Functions	Chemical Functions
Mouth	Chewing reduces large food particles to smaller ones. Saliva moistens food and prepares it for swallowing.	Cooked starch is changed first to dextrin and then to maltose by the salivary enzyme, ptyalin (amylase).
Esophagus	Peristaltic constrictions send food from mouth into fundus, or storage portion of the stomach.	
Stomach (empties in 2 to 6 hours)	Fundus acts as a temporary storage place for food. Food is kept in motion by the muscular walls to bring it into contact with the gastric juice secreted by stomach cells. Reduces food to semiliquid state (chyme) and passes it to small intestine. Presence of food in the stomach stimulates	Complex proteins are partially digested by gastric juice enzyme pepsin (protease). Milk protein is coagulated by gastric juice enzyme rennin, and then partially digested by pepsin. Emulsified fats are digested to fatty acids and glycerol by gastric juice enzyme lipase. Hydrochloric acid aids digestive enzymes of

Parts of Digestive Tract	Mechanical Functions	Chemical Functions
	functions of the digestive tract.	gastric juice in their work; increases solubility of Ca and Fe.
Small Intestine Parts: Duodenum Jejunum Ileum 20 feet long Food mass remains in intestine 3 to 8 hours	Chyme mixes with the digestive juices of small intestine: pancreatic and intestinal juices and bile, which is manufactured in liver and stored in gallbladder. Digested food moves in peristaltic waves through small intestine. Any unused food, waste materials, and water move to large intestine.	Alkaline juices neutralize chyme. Bile excreted into duodenum by liver prepares unemulsified fats for digestion. Digestion is completed: pancreatic enzymes complete starch digestion, digest fats, and partially digest proteins; intestinal enzymes complete protein digestion and carbohydrate digestion.
Large Intestine Parts: Cecum Colon Rectum Anal canal	Water absorbed from contents of large intestine. Solid feces formed. Waste is eliminated: indigestible residue, undigested food particles, meat fibers, decomposition products.	No enzymes produced in the large intestine so no digestion here.

SUMMARY

DIGESTION, ABSORPTION, METABOLISM

Carbohydrates

In the mouth	In the stomach	In the small intestine		Absorption Small intestine	Fate in metabolism
Starch ↓ Dextrin ↓ Maltose by action of ptyalin	No action except continued action of ptyalin until destroyed by HCl	Starch ↓ Dextrin ↓ Maltose by action of pancreatic enzyme	Sucrose Lactose Maltose ↓ Glucose by action of sucrase lactase maltase	In the form of glucose	Oxidized for energy to carbon dioxide and water Changed to glycogen and stored in liver Changed to fat and stored as fatty tissue

SUMMARY

DIGESTION, ABSORPTION, METABOLISM

(Continued)

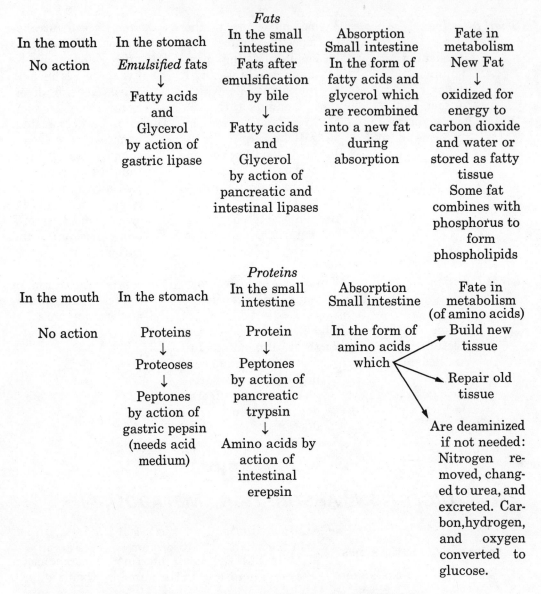

Fats

In the mouth	In the stomach	In the small intestine	Absorption Small intestine	Fate in metabolism
No action	*Emulsified* fats ↓ Fatty acids and Glycerol by action of gastric lipase	Fats after emulsification by bile ↓ Fatty acids and Glycerol by action of pancreatic and intestinal lipases	In the form of fatty acids and glycerol which are recombined into a new fat during absorption	New Fat ↓ oxidized for energy to carbon dioxide and water or stored as fatty tissue Some fat combines with phosphorus to form phospholipids

Proteins

In the mouth	In the stomach	In the small intestine	Absorption Small intestine	Fate in metabolism (of amino acids)
No action	Proteins ↓ Proteoses ↓ Peptones by action of gastric pepsin (needs acid medium)	Protein ↓ Peptones by action of pancreatic trypsin ↓ Amino acids by action of intestinal erepsin	In the form of amino acids which	Build new tissue → Repair old tissue → Are deaminized if not needed: Nitrogen removed, changed to urea, and excreted. Carbon, hydrogen, and oxygen converted to glucose.

WHAT FACTORS AFFECT DIGESTIBILITY OF FOODS?

The term "digestibility" of food refers to the rapidity and ease of digestion, as well as to its completeness. Thoroughly masticated solid foods and liquid foods are more rapidly digested than food left in large pieces. The amount and type of food eaten at one time also affects rapidity of digestion. Of the three organic nutrients, carbohydrates are digested and leave the stomach most rapidly, proteins less rapidly, and fats require the longest time for digestion. The flow of digestive juices is retarded by fatty food. Proteins or starches coated or mixed with fat require a longer time than either alone. Foods containing a large amount of cellulose are digested more slowly than the same foods with cellulose removed (seeds and tough fibers are not digested); a limited amount of cellulose or fiber is good, however.

Concentrated foods such as cheese require a long time to digest but are completely digested. Because of the completeness of digestion, cheese is often thought of as a constipating food. Serving cheese with fruit or vegetable or salad assures adequate fiber to go with it.

No matter how digestible a food combination may be or how well the food has been prepared, mental factors may and do interfere, favorably or unfavorably, with proper digestion. Such factors as violent emotion, excitement, anger, excessive fatigue, fear, worry, or strain of any kind may slow down or even suspend it temporarily. Good digestion is also influenced by and depends upon regularity of meals, slow eating, thorough mastication, eating lightly at times, a cheerful frame of mind, and pleasant and happy conditions at meal time. "Appetite juice," the so-called psychic secretion, also aids digestion. This juice is secreted at the thought, sight, smell, and taste of appetizing food, attractively served, and plays a considerable part in initiating the flow of true digestive juices. Certain of the vitamins influence appetite and proper functioning of the digestive tract.

Certain disorders of the digestive tract and hereditary disease characterized by absence of digestive enzymes (discussed in Section Two) reduce completeness of digestion.

TERMS TO UNDERSTAND

Digestive system	Absorption	Catabolism	Hormone
Digestion	Metabolism	Enzyme	Villi
Peristalsis	Anabolism	Bile	Osmosis

STUDY QUESTIONS AND ACTIVITIES

1. What are the parts of the digestive system?

2. What is the purpose of digestion?

3. What is absorption? Where does it take place?

4. In what form are all carbohydrates absorbed? All fats? All proteins?

5. Why might taking baking soda for "indigestion" retard stomach digestion?

6. How does anger affect digestion?

7. Why is well prepared food, attractive in appearance, and attractively served important to good digestion?

8. How does bile aid in the digestive process?

SUPPLEMENTARY READING

Bogert: Chapters 18, 19, 20   Howe: Chapter 7   Mowry: Chapter 8
                                                        Robinson: Chapter 3

Unit Three

FOODS AND MEALS FOR GOOD NUTRITION

PART 1.   FOODS IN THE FOUR FOOD GROUPS

PART 2.   FOOD PLANS FOR FAMILY NUTRITION

PART 3.   MEAL PLANNING FOR THE FAMILY

Object

To study the foods included in each of the Four Food Groups: varieties, ways to use, nutritional contributions, daily servings, selection and care, and principles of preparation and serving; food budgets, food plans, and economics of family feeding; and the combination of the daily foods into palatable and satisfying meals to fit the family budget, the ages and tastes of family members, and the cooking skill of the person preparing the meals.

PART 1.   FOODS IN THE FOUR FOOD GROUPS

HOW CAN DAILY FOOD SELECTION HELP GOOD NUTRITION?

In Units One and Two the relation of nutrition to good health and the functions, recommended daily allowances, and food sources of each of the essential nutrients were discussed. Now it is necessary to learn how to choose the daily foods and learn the basic principles of food preparation to insure an adequate daily intake of the essential nutrients. In other words, we are now ready to learn to apply the basic principles of nutrition to daily food selection and meal planning. At the close of Part 1 you will find a table showing how a daily foundation diet pattern based on the Four Food Groups can meet daily nutritional needs of an adult man and woman.

"For health and buoyancy, it is necessary to eat wisely every day—not to overeat or undereat. Certain food nutrients are leaders in the day-by-day nourishment and upkeep of the body. Eating well-chosen foods in the right amounts regularly helps keep one—and one's family—strong and healthy. A food plan, followed faithfully, supplies the foods needed by the body. It provides food for energy—food for growth and repair—food to regulate body processes—and food to keep the body parts functioning efficiently. You can put nutrition to work for yourself and family by making sure daily meals include the key nutrients in the Four Food Groups on the Daily Food Plan."[1]

"The daily food guide [see page 29] points out the main kinds of foods to include in our meals each day. The pattern of choices suggested are based on what we know about people's needs for vitamins, minerals, proteins, and other nutrients. Foods valuable for these nutritional essentials are grouped into four main classes according to their major contributions of nutrients. The number of servings that it will take to add up to a good diet is listed. There is ample choice within groups to allow for varied meals from day to day. Choices within groups allow us to select favorite foods, foods within the family budget, and those in season.

"The foods grouped together furnish about the same nutrients, but they vary in the amounts they provide in a serving. They are enough alike that we can make different selections from a group with the assurance that our choices will contribute their share of nutrients toward a good diet."[2]

Since foods can lose much of their nutrient value as well as flavor, color, texture, and palatability by improper care and cooking, it is also necessary to learn how to select, care for, prepare, cook, and serve food properly.

I. MILK GROUP

Foods Included[3]

Milk .....fluid whole, evaporated, skim, dry, buttermilk.

Cheese ...cottage; cream; cheddar-type—natural or processed.

Ice cream.

Contribution To Diet

Milk is our leading source of calcium, which is needed for bones and teeth. It also provides high-quality protein, riboflavin, vitamin A, and many other nutrients.

Homogenized and evaporated milk may be vitamin D fortified.

Amounts Recommended

Some milk every day for everyone.

Recommended amounts are given below in terms of whole fluid milk:

8-ounce cups

Children under 9... 2-3 cups

8-ounce cups

Children 9–12 ....3 or more
Teen-agers ....4 or more
Adults ....2 or more
Pregnant women ......3 or more
Nursing mothers ......4 or more

Part or all of the milk may be fluid skim milk, buttermilk, evaporated milk, or dry milk. Package label will indicate any vitamin or other fortification.

Cheese and ice cream may replace part of the milk. The amount of either it will take to replace a given amount of milk is figured on the basis of calcium content. Common portions of various kinds of cheese and of ice cream and their milk equivalents in calcium are:

1-inch cube cheddar- = 1/2 cup type cheese milk

1/2 cup cottage cheese = 1/3 cup milk

---

[1] *Family Food Budgeting.* Home and Garden Bulletin No. 94. Washington, D. C., U. S. Department of Agriculture, 1971. p. 14.

[2] *Food, The Yearbook of Agriculture.* Washington, D. C., U. S. Department of Agriculture, 1959. p. 267.

[3] For each of the four food groups in this section, the "Foods Included," "Contribution to Diet" and "Amounts Recommended" are taken from *Food for Fitness, A Daily Food Guide.* Leaflet no. 424. Washington, D. C., Institute of Home Economics, U. S. Department of Agriculture. Revised 1967.

2 tablespoons cream = 1 table-
cheese   spoon
                             milk

1/2 cup ice cream   = 1/4 cup
                             milk

Care of Milk

Rule of 3 C's and a D: Clean, Cold,
Covered, Dark.

Store in bottle or carton in which
delivered (wash and dry container).

Store in coldest part of refrigerator.

Remove from refrigerator only as
needed.

Protect milk from strong light especially if in glass bottles.

Ways of Using[4]

Basis for many solid and liquid foods.

Drinking—plain or in flavored beverages, hot or cold.

On cereals or cereals cooked in milk

Foods prepared with milk—each
serving provides:

1/2–1 cup milk—soups and
chowders.

1/4–1/2 cup milk—scalloped or
creamed vegetables, meat, fish,
eggs, or souffles.

1/4–2/3 cup milk—desserts such
as ice cream, puddings, custards,
cream pies.

4 Tbsp. dry milk added to each
cup of fluid milk in a recipe doubles
the milk content of a dish; may be
added also to beverages, cereals,
mashed potatoes.

Homemade pudding mixes made with
nonfat dry milk.

Puddings and pie fillings made with
evaporated milk carry more milk
when evaporated milk is diluted
2 parts to 1 part water instead
of equal parts.

Cheese adds milk value to meals: 1
ounce equals about 3/4 cup fluid
milk.

Cooking Principles

Use moderately low, even temperatures when heating milk, to prevent scorching.

Cover or stir milk while heating to
prevent scum formation. (Scum is
coagulated protein with enmeshed
fat and calcium.)

Use slow oven for milk dishes.

To prevent curdling when cooking
with milk, thicken milk first, add
other ingredients to milk gradually, avoid overheating.

Milk Use Economies

Milk is an excellent buy for the money.

Milk is least expensive source of
calories, protein, calcium, and
riboflavin.

Buy several quarts at a time to get
any discount offered.

Buy milk in larger sized containers
whenever possible.

Milk purchased at store may be
cheaper than milk delivered.

Milk in bottles may be cheaper than
in disposable containers.

Use top milk of whole milk or evaporated milk in place of cream.

Substitute evaporated or dry milk
for fresh in cooking.

CHEESE

Importance As Food

Excellent protein, calcium, phosphorus, riboflavin, vitamin A. (No
A in cottage.)

Value depends on kind of milk used
—skim or whole.

Generally digested easily and completely (leaving no residue).

Not desirable for certain ill persons
because of high fat content and
strong flavor.

Varieties Commonly Used

Hard: Cheddar, Edam, Gouda, Swiss,
Parmesan.

Semi-hard: Muenster, Roquefort,
Gorgonzola.

---

[4] *Food, The Yearbook of Agriculture.* Washington, D. C., U. S. Department of Agriculture, 1959,
p. 520.

Soft: Cottage, Cream, Limburger, Camembert.

Processed: Blend of American cheese with other cheeses and pasteurized with an emulsifying agent added.

Ways of Using

Milk and cheese make many inexpensive main dishes: cheese in souffles, fondues, casseroles; cheese sauce on toast, on vegetables, or for scalloped dishes; spaghetti, rice, or macaroni and cheese (served for four in place of meat requires 1 pint milk and 1/2 pound cheese).

Sandwich fillings—open or closed or grilled.

Grated cheese on various dishes and soups.

Stuffing for celery, tomatoes, green peppers.

Cheese and crackers for dessert.

On fruit and relish trays.

Place in Diet

Acceptable and economical meat substitute because of high protein content.

Should have prominent place in diet.

Can supplement a meal otherwise low in protein or where protein is of poor quality.

1/2 pound cheese equals approximately 1 pound of meat with moderate bone and fat.

Cottage cheese an inexpensive animal protein: costs 1/4 to 1/2 as much as meat, has no waste and requires no cooking.

Economies and Care

American Cheddar-type and a few processed and soft cheeses are comparatively inexpensive.

Many Cheddar-type cheeses may cost less than meat.

Less expensive: domestic varieties, mild Cheddar, simple packs, larger packs, wedges or blocks.

Wrap cheese in plastic or waxed paper.

Store cheese in cool place.

Use hardened Cheddar by grating or grinding.

Cooking Principles

Low temperatures and short cooking periods to prevent toughening.

Double boiler for top stove cooking.

Dish placed in pan of water for oven cooking.

Cheese blends more readily with sauces if grated.

As short a period as possible when broiling cheese sandwiches at high temperature.

II. MEAT GROUP

"The minimum of two daily servings of foods from the meat group is easily taken care of by our usual pattern of eating. Meat, poultry or fish, with dry beans or peas, nuts, or eggs as an occasional alternate, is commonly the main dish at our noon and evening meals. Eggs appear often on our breakfast tables, too, sometimes with ham, bacon, or sausage.

"Some of our favorite main dishes are combinations of meat, poultry, or fish with vegetables, milk, or cereals—in stews, salads, creamed or scalloped dishes, and casseroles. These combinations offer many ways to get variety into meals—and they often are frugal dishes that make good use of leftovers and help balance the food budget.

"Meal planning usually starts with the main dish—meat or a meat alternate— and the rest of the meal is built around it."[5]

---

[5] *Food, The Yearbook of Agriculture.* Washington, D. C., U. S. Department of Agriculture, 1959, p. 525.

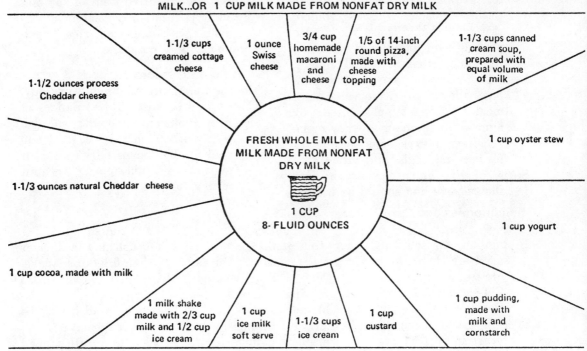

GETTING A DAY'S SUPPLY OF MILK

Everyone needs milk every day

8-fluid-ounce cups

Children under 9...2 to 3.
Children 9 to 12...3 or more.
Teenagers.......4 or more.

Adults..........2 or more.
Pregnant women...3 or more.
Nursing women....4 or more.

THESE MILK PRODUCTS AND MILK–RICH FOODS GIVE ABOUT AS MUCH CALCIUM AS 1 CUP OF FRESH WHOLE MILK...OR 1 CUP MILK MADE FROM NONFAT DRY MILK

FRESH WHOLE MILK OR MILK MADE FROM NONFAT DRY MILK

1 CUP
8- FLUID OUNCES

1-1/3 cups creamed cottage cheese

1 ounce Swiss cheese

3/4 cup homemade macaroni and cheese

1/5 of 14-inch round pizza, made with cheese topping

1-1/3 cups canned cream soup, prepared with equal volume of milk

1-1/2 ounces process Cheddar cheese

1 cup oyster stew

1-1/3 ounces natural Cheddar cheese

1 cup yogurt

1 cup cocoa, made with milk

1 milk shake made with 2/3 cup milk and 1/2 cup ice cream

1 cup ice milk soft serve

1-1/3 cups ice cream

1 cup custard

1 cup pudding, made with milk and cornstarch

SMART SHOPPER

U S DEPARTMENT OF AGRICULTURE • CONSUMER AND MARKETING SERVICE • FOOD TRADES STAFF • PF.493.E6

II. MEAT GROUP

Foods Included

Meat	*Poultry*	*Fish*
Beef, veal, lamb or mutton, pork.	Chickens: broilers, fryers, roasters, hens.	Lean fish: haddock, cod, halibut, perch, flounder, whiting.
Variety meats: tongue, liver, kidneys, sweetbreads, heart, tripe, and brains.	Duck Geese Turkeys	Fat fish: shad, salmon, mackerel, lake trout, tuna, herring.
As alternates—dry beans,		Shellfish:

| *Meat* | *Poultry* | *Fish* |

dry peas, lentils, nuts, peanuts, peanut butter.

Mollusks: clams, oysters, scallops.
Crustaceans: crabs, lobsters, shrimp.

Contribution to Diet

Foods in this group are valued for their protein, which is needed for growth and repair of body tissues—muscle, organs, blood, skin, and hair. These foods also provide iron and the B vitamins, thiamine, riboflavin, and niacin.

Legumes and nuts have good protein but of lower nutritive value than meat. When supplemented by more milk in the meal they make excellent inexpensive sources of protein, minerals, and vitamins.

Some of the glandular organs are inexpensive and should be included for their excellent protein, vitamins, and certain minerals.

Meat is an expensive item in the diet so it is frequently "extended" in dishes with macaroni, rice, vegetables, and potatoes.

Amounts Recommended

Choose 2 or more servings every day.

Count as a serving: 2 to 3 ounces of lean cooked meat, poultry, or fish —all without bone; 2 eggs; 1 cup cooked dry beans, dry peas, or lentils; 4 tablespoons peanut butter.

Economies and Care

| *Meat* | *Poultry* | *Fish* |

Meat

Best guides for selecting meat are U. S. D. A. grades: Prime, Choice, Good, and Commercial.

Federal grade name appears in purple on retail cuts.

Round purple stamp indicates meat has been inspected for wholesomeness.

Choose cuts giving the most lean for the money.

Buy grade best suited to use: lower grades for pot roast, meat loaf, stews, hamburger.

Store poultry, fish, and unsmoked meats loosely covered in refrigerator.

Store ground fresh meat and variety meats loosely wrapped and use within 2 days.

Poultry

For top quality, choose well fleshed birds with well distributed fat and skin with few blemishes.

Larger well fleshed birds are better buys than smaller ones (have more meat in proportion to bone).

Less heavy ducks are less fatty.

Poultry may be more expensive than meat because of bone.

Fish

Whole fish may be cheaper than fillets or steaks.

Most fish have little waste.

Less familiar fish may be less expensive.

Food value of all canned fish the same; lower grades and flaked forms will be less expensive.

Buy canned fish according to use: top grades where flavor and appearance count; low grades in cooked and baked dishes and salads.

Use oil from canned fish.

Fish a high quality protein food and should be used more often and is economical.

Keep uncooked fish in coldest part of refrigerator.

Meat

Store smoked meats tightly wrapped.

Store cooked meat, poultry, fish, broth and gravies covered in refrigerator.

Federal inspection stamp. (Courtesy U.S. Dept. of Agriculture, Bureau of Animal Industry.)

Government Meat Grades

Cooking Principles

Moderate heat best for all meat cookery—top of stove, oven, or broiler.

Cook frozen meats with or without thawing.

Purpose: to improve flavor and appearance, increase digestibility, destroy harmful bacteria.

Broil, pan fry or roast tender meat cuts.

Braise, pot roast, or simmer less tender cuts of meat.

See meat cooking guides in standard cook books.

Age, weight, quality, and fatness determine method of cooking.

Broil, fry or roast plump, young birds.

Braise, stew or steam older birds or lean ones.

Cook at low to moderate temperatures.

Do not overcook.

Cook uncovered when frying and roasting to retain juice and prevent shrinkage.

Thaw frozen birds just ahead of cooking.

Stuff birds just before roasting.

Fat content determines method of cooking.

Bake or broil salmon, shad, mackerel, lake trout, and whitefish.

Cook in water or bake or broil and baste with melted fat: cod, flounder, haddock, pike, sea bass, perch, carp.

Fry either fat or lean fish.

Cook just until flesh can be easily flaked.

Do not overcook.

Exhibit: Commonly used cuts of meat (or models or posters). Commonly used fish: whole, steaks, fillets. A field trip to a supermarket where meat cuts and fish are sold could be substituted for this exhibit.

Demonstration: Preparation of oven roast, pot roast, scraped beef, gravy making. Stuffing and roasting poultry, frying chicken, cooking fowl.

EGGS

Importance as Food

Excellent amount and quality of protein.

Excellent source of iron.

Good vitamin A and riboflavin.

Small amounts of thiamine.

Vitamin D variable.

Most of food value except protein in the yolk.

Rank close to milk in valuable nutrients but much richer in iron.

Easily digested and absorbed—raw or cooked.

Place in Diet

Economical everyday food most of the year.

Some form in the diet every day with a minimum of 4 eggs weekly.

Use in Cooking

Combined with other foods in preparation of beverages, cakes, desserts, salads, and dressings, sandwiches, sauces, vegetables in addition to providing nutritive value, flavor and color.

In cookery, eggs

thicken custards and puddings, sauces, boiled salad dressings.

leaven cakes, souffles, omelets.

bind and coat croquettes, meat loaves, cookies, muffins.

form framework in popovers.

clarify soups and coffee.

emulsify salad dressings.

garnish canapes, salads, soups.

Use in Diet

Reinforcing beverages.

Breakfast dishes: poached, scrambled, soft cooked, omelets, etc.

Luncheon and supper: casseroles, souffles, scalloped dishes, salads, sandwich fillings, creamed, with hash.

Desserts: baked and soft custards, sweet souffles, sauces, in puddings and pie fillings.

Economies and Care

All eggs, regardless of color, size, and grade, have the same food value.

Buy refrigerated eggs.

Store eggs clean (do not wash), cold, and covered.

Use top grades for table use; lower grades for cooking and baking.

Cooking Principles

Low temperatures and short cooking periods for delicate and tender texture and attractiveness and to prevent discoloration, curdling and shrinkage.

Simmering for poached and hard and soft cooked eggs, slow oven for custards, souffles (dish may be placed in pan of water), double boiler for soft custards.

Eggs beat up faster and to greater volume when brought to room temperature.

In combining hot mixtures and eggs as in custards, cream fillings, etc., pour hot mixture slowly into beaten egg with constant stirring.

III. VEGETABLE-FRUIT GROUP

"Vegetables and fruits—fresh, frozen, canned, dried—offer a wide range of choice in planning for the four or more servings recommended daily.

"The needed serving of vitamin C rich food is furnished much of the time in many homes by the citrus fruit or juice that is part of the breakfast pattern customary among many families. Ample variety for a serving at least every other day of a vegetable or fruit rich in vitamin A is provided by the many dark-green and deep-yellow kinds available in our markets and gardens. And there are plenty of other vegetables and fruits to choose from to make up the two or more additional servings without frequent repetition.

"A cooked vegetable is a standby for serving with the main dish at the noon or evening meal. Raw vegetables in salads or on the relish plate and noon or evening meal. Raw vegetables in salads or on the relish plate and vegetables in stews and other combinations all count toward the day's quota, too.

"Most fruits are at their best when simply prepared. Many people prefer them raw, either whole or sliced or diced and perhaps slightly sweetened, or in fruit cups and salads. Stewed and baked fruits are popular too—at breakfast, with the main course at lunch or dinner, or as a dessert. For a change, there are fruit pies and puddings in wide variety."[6]

Foods Included

All vegetables and fruit. The food guide emphasizes those foods that are valuable sources of vitamin C and vitamin A.

Classes

Root: carrots, beets, sweet potatoes, turnips.
Thiamine and vitamin A in yellow vegetables.
Bulb: onions. Fair for vitamin C.
Stalk or stem: celery and asparagus.
Vitamin A and iron in green types.
Green leafy: calcium and iron, vitamin A, riboflavin, ascorbic acid, cellulose.
Seeds (legumes): peas, beans, lentils. Contain protein, iron and thiamine.
Flowers: cauliflower, broccoli.
Vitamin A, ascorbic acid, and iron in green types.
Fruits used as vegetables: tomatoes, egg plant, peppers, cucumbers, squash.
Ascorbic acid in tomatoes and peppers.

Good Sources of Vitamin C:
Grapefruit or grapefruit juice; orange or orange juice; cantaloup; guava; mango; papaya; raw strawberries; broccoli; green pepper; sweet red pepper.

Fair Sources of Vitamin C:
Honeydew melon; tangerine or tangerine juice; watermelon; asparagus tips; raw cabbage; collards; garden cress; kale; kohlrabi; mustard greens; potatoes and sweet potatoes cooked in the jacket; spinach; tomatoes or tomato juice; turnip greens.

Sources of Vitamin A: Dark-green and deep-yellow vegetables and a few fruits, namely apricots, broccoli, cantaloup, carrots, chard, collards, cress, kale, mango, persimmon, pumpkin, spinach, sweet potatoes, turnip greens and other dark green leaves, winter squash.

Contribution to Diet

Fruits and vegetables are valuable chiefly because of the vitamins and minerals they contain. They also provide color, flavor, texture and palatability; add variety to menu; fiber or bulk stimulates peristalsis.
Good for minerals and vitamins but individual vegetables vary in kind and amount.
Easily digested.
Alkaline ash.
Low calories.
Food value similar in fresh, frozen or canned forms.
Food value depends on the vegetable variety, growing conditions, storage, and method of preparation.

Amounts Recommended

Choose 4 or more servings every day, including:
1 serving of a good source of vitamin C or 2 servings of a fair source. 1 serving, at least every other day, of a good source of vitamin A. If the food chosen for vitamin C is also a good source of vitamin A, the additional serving of a vitamin A food may be omitted.

The remaining 1 to 3 or more servings may be of any vegetable or fruit, including those that are valuable for vitamin C and vitamin A.

Count as 1 serving: 1/2 cup of vegetable or fruit; or a portion as ordinarily served, such as 1 medium apple, banana, orange, or potato, or half of a medium grapefruit or cantaloup, or the juice of 1 lemon.

---

[6] *Food. The Yearbook of Agriculture.* Washington, D. C., U. S. Department of Agriculture, 1959, p. 542.

Economies and Care

Buy vegetables which are kept in a cool place.

Choose vegetables that are firm, crisp, free from decay and bright in color.

Avoid buying dirty vegetables.

The larger the amount of waste, the more expensive the vegetable.

Usually, a vegetable is lowest in price and highest in quality when it is plentiful locally.

Wash and dry perishable vegetables and store in covered containers in the refrigerator.

Store small quantities of non-perishable vegetables such as potatoes and onions so that dry, cool air circulates through them.

Reasons for Cooking

Makes some vegetables more digestible by softening cellulose and bursting starch cells.

Improves flavor and palatability of some vegetables.

Cooking Methods[7]

Boiling: See suggestions opposite page.

Baking: potatoes, onions, carrots, tomatoes.

Steaming: white, yellow, and red vegetables.

Broiling: raw and leftover cooked.

Pressure saucepan cooking: dried beans, fibrous and mature vegetables, whole beets, whole potatoes.

Braising and panning: carrots, celery, beets, cabbage, cauliflower, spinach, and other greens.

Pan and deep-fat frying: potatoes, cauliflower, eggplant, onions.

Waterless cooking.

Cooking Principles[8]

Vitamin C as well as other vitamins, minerals, and flavors can be lost through improper cooking. The following general procedures will help to retain the nutritive value of vegetables and, at the same time, make them taste their best.

1.   Use fresh vegetables which have been properly stored. Whenever possible, pare, cut, or otherwise prepare the vegetable just before cooking.

2.   Use as little water as possible, if the cooking method calls for water. Minerals, certain vitamins, and the natural vegetable sugar essential to flavor dissolve in the water. When you throw away the water in which the vegetables have been cooked, some of these vitamins, minerals, and flavoring materials go with it.

3.   Cook vegetables only until fork-tender. They should still hold their shape and color. Overcooking impairs their flavor, color, and texture.

4.   Cook vegetables with all possible speed. If you are boiling a vegetable, start it in boiling water. Covering the pan will not injure the color or flavor.

5.   Cook vegetables in skins whenever possible. Some of the nutrients are removed with the skin when a vegetable is pared. If you must pare them, use a vegetable peeler or some other instrument which will remove only a *small* part of the vegetable with the skin.

6.   Use a sharp knife to cut vegetables. A dull knife bruises the vegetable and hastens the loss of valuable nutrients.

7.   Do not add soda to vegetables, except in some cases for dried peas and beans. Soda is apt to make vegetables mushy, may impair flavor and destroy certain vitamins.

8.   Serve vegetables immediately after cooking. Do not try to keep them hot for long periods of time. If you must postpone a meal, it is better to let the vegetables cool and then reheat them quickly before serving.

[7,8] *How to Cook Vegetables.* From research material compiled at New York State College of Human Ecology, Cornell University, adapted.

How to Boil Vegetables

1. Use very little water. The amount depends upon the size of the pan and the amount of vegetables to be cooked. In general, use from 1/4 inch to 1 inch of water in the pan. More boiling water may be added later in cooking if necessary.

2. To shorten cooking time, bring water to boil before adding the vegetables.

3. Salt the water, allowing 1/2 to 3/4 teaspoon salt for each pound of vegetable. Salting may be done at end of cooking.

4. Add the vegetable.

5. Use a tight fitting lid that will keep steam in pan. Most of the vegetable must cook in steam.

6. Quickly bring the water to boiling point again.

7. Lower heat so water boils gently.

8. Try to cook vegetables so that there is no liquid left in the pan. You may leave cover of the pan off the last few minutes of cooking to allow remaining water to evaporate.

To Prevent Color Changes

1. Be careful not to overcook vegetables as excessive heat will change the pigment which gives them their attractive color.

2. Cook the vegetable in an uncovered or partially covered pan for at least the first part of the cooking period. This allows the mild acids to go off in the steam as cooking progresses; otherwise they stay in pan and change green color to olive-green. Spinach and nearly all frozen vegetables cook quickly so they can be cooked in a covered pan.

To Prevent Strong Flavors Developing

1. Cook vegetables such as cabbage, cauliflower, broccoli, Brussels sprouts, or turnips in an uncovered pan to allow the substances which may develop strong flavors to go off in steam.

2. Cook just until the vegetable is done, as strong flavors develop with long cooking.

Fruits

Importance in the Diet

Minerals, varying amounts of vitamins A and B complex; especially ascorbic acid.

Fruit acids (which give characteristic flavor) by leaving alkaline ash on oxidation aid in maintenance of neutrality of body fluids.

Indigestible fruit cellulose stimulates intestinal function.

Easily digested (ripe fruits).

Stimulate appetite with color, aroma, texture, tart taste.

Minimum daily serving: 1 citrus and 1 other fruit.

Place in Menu

Raw, juice, cooked, pureed.

Breakfast fruit: raw, juice, cooked alone or combined with cereals.

Fruit cups: beginning or ending of luncheon or dinner menu.

Salads, garnishes.

Desserts: raw, cooked, in pies, cakes, ices, whips, gelatin, etc.

Between meal snacks.

Therapeutically as juice:
force fluids, quench thirst, easily digested fuel. Alkaline ash.

Preparing and Serving

Raw.

Wash carefully and remove blemishes.

Chill (except bananas and pineapple).

Serve different ways for variety.

Cut just before serving.

Juice fruits just before serving.

Whole citrus fruits have more nutritive value than fruits juiced and strained.

Store fruit juices covered and chilled.

Thaw frozen fruits just before serving and do not refreeze.

Cooked.

Cook slowly but no longer than necessary.

Cooking lessens tart flavor, causes some color changes, softens cellulose, inverts some sugars to less sweet ones.

Simmer rather than boil to lessen loss of volatile flavors.

Cook dried fruits in same water in which they were soaked.

Fruit desserts. Types:

Whips — sweetened fruit pulp and beaten egg white.

Souffles — whips baked at low temperatures.

Baked fruit puddings:

Fruit Betty — fruit combined with bread.

Fruit crisp — fruit topped with crumb mixture.

Fruit cobbler — fruit topped with biscuit or pastry.

Fruit pudding — fruit combined with uncooked batter before baking.

Gelatin desserts — unflavored gelatin plus fruit juices with or without the addition of fruit, nuts, marshmallows, whipped cream, etc. Flavored gelatin may be used as the base. May also serve as salad when placed on greens.

Frozen — frozen fruit juices called ices; plus beaten egg white or milk called sherbets.

Fruit tapioca.

Salads

Nutritive Value

Excellent way to introduce fruits and vegetables in the diet, especially raw ones.

Enhance the meal in attractiveness because of flavor, color, and texture.

Add bulk (cellulose) to diet.

Low in calories when served without dressing.

Green and yellow vegetables and yellow fruits provide vitamin A.

Leafy green vegetables, tomatoes, citrus fruits, strawberries, cantaloup, and raw cabbage provide vitamin C.

Green vegetables, especially leafy ones, provide iron.

Salads of meat, poultry, fish, cheese, or eggs provide good protein.

Can be made a source of additional calories with dressings.

Greens Used

Lettuce: iceberg, Boston, leaf.

Escarole, romaine, endive, chicory.

Miscellaneous: beet and celery tops, parsley, watercress, green pepper, spinach.

Cabbage: Chinese or celery, regular, red.

Other materials: white turnip slivers, cucumbers, raw cauliflower, carrots, tomatoes, radishes.

Place in Diet

Appetizer or first course: fruit salads or salad plates and green salads.

Meal accompaniment: cole slaw, salad bowl, tossed, gelatin—any light fruit or vegetable, depending on rest of meal.

Main part of meal: meat, chicken, fish, eggs, or cheese as protein base.

Separate course: fruit or vegetable.

Dessert: frozen salads, jellied salads, salad plate or bowl.

Light refreshment.

Relish dish or plates; served with first course or with main course.

Salad Dressings

French: oil, vinegar or lemon juice or fruit juice and seasonings in temporary emulsion.

Mayonnaise: egg, oil, acids, seasonings in permanent emulsion.

Cooked: egg or flour, or both, used as a thickening agent with added acid.

Sour cream: alone or with variations as desired.

Main dish salads usually served with mayonnaise type or cooked dressing; some with tart French dressing.

Vegetable and vegetable fruit salads usually served with tart French dressing; some with mayonnaise or cooked dressing.

Fruit salads usually served with sweet clear French dressing; mixtures sometimes with mayonnaise and whipped cream or with thinned fruit juice.

Garnishes for Meat and Vegetable Salads

Keep simple and few in number.

Flavor of garnish should add to salad.

Lettuce cup edge dipped in paprika.

Sliced cucumber—scored or plain—peeled or unpeeled.

Tomatoes—quartered or sliced.

Radishes—plain, roses, or fans.

Green or red pepper strips—or rings.

Carrots—sticks or curls.

Hard cooked eggs—quartered or sliced.

Garnishes for Fruit Salads

Maraschino cherries.

Mint leaves.   Coconut.

Strawberries.   Nuts.

Dark fruits (plums, cherries, cooked prunes).

Cream cheese balls.

Preparation Principles

Keep salad ingredients cold, crisp, fresh, and colorful.

Put tossed salads together with a light touch.

Arrange individual salads simply.

Use clean, chilled, crisp salad greens.

Choose ingredients that provide a variety of color, flavor, shape, and texture.

Have pieces large enough to keep the food's identity.

Chill and drain canned fruits and vegetables.

Save vitamin C in vegetables by using a sharp knife for shredding, and toss with a wooden spoon and fork or two silver forks.

Prevent discoloration of fruits by dipping them in citrus or pineapple juice.

Prepare salads just ahead of serving time for best appearance, texture, flavor and vitamin value.

Do not shred or grate ingredients ahead of time.

Add dressings just at serving time.

Do not soak prepared relishes in cold water too long.

Exhibit. Unusual greens and raw vegetables used in salads. Attractive relish tray. Cheese and cracker tray to accompany salad service.

Serving Salads

Salads may be served on individual plates, in wooden bowls, on a large platter or plate, or in an attractive serving bowl.

Chill serving dishes.

For individual or platter salads, lettuce or other greens may form a cup to hold salad, or greens may be shredded and the salad placed on top. Greens should not extend over rim of plate.

Add the salad dressing to the salad just before serving except when ingredients are to be marinated or when the dressing is needed to help prevent fruits from discoloring.

Dressing may be passed at the table.

Use the appropriate dressing for the salad.

Gelatin salads should be tender and firm—not rubbery or runny.

Use attractive and appropriate garnishes when needed.

Choose salad appropriate to purpose for

which used and in relation to other foods.

Demonstration. Preparation of lettuce for salads. Preparation of garnishes—radish roses, carrot curls, etc. Tossing a salad with oil, vinegar, and seasonings. Peeling tomatoes; peeling and sectioning citrus fruits; cutting fresh pineapple.

IV. BREAD-CEREAL GROUP

"The four daily servings from the bread-cereal group may come from many different grain products, used in many different ways.

"The bread need not always be a slice of yeast bread, nor must the cereal necessarily be a breakfast cereal. For variety, there are biscuits, muffins, pancakes, and many other hot breads, and quick loaf breads such as date or nut bread. All of them can be counted, provided they are made with whole grain or enriched flour or meal. Half to three fourths of a cup of rice, grits, spaghetti, noodles or other similar products may be counted as a serving of cereal if the product is enriched.

"Part of the day's quota from the bread-cereal group may be in combination dishes. Bread is often an important ingredient in stuffing for meat, poultry, and fish, and in scalloped dishes and puddings. A serving of cereal can come from a combination such as macaroni and cheese, spaghetti and meat sauce, or Spanish rice.

"Enriched or whole-grain flour or cereal in cakes, cookies, pastries, and other sweet baked goods used primarily to round out meals and to satisfy the appetite also may count toward the quota."[9]

Enrichment of Cereal Products

Whole grains contribute not only considerable amounts of carbohydrate to the diet but also some protein and appreciable amounts of certain minerals and vitamins. When whole grains are milled to produce a whiter product with better keeping qualities (by removal of bran layers and germ), most of the iron, and thiamine, riboflavin, and niacin (Vitamin B Complex vitamins) are lost.

In an effort to improve nutrition in the United States during World War II, when many diets were poor in the B Complex vitamins and iron, an enrichment program was established to replace in cereal products the nutrients lost in the milling process. This program had the approval of the American Medical Association, the National Research Council, and milling and baking industries. The U. S. Food and Drug Administration set up standards for enrichment. Today 30 or more states and Puerto Rico have legal requirements for flour and bread enrichment, and a number of southern states for corn and rice enrichment also. It is estimated that 80–90 percent of all white flour and bread are now enriched as well as some pasta products such as macaroni, noodles, and spaghetti; also, more and more crackers are being made with enriched flour. Read labels and choose the enriched products.

Enrichment means the addition of thiamine, riboflavin, niacin and iron to cereal products to replace those nutrients removed in the milling, bringing the level up to that of natural grains. It is generally agreed by nutrition experts that this enrichment program has contributed in large measure to better health and nutrition in the United States over the years.

---

[9] *Food, The Yearbook of Agriculture.* Washington, D. C., U. S. Department of Agriculture, 1959, p. 549.

Foods Included

All breads and cereals that are whole grain, enriched or restored; *check labels to be sure.*

Specifically, this group includes: Breads; cooked cereals; ready-to-eat cereals; cornmeal; crackers; flour; grits; macaroni and spaghetti; noodles; rice; rolled oats; and quick breads and other baked goods if made with whole-grain or enriched flour. Bulgur and parboiled rice and wheat may also be included in this group. "Converted" rice is treated to reduce thiamine loss during polishing and washing.

Contribution to Diet

Supply variety of nutrients:
   Important source of calories.
   Considerable protein.
   Whole grains: starch, protein, minerals, iron, B-vitamins, cellulose, small amount fat.
   Refined forms (germ and bran layers removed): starch, protein.
   Bran stimulates intestinal tract.
   Easily digested, economical.
   Use of milk with cereals important.
   Good base for extension of meat and cheese dishes.

Amounts Recommended

Choose 4 servings or more daily. Or, if no cereals are chosen, have an extra serving of breads or baked goods, which will make at least 5 servings from this group daily.

Count as 1 serving: 1 slice of bread; 1 ounce ready-to-eat cereal; 1/2 to 3/4 cup cooked cereal, cornmeal, grits, macaroni, noodles, rice, or spaghetti.

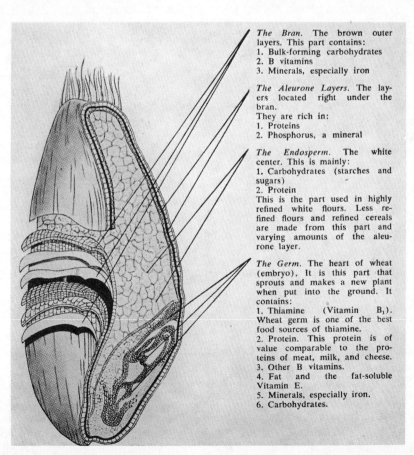

The Bran. The brown outer layers. This part contains:
1. Bulk-forming carbohydrates
2. B vitamins
3. Minerals, especially iron

The Aleurone Layers. The layers located right under the bran.
They are rich in:
1. Proteins
2. Phosphorus, a mineral

The Endosperm. The white center. This is mainly:
1. Carbohydrates (starches and sugars)
2. Protein
This is the part used in highly refined white flours. Less refined flours and refined cereals are made from this part and varying amounts of the aleurone layer.

The Germ. The heart of wheat (embryo). It is this part that sprouts and makes a new plant when put into the ground. It contains:
1. Thiamine (Vitamin B₁). Wheat germ is one of the best food sources of thiamine.
2. Protein. This protein is of value comparable to the proteins of meat, milk, and cheese.
3. Other B vitamins.
4. Fat and the fat-soluble Vitamin E.
5. Minerals, especially iron.
6. Carbohydrates.

Whole wheat—cross section of grain. *(Courtesy of the Ralston Purina Company, St. Louis, Mo.)*

Reasons for Cooking

To soften and rupture cell walls.
To improve digestibility.
To improve flavor.

Cooking and Serving Cereals

Follow manufacturer's directions for proportions of water and cereal and method of combining.
Use direct heat or double boiler.
Quick cooking helps to conserve thiamine.

Cook in milk for extra food value.
Finished product should be free from lumps, neither too thick nor too thin, well flavored, served hot. May be cooked or served with dried or fresh fruit, butter and brown sugar.

Exhibit: Various cereals and breads or their labels for study and comparison.

Sandwiches

Kinds

Hearty: serve as main dish of meal hot or cold, knife and fork or finger style, of meat, cheese, fish, poultry, eggs.
Less hearty: to serve with soup course, salad, tea.
Canapes: open sandwiches, specially garnished.
Tea: dainty sandwiches cut in various shapes and with bread crusts removed.
Sandwich fillings: sliced meat, chopped or grated vegetables, peanut butter, baked beans, tasty chopped mixtures of meat, fish, poultry, eggs, etc.
French toasted sandwiches; many types may be French toasted.

Preparation Points

Use day old bread except for rolled sandwiches.
Slice thinly for dainty tea sandwiches and canapes; thicker for main dish sandwiches.
Remove crusts for dainty sandwiches (plan to use crusts for croutons, crumbs, or in puddings).
Spread sandwiches with softened (not melted) butter.
Cut in different shapes for eye appeal.
Have fillings fresh and crisp.
Use variety of breads: white, whole wheat, rye, nut, raisin, fruited.
Use appropriate garnish for sandwich service when desired.

Quick Breads

Quick breads: made with quick acting leavenings such as baking powder, soda and sour milk, or steam. Ratio of liquid to flour varies.
Pour batters: popovers, griddle cakes, waffles.
Drop batters: muffins, cakes.
Stiff doughs: pastry, cookies.
Oven-baked: biscuits, muffins, corn breads, quick loaf breads.
Griddle baked: griddle cakes, waffles.
Steamed: dumplings, brown bread.
Deep fat fried: doughnuts, fritters.
Commercial mixes.

Cakes

Shortened or butter cakes: contain shortening.
Unshortened cakes: sponge and angel food contain no fat and depend chiefly upon the air which is beaten into the egg whites to leaven the cake. The air expands during baking and causes the cake to rise.
Commercial mixes.

Other Foods

To round out meals to meet energy needs, and to satisfy the appetite almost everyone will use some foods not specified—butter, margarine, other fats, oils, sugars; unenriched, refined breads, cereals, and flours. These are often ingredients in baked goods and mixed dishes, Fats, oils, and sugars are

SOURCES OF FAT

Visible	Invisible	** Oils	Vegetable Sources
** Lard	Milk	Cottonseed	Avocados
* Butter	Cream	Soybean	Coconut
** Beef suet	Cheese (whole milk)	Coconut	Chocolate
** Poultry fat	Meats	Corn	Nuts
Fish liver oils	Fatty fish	Peanut	Olives
** Bacon fat	Egg yolk	Olive	
* Margarine		Hydrogenated fat made from above oils	

* Used as table fats.   ** Used in cooking and oils in salad dressings.

also added to foods during preparation or at the table. Try to include some vegetable oil among the fats used.

These "other" foods supply calories and can add to total nutrients in meals.

Care of Fats

Avoid rancidity caused by air, light, and high temperatures (destroys vitamin A, if present). Antioxidant may be added to some fats by manufacturer.

Keep tightly covered containers away from strong odors and flavors.

Read labels to see if refrigeration is necessary.

Use In Cooking

Frying medium.

Shortening agent for flavor and texture.

Basis for salad dressings.

Flavoring agent (butter).

Cream (White) Sauces

Standards

Right thickness for purpose.

Smooth, well seasoned.

Thoroughly cooked starch.

Uses

Creamed soups, sauces, scalloped dishes.

Basis for croquettes, souffles.

Introduces milk into diet.

Promotes variety in menu.

Cooking Rules

Measure accurately.

Blend melted fat and flour to separate starch grains.

Add liquid slowly to prevent lumping.

Cook slowly at low temperature to prevent scorching and cook starch thoroughly.

Stir frequently to prevent lumping.

Very thin: cream soups from starchy foods.

Thin: cream soups from non-starchy foods.

Medium: creamed dishes, scalloped dishes, gravies.

Thick: souffles.

Very thick: croquettes.

TERMS TO UNDERSTAND

Pasteurized milk	Organ or glandular meat	Enriched cereal
Homogenized milk	Meat alternates	Variety meats
Nonfat dry milk	Meat extender	Modified skim milk
Vitamin D milk	Refined cereal	Fortified milk

SUPPLEMENTARY READING

Bogert: Chapters 16, 17   Peyton: Section III, Chapters 30–38
Howe: Section III   Robinson: Chapter 16

Special Home and Garden Bulletins, U. S. Department of Agriculture. Available from Superintendent of Documents, U. S. Government Printing Office, Washington, D. C.

HG 112 Cheese in Family Meals
    127 Milk in Family Meals
     27 Meat for Thrifty Meals
     36 Peanut and Peanut Butter Recipes
    103 Eggs in Family Meals
    110 Poultry for Family Meals
    118 Beef and Veal in Family Meals
    124 Lamb in Family Meals
    160 Pork in Family Meals
        Meat and Poultry:
    170 Wholesome for You
    172 Labeled for You
    173 Clean for You
    174 Care Tips for You
    176 Nuts in Family Meals
   L326 Dry Beans, Peas, Lentils
    186 Bread, Cakes and Pies in Family meals

HG   33 Root Vegetables in Everyday Meals
     41 Green Vegetables for Good Eating
     55 Potatoes in Popular Ways
    105 Vegetables in Family Meals
   1276 Tomatoes on Your Table
   L293 Sweet Potato Recipes
    125 Fruits in Family Meals
    161 Apples in Appealing Ways
    150 Cereals and Pasta in Family Meals
     69 Home Care of Purchased Foods
     78 Storing Perishable Foods in the Home
     90 Conserving Nutritive Values in Foods
    162 Keeping Food Safe to Eat

Consumers All—U. S. D. A. Yearbook, 1965—pages 391–440
Food for Fitness—A Daily Food Guide, U. S. D. A. Leaflet No. 424
Food for Us All—U. S. D. A. Yearbook, 1969—pages 94, 117, 127, 139, 146, 160, 174, 196, 205, 213, 226, 232

HOW DOES A BASIC OR FOUNDATION DIET PLAN MEET ADULT RECOMMENDED DIETARY ALLOWANCES?

As you already are aware, the Daily Food Guides (pages 29 and 118) specify definite amounts of foods from each of the Four Food Groups as a basic or foundation diet plan. With careful selection of foods within each group, this diet plan may actually provide complete or almost complete allowances for all essential nutrients except calories (which can be met with more foods from all groups) and possibly iron (for the woman) which can be supplied by paying attention to special foods.

On page 117 is shown a nutritive evaluation of a basic diet pattern compared with the RDA for an adult man and woman. What suggestions do you have for making adequate any nutrients falling short of RDA in each case?

EVALUATION OF THE FOUNDATION OF AN ADEQUATE DIET FOR AN ADULT[10]

FOOD	Household Measure	Weight Gm.	Calories	Protein gm.	Fat gm.	Carbohydrate gm.	Calcium Mg.	Iron Mg.	A. (I.U.)	Ascorbic Acid Mg.	Thiamine Mg.	Riboflavin Mg.	Niacin Mg.
Milk (whole or equivalent)	1 pt.	488	320	18	18	24	576	.2	700	4	.14	.82	.4
Meat group													
Eggs	1	50	80	6	6	tr.	27	1.1	590	–	.05	.15	tr.
Meat, poultry, fish	3 oz. (cooked)	85	274	21	21	0	9	2.1	20	0	.09	.20	4.4
Vegetable-fruit group													
Vegetables:													
Deep green or yellow[2]	1 salad or cooked	50 raw or 75 cooked	26	1.2	tr.	5.8	34	.6	3440	6	.04	.08	.4
Other cooked[3]	½ cup	80	43	2.8	tr.	7.8	15.3	1	220	11	.12	.06	.2
Potato peeled, boiled	1 medium	122	80	2	tr.	18	7	.6	tr.	20	.11	.04	1.4
Fruits:													
Citrus[4]	1 Serving	125	53	1	tr.	13	48	.4	210	52	.05	.03	.3
Other (fresh and canned)[5]	1 Serving	150	97	.6	tr.	25	8	.6	180	5	.04	.04	.5
Bread-cereal group													
Cereal (whole grain and enriched)[6]	½ cup cooked	28 (dry)	58	1.8	tr.	11	7	.5	0	0	.08	.02	.2
Bread (whole grain and enriched)	3 slices 1 whole wheat 2 white	75	205	7	3	40	66	2.0	tr.	tr.	.21	.13	2.0
Totals[7]			1236	61.4	48	144.6	797.3	9.1	5360[8]	98	.93[9]	1.57	9.8[10]
Recommended Daily Dietary Allowances*													
Man (Age 35–55; wt., 154 lb., ht., 68 in.)			2600	65			800	10	5000	60	1.3	1.7	17[11]
Woman (Age 35–55; wt., 128 lb., ht., 63 in.)			1850	55			800	18	5000	55	1.0	1.5	13[11]

Evaluation based on Nutritive Value of Foods, Home and Garden Bulletin No. 72, U. S. Department of Agriculture, 1970

[1] Evaluation based on figures for cooked (lean and fat) beef, lamb, and veal.

[2] Evaluation based on lettuce, cooked carrots, green beans, winter squash and broccoli.

[3] Evaluation based on average for cooked peas and beets.

[4] Evaluation based on Florida orange and white and pink grapefruit; whole and juice.

[5] Evaluation based on canned peaches, applesauce, raw pears, apples and bananas.

[6] Evaluation based on oatmeal and cornflakes.

[7] With the addition of more of the same foods, or other foods, to meet calorie requirement, the totals will be increased.

[8] With the use of liver this figure will be markedly increased.

[9] With the use of pork, legumes and liver this figure will be markedly increased.

[10] The average diet in the United States, which contains a generous amount of protein, provides enough tryptophan to increase the niacin value by about a third.

[11] These figures are expressed as niacin equivalents, which includes dietary sources of the preformed vitamin and the precursor, tryptophan.

* Recommended Dietary Allowances. Washington, D. C., National Research Council, Publication 1694, 1968.

[10] M. V. Krause: Food, Nutrition and Diet Therapy, 4th edition, Philadelphia, W. B. Saunders Company, 1966, page 123, adapted.

A Guide to Good Eating

Use Daily:

Milk Group

3 or more glasses milk — Children
smaller glasses for some children under 8

4 or more glasses — Teen-agers

2 or more glasses — Adults

Cheese, ice cream and other milk-made foods can supply part of the milk

Meat Group

2 or more servings

Meats, fish, poultry, eggs, or cheese—with dry beans, peas, nuts as alternates

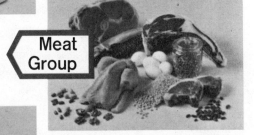

Vegetables and Fruits

4 or more servings

Include dark green or yellow vegetables; citrus fruit or tomatoes

Breads and Cereals

4 or more servings

Enriched or whole grain Added milk improves nutritional values

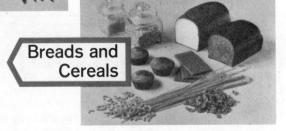

This is the foundation for a good diet. Use more of these and other foods as needed for growth, for activity, and for desirable weight.

The nutritional statements made in this leaflet have been reviewed by the Council on Foods and Nutrition of the American Medical Association and found consistent with current authoritative medical opinion.

National Dairy Council, Chicago, 1970, 3rd edition.

PART 2. FOOD PLANS FOR FAMILY NUTRITION

WHY IS FAMILY FOOD PLANNING IMPORTANT?

Feeding a family well is a homemaker's major responsibility. A task so vital to family health and important to happines requires her to serve meals which are both nutritionally adequate and enjoyable, to practice thrift as necessary, and to save time and energy where she can. Planning and buying food for one's family presents a real challenge to the manager-homemaker. "To shop wisely in today's supermarket takes knowledge, good judgement, and a keen sense of food values in relation to food costs."

WHAT GUIDES ARE AVAILABLE FOR FAMILY FOOD BUDGETING?

Following some plan is the only way a homemaker can be sure to provide each important kind of food and enough of it to see that her family is well fed. When families in this country are poorly fed, the foods they neglect most often are milk and milk products, and vegetables and fruits—especially the leafy, green and yellow vegetables and the citrus fruits. These foods need to be watched in careful planning.

Five ready-made food plans which are workable and up-to-date guides to family food budgeting at different cost levels have been prepared by nutritionists in the U.S. Department of Agriculture to help in the choice of the right foods, in the right amounts, and at the desired price level. Each plan lists the weekly amounts of different groups of foods that together supply an adequate diet for different age, sex, and activity groups within a family. For convenience the Four Food Groups have been enlarged to 11 groups.

WHAT ARE FOOD PLANS AT DIFFERENT COST LEVELS?[11]

Economy Plan
Least expensive. For temporary or emergency use when funds low. Food costs about 20 percent less than Basic Low-cost plans. Less nutritious but will meet needs of most families. Less milk, meat, poultry, fish, eggs, fruits, vegetables. Larger share of nutrients from cereal products. Vitamin C adequate in fruits and vegetables. A serving of liver or extra servings of dark green vegetables weekly provides adequate iron for adolescent girls and women.

Low-cost Plan
Basic Low-cost plan meets needs of most U. S. families on low-cost diet. (A second less expensive, low-cost plan is available for family food habits in the southeastern section of the U. S., where more cereal products and less potatoes are consumed). Both plans provide adequate nutrition for each family member.

Moderate-cost Plan
Costs 30 to 35 percent more to follow than Basic Low-cost plan. Permits

---

[11] *Family Food Budgeting for Good Meals and Good Nutrition.* Home and Garden Bulletin no. 94. Washington, D. C., U. S. Department of Agriculture, 1971, adapted.

BASIC LOW-COST FAMILY FOOD PLAN

Weekly quantities of food[1] for each member of family

Sex-age group	Milk, cheese, ice cream[2] (Qt.)	Meat, poultry, fish[3] (Lb. oz.)	Eggs (No.)	Dry beans, peas, nuts (Lb. oz.)	Flour, cereals, baked goods[4] (Lb. oz.)	Citrus fruit, tomatoes (Lb. oz.)	Dark-green and deep-yellow vegetables (Lb. oz.)	Potatoes (Lb. oz.)	Other vegetables and fruits (Lb. oz.)	Fats, oils (Lb. oz.)	Sugars, sweets (Lb. oz.)
Children:											
7 months to 1 year	5½	1 0	5	0 0	0 12	1 8	0 2	0 8	1 0	0 1	0 2
1–3 years	5½	1 4	5	0 1	1 4	1 8	0 4	0 12	2 4	0 4	0 4
4–6 years	5½	1 8	5	0 2	2 0	1 12	0 4	1 4	3 4	0 6	0 6
7–9 years	5½	2 0	6	0 4	2 4	2 0	0 8	2 0	4 4	0 8	0 10
10–12 years	6½	2 4	6	0 6	3 0	2 4	0 8	2 8	5 0	0 8	0 12
Girls:											
13–15 years	7	2 8	6	0 4	3 0	2 4	0 12	2 8	5 0	0 10	0 12
16–19 years	7	2 8	6	0 4	2 12	2 4	0 12	2 4	4 12	0 6	0 10
Boys:											
13–15 years	7	2 8	6	0 6	4 4	2 8	0 12	3 4	5 4	0 12	0 12
16–19 years	7	3 4	6	0 8	5 4	2 8	0 12	4 12	5 8	0 14	0 14
Women:											
20–34 years	3½	2 8	5	0 4	2 8	2 0	0 12	2 0	5 0	0 6	0 10
35–54 years	3½	2 8	5	0 4	2 8	2 0	0 12	1 8	4 8	0 4	0 10
55–74 years	3½	2 8	5	0 4	2 4	2 0	0 12	1 4	3 8	0 4	0 6
75 years and over	3½	2 8	5	0 4	2 0	2 0	0 12	1 4	3 0	0 4	0 6
Pregnant	7	2 8	7	0 4	2 8	3 8	1 8	2 0	5 8	0 6	0 8
Nursing	10	3 4	7	0 4	3 0	4 8	1 8	3 4	5 8	0 8	0 10
Men:											
20–34 years	3½	3 12	6	0 6	4 4	2 4	0 12	3 4	5 8	0 12	1 0
35–54 years	3½	3 8	6	0 6	3 12	2 4	0 12	3 0	5 0	0 10	0 12
55–74 years	3½	3 4	6	0 4	3 8	2 0	0 12	2 8	4 12	0 10	0 10
75 years and over	3½	3 4	6	0 4	3 4	2 0	0 12	2 4	4 8	0 8	0 10
Total											

[1] Food as purchased or brought into the kitchen from garden or farm.

[2] Fluid whole or its calcium equivalent in cheese, evaporated milk, dry milk, ice cream.

[3] Bacon and salt pork should not exceed ⅓ pound for each 5 pounds of meat group.

[4] Weight in terms of flour and cereal. Count 1½ pounds bread as 1 pound flour.

From *Family Food Budgeting for Good Meals and Good Nutrition.* Home and Garden Bulletin No. 94. Washington, D. C., U. S. Department of Agriculture, 1971.

1. Food as purchased or brought into the kitchen from garden or farm.
2. Fluid whole or its calcium equivalent in cheese, evaporated milk, dry milk, ice cream. (See p. 100.)
3. Bacon and salt pork should not exceed ⅓ pound for each 5 pounds of meat group.
4. Weight in terms of flour and cereal. Count 1½ pounds breads as 1 pound flour.

MODERATE-COST FAMILY FOOD PLAN

Weekly quantities of food [1] for each member of family

Sex-age group	Milk, cheese, ice cream [2] (Qt.)	Meat, poultry, fish [3] (Lb. Oz.)	Eggs (No.)	Dry beans, peas, nuts (Lb. Oz.)	Flour, cereals, baked goods [4] (Lb. Oz.)	Citrus fruit, tomatoes (Lb. Oz.)	Dark-green and deep-yellow vegetables (Lb. Oz.)	Potatoes (Lb. Oz.)	Other vegetables and fruits (Lb. Oz.)	Fats, oils (Lb. Oz.)	Sugars, sweets (Lb. Oz.)
Children:											
7 months to 1 year	6	1 4	6	0 0	0 12	1 8	0 2	0 8	1 8	0 1	0 2
1–3 years	6	1 12	6	0 1	1 0	1 8	0 4	0 12	2 12	0 4	0 4
4–6 years	6	2 4	6	0 1	1 12	2 8	0 4	1 0	4 12	0 6	0 10
7–9 years	6	3 0	7	0 2	2 0	2 4	0 8	1 12	4 8	0 10	0 14
10–12 years	6½	4 0	7	0 4	2 12	2 8	0 12	2 4	5 8	0 10	0 14
Girls:											
13–15 years	7	4 8	7	0 2	2 12	2 8	0 12	2 4	5 12	0 12	0 14
16–19 years	7	4 4	7	0 2	2 8	2 8	0 12	2 0	5 8	0 10	0 12
Boys:											
13–15 years	7	4 12	7	0 4	4 0	2 12	0 12	3 4	6 0	0 14	1 0
16–19 years	7	5 8	7	0 6	5 0	3 0	0 12	4 4	6 4	1 2	1 2
Women:											
20–34 years	3½	4 4	6	0 2	2 4	2 8	0 12	1 8	5 12	0 8	0 14
35–54 years	3½	4 4	6	0 2	2 0	2 8	0 12	1 4	5 4	0 8	0 12
55–74 years	3½	4 4	6	0 2	1 12	2 4	0 12	1 4	4 4	0 6	0 8
75 years and over	3½	3 12	6	0 2	2 12	2 8	0 12	1 0	3 12	0 6	0 8
Pregnant	7	4 4	7	0 2	2 4	3 8	1 8	1 8	5 12	0 8	0 12
Nursing	10	5 0	7	0 2	2 12	5 0	1 8	2 12	6 4	0 12	0 12
Men:											
20–34 years	3½	5 8	7	0 4	4 0	2 12	0 12	3 0	6 8	1 0	1 4
35–54 years	3½	5 4	7	0 4	3 8	2 12	0 12	2 8	5 12	0 14	1 0
55–74 years	3½	5 0	7	0 2	3 4	2 12	0 12	2 4	5 8	0 12	0 14
75 years and over	3½	5 0	7	0 2	2 12	2 8	0 12	2 0	5 4	0 10	0 12
Total											

[1] Food as purchased or brought into the kitchen from garden or farm.
[2] Fluid whole or its calcium equivalent in cheese, evaporated milk, ice cream.
[3] Bacon and salt pork should not exceed ⅓ pound for each 5 pounds of meat group.
[4] Weight in terms of flour and cereal. Count 1½ pounds bread as 1 pound flour.

From *Family Food Budgeting for Good Meals and Good Nutrition.* Home and Garden Bulletin No. 94. Washington, D. C., U. S. Department of Agriculture, 1971.
1. Food as purchased or brought into the kitchen from garden or farm.
2. Fluid whole or its calcium equivalent in cheese, evaporated milk, dry milk, ice cream. (See p. 100)
3. Bacon and salt pork should not exceed ⅓ pound for each 5 pounds of meat group.
4. Weight in terms of flour and cereal. Count 1½ pounds breads as 1 pound flour.

more variety in meals and less home preparation. Larger quantities of milk, eggs, fruits, vegetables.

Liberal Plan

Costs 10 to 20 percent more than Moderate-cost plan. Quantities of food about same but allows more variety and varied food choices, out-of-season, and speciality foods.

Note: Large families can buy food more economically. Allowance is made for this in estimating food costs. See pages 120 and 121 for Basic Low-cost and Moderate-cost Family Food Plans and see below for weekly food cost of Food Plans.

WHAT ARE WEEKLY FOOD COSTS FOR FAMILY FOOD PLANS AT DIFFERENT COST LEVELS?

COST OF FOOD AT HOME: SEPTEMBER 1971 U.S. AVERAGE[12]

Sex-age groups	Cost for 1 week		
	Low-cost plan	Moderate-cost plan	Liberal plan
	$	$	$
FAMILIES			
Family of 2:			
20 to 35 years	18.80	24.00	29.50
55 to 75 years	15.30	19.90	24.10
Family of 4:	—		
Preschool children	27.20	34.70	42.30
School children	31.70	40.50	49.80
INDIVIDUALS*			
Children, under 1 year	3.60	4.60	5.10
1 to 3 years	4.60	5.80	7.00
3 to 6 years	5.50	7.10	8.50
6 to 9 years	6.70	8.60	10.80
Girls, 9 to 12 years	7.60	9.90	11.60
12 to 15 years	8.40	11.00	13.30
15 to 20 years	8.60	10.90	13.00
Boys, 9 to 12 years	7.90	10.10	12.20
12 to 15 years	9.20	12.10	14.40
15 to 20 years	10.60	13.50	16.30
Women, 20 to 35 years	7.90	10.10	12.20
35 to 55 years	7.60	9.70	11.70
55 to 75 years	6.40	8.30	10.00
75 years and over	5.80	7.40	9.10
Pregnant	9.40	11.80	13.90
Nursing	11.00	13.60	15.90
Men, 20 to 35 years	9.20	11.70	14.60
35 to 55 years	8.50	10.80	13.30
55 to 75 years	7.50	9.80	11.90
75 years and over	7.00	9.40	11.40

* Costs given for persons in families of 4. Adjustments for individuals in other size families: 1 person family, add 20%; 2 person family, add 10%; 3 person family, add 5%; 5 person family, subtract 5%; 6 or more person family, subtract 10%.

[12] Family Economics Review, ARS 62–5, Consumer and Food Economics Research Division. ARS, U.S. Department of Agriculture, December 1971, page 25.

HOW DOES THE COST OF FOOD FOR YOUR FAMILY COMPARE WITH THE AVERAGE? (See previous page)

Using either the basic or moderate-cost table, find what the average weekly food cost would be for each member of *your* family according to his sex and age. Add these figures. If your family has more or less than four members, correct the total by the percentages given at the end of the table.

How does the amount you actually spend for food compare with this average? "If the amount varies greatly it may be because these figures are averages for the entire United States, and the families making up the averages differ widely. Families with the same income spend different amounts for food, and families with different incomes spend the same amount. In general, as income increases the amount spent for food increases, but the percentage of income used for food decreases."[13]

The cost of food varies from time to time. These figures were compiled for September 1971. Also, do not forget to deduct from your food bill the cost of any non-food items you may buy at the supermarket—cigarettes, pet food, household supplies, clothes, etc.

WHAT ARE THE STEPS IN FOLLOWING A FOOD PLAN?[14]

1. Select either the basic low-cost plan or the moderate-cost plan—whichever fits your family situation and the amount you are able to spend for food weekly. (If you wish to use one of the other plans, your instructor can provide the data for you.)

2. Write down the name of each person who eats at your family table: use the blank lines at the bottom of the table, one line to a name.

3. Find the line on the food plan which describes each person. The quantities of foods for adults are based on the needs of "moderately active" persons. If your activities or those of your family are more or less than those specified, food quantities may need to be increased or decreased accordingly. Adjustments in the quantities of fats and oils and in sugars and sweets are easily made to take care of minor variations in activity.

4. Fill in each person's needs in blank spaces opposite his name, taking each in turn, and total each column. This could serve as a shopping list. These plans provide for 3 meals a day, 21 meals a week for each family member, including any lunchbox meals. If any member regularly eats one of the day's meals away from home, you will buy that much less.

5. Keep records of foods used from each group. Remember the weight or measure of food you record is as it was purchased, not after it has been prepared for serving.

6. Compare quantities and costs of foods used with your family food plan. If quantities are similar and cost is much more or less than estimated, the cost difference may be due to:

Choices of foods within the groups that are more or less expensive than the average assumed for the plans.

Local food prices that are higher or lower than estimated in plans.

Use of large amounts of home produced foods for which you assumed no cost.

---

[13] *Feeding the Family—A Marketing and Management Challenge.* Cornell Extension Bulletin no. 1135. Ithaca, N. Y., New York State College of Human Ecology, 1965, adapted.

[14] *Family Food Budgeting for Good Meals and Good Nutrition.* Home and Garden Bulletin no. 94. Washington, D. C., U. S. Department of Agriculture, 1971, adapted.

Changes in cost of food since September 1971.

Inclusion of non-food items in food bill. You should remember to subtract such items from the supermarket sales slip.

If the quantities of any food group are much less than in the plan or if any group is left out entirely, your family's meals may be inadequate. Meals are likely to be unbalanced if the neglected food groups are:

Milk, cheese, ice cream

Dark-green, deep-yellow vegetables

Citrus fruits and tomatoes

Flour, cereals, baked goods, enriched or whole-grain

The above may be made an individual class activity with each student determining the weekly food needs of her family according to the chosen cost plan. Or it may be used as a class problem for a family chosen by the class with the desired number of family members or a real family known to the whole class.

WHAT ARE SOME "FOOD-COST CUTTERS"?[15]

"Although food is usually the largest single expense in a family budget, you can generally reduce the amount you spend for food by—

Checking weekly specials in food store advertisements.

Preparing a grocery list before you shop.

Comparing costs and buying food in the form—fresh, frozen, or canned—or the weight of package—that gives the most servings for the money. To make an intelligent choice among brands of the same product, test different ones to see which one gives the greatest quality and number of servings for the money.

Shopping carefully for low-cost foods within each food group.

Using grades in making your food purchases. Government grades will enable you to be sure of the quality of the food you buy, and you are then better able to compare prices asked.

Taking advantage of seasonal abundances. Radio, television, and newspapers call attention to foods in plentiful supply, as listed each month by the USDA. These foods will be at their peak of quality, and sometimes will be offered at lower prices.

Limiting perishable food purchases to amounts that can be used while they are in top quality.

Preventing food waste by proper storage and by cooking methods that conserve nutrients.

Increasing skills in cookery.

Considering family likes and dislikes when food shopping. Thrifty food buys pay off only if your family eats and enjoys the food.

Here are suggestions that may help you get more food value for your dollars:

When buying meat, consider the amount of lean meat in the cut, not the cost per pound. Some cuts contain bone, gristle, and fat waste, For example, ground beef and beef short ribs may cost the same per pound but ground beef will give twice as many servings or more per pound as short ribs. Bacon, which is largely fat, is one of the most expensive foods you can buy in terms of protein value.

Chicken and turkey have a large proportion of bone to lean, but are often bargains compared with other meats. Fish is high in nutrients; often low in cost.

---

[15] *Family Food Budgeting for Good Meals and Good Nutrition.* Home and Garden Bulletin no. 94. Washington, D. C., U. S. Department of Agriculture, 1971, pp. 12, 13.

Eggs are usually a less expensive source of nutrients than most meats. Dry beans and peanut butter are inexpensive alternates for meat.

Beef, lamb, and pork liver give unusually high nutritive returns for money spent.

Study bread labels before you buy. Choose bread for weight and food value, not by the size of loaf. Look for bread that is whole-grain or enriched and that contains milk.

Buy packaged cereals or any other packaged food by weight, not by the size of the package. To compare prices, first look for the weights listed on the labels and note the prices. Then figure the costs for an ounce or a pound.

Ready-to-serve cereals in multipacks of small boxes may cost two or three times more per ounce than the same cereal in a larger box. Sugar-coated, ready-to-serve cereals cost more, per ounce, than many common, unsweetened ones, and furnish more calories, but less other food value.

Cereals you cook yourself (particularly the kinds that take longer to cook) are nearly always less expensive than the ready-prepared ones.

Baked goods made at home usually cost less than ready-baked ones.

Nonfat dry milk and evaporated milk cost considerably less per quart when reconstituted than whole fluid milk, and supply comparable amounts of calcium and protein. Reconstituted nonfat dry milk is an excellent beverage for most persons and generally can be substituted for whole fluid milk in cooking. For baking and preparing many other foods, nonfat dry milk does not need to be reconstituted before using. A glass of whole fluid milk usually costs three times as much as a glass of reconstituted nonfat dry milk. Count the following as equivalent in calcium to a quart of fluid whole milk: evaporated milk, 16 ounces; nonfat dry milk, 3 ounces; cheese, Cheddar type, processed, 6 ounces; cheese, cottage, creamed, 2–1/2 pounds; ice-cream, 1–2/3 quarts.

Be sure to read labels on all cartons of milk other than those containing the usual fresh fluid milks. Substitutes which appear in dairy cases similarly packaged under various names cost less but may not be nutritionally equivalent to fresh cow's milk. There are two types of such products; "filled" milk made of a combination of skim milk and vegetable oils and "imitation" or simulated milk which does not contain any milk products, being made from a combination of water, sugar, vegetable fat and some source of protein.

Choose the type of pack or grade in a canned product that is appropriate to your cooking method. It is thrifty to buy canned tomatoes of low market grade for stews and sauces. A can of solid white meat tuna costs more than the same size can of grated light meat tuna. You may prefer the solid pack for a salad and the grated pack for casseroles and sandwich fillings.

Consider your time and the quality of the finished product in deciding between convenience foods (those with more than usual services added) and unserviced ones. Compare prices to see if it pays to prepare a product yourself from basic ingredients. Sometimes it does not. How much you enjoy cooking and how much time you can spend will influence your choice."

Special References, U. S. D. A. Bulletins. Available from Superintendent of Documents, Government Printing Office, Washington, D. C.

A Guide to Budgeting for the Family, HG No. 108, 1968

Food for the Family with Young Children, HG No. 5, 1969

Food for the Young Couple, HG No. 85, 1971

Your Money's Worth in Foods, Hg No. 183, 1970

How to Buy Food, A series of booklets (currently about 12); 1969.

Be a Good Shopper, Leaflet

PART 3. MEAL PLANNING FOR THE FAMILY

WHY IS SOME PLAN FOR DAILY MEALS DESIRABLE?

Without some kind of plan for choosing and combining into meals the foods needed daily for good nutrition, the meals of many families may be found wanting in both nutrition and satisfaction. Any plan needs to be flexible enough to take advantage of sales and other specials in the market, seasonal foods, family tastes and desires, holidays, special family occasions and guests. A plan will also prove a time, work, and money saver and a good way to avoid uninviting, unpalatable, and unsatisfying meals. A plan is especially important when the food allowance is low, to insure sufficient and nutritionally adequate food.

The Four Food Groups on the Daily Food Plan, referred to frequently (see pages 29 and 98) provide a framework for the daily meals. The foods on this guide fit easily into our three-meals-a-day way of eating, safeguard the nutritional quality of the diet, and permit the addition of other foods as desired (if consistent with maintenance of normal weight) to supplement the basic foods.

The same basic foods are needed by every person in the family; the amount depends upon the age, activity, physical condition, and special needs of the individual. Except for milk, children will require less of foods than adults—smaller helpings rather than fewer foods—and sometimes prepared differently. Variety in the type of servings helps in the establishment of good eating habits. Even weight watchers in the family need the same basic foods, with calories being cut by substituting skim and buttermilk for whole milk, skim milk cheese for whole milk cheese, uncreamed cottage cheese for creamed type, using only meat trimmed of fat, using broiled and roasted instead of fried meats, vegetables without butter or cream sauce and fruits without sugar and cream, and avoiding sweets.

WHAT ARE ADDITIONAL CONSIDERATIONS IN MEAL PLANNING?

Good meal planning is both a science and an art: *science* dictates what foods should be included in meals to *nourish our bodies* and *art* is involved in the combination of the needed foods into meals that are *attractive, appetizing* and *satisfying* in all ways or which have appeal to the senses. Many factors affect our acceptance of food—individual and family attitudes toward food, individual tastes and preferences, racial, regional, and religious customs and, very importantly, how foods look and taste.

Appearance of Food:

Color: attractive and appealing; natural food colors are the most attractive; no predominance of white, neutral or single color; colorful combinations; avoidance of too intense colors (or of too much artificial color, if used).

Contrast: in *shape,* form and size (slices, strips, wedges, diced, round), and *type* of food (concentrated and bulky, with neither predominating), a pleasant balance between simple and richer dishes; in *texture,* assortment among hard and soft, moist and dry, no overcooked foods (mushy).

Arrangement of Foods:

On dining table to be served; on plates as served, uncrowded, suitably garnished; on trays without crowding; simple but attractive table appointments to complement food; serving area free from disagreeable odors.

Taste and Flavor:

Contrast: pleasing balance between bland and sharp, sweet and sour, distinct and mild, with none predominating.

Method of preparation: balance between creamed, fried and baked without repetition of same method.

Seasoning: used with care.

Variety: no repetition of same food or preponderance of one type of food in a meal.

Temperature: "hot foods hot" and "cold foods cold" or at room temperature depending on food; some hot and some cold food in each meal is desirable.

Food Costs   (see Food-Cost cutters, page 124).

Racial, Regional and Religious Food Tastes and Customs   (see page 131).

Time and Effort Involved in Preparation:

Planning meals ahead with the help of the Daily Food Guide (page 29) and the Daily Meal Pattern (page 130) from which shopping lists may be made can be a real timesaver in shopping (with more food for every food dollar), in meal preparation (with better use of storage and equipment facilities and more efficient work habits), as well as in better meals for the family.

Familiarity with basic recipes and standard proportions, and the use of standardized recipes and accepted methods of food preparation can produce high quality foods with ease and efficiency. Adequate equipment for meal preparation, with a supply of basic foods and emergency items on kitchen shelves and in refrigerator and freezer, aids in shopping and quick food preparation.

Start meal planning with the main dish and then choose appropriate accompaniments. Plan the salad (or appetizer or both) and dessert next to avoid repetition of the same foods and flavors in a meal; certain salads may serve as both salad and dessert. Serve a light dessert with a heavy main course, a heavier dessert with a lighter main course. Try to have meat, poultry, fish, eggs, cheese, or milk at each meal. Fruit may sometimes be used in place of a vegetable.

WHAT ARE SPECIAL CONSIDERATIONS IN PLANNING LOW-COST MEALS?[16]

An easy to make, hearty, and economical main dish is the core around which the rest of the meal is built—usually it is the main source of protein. The average family in the United States spends well over a third of each food dollar for foods commonly used in main dishes—meat, poultry, fish—and other foods such as eggs, cheese, dry beans, and dry peas.

Main dish should provide about one-fourth of the day's need for protein. If it furnishes less, additional protein foods should be included in the meal. Or, the amount of protein-rich food may be increased in the main dish. The rest of the

---

[16] *Money-saving Main Dishes,* Home and Garden Bulletin No. 43, Washington, D. C., U. S. Department of Agriculture, February 1970, adapted.

protein for the day will come from milk as a beverage, and from cereals, bread, and other foods eaten as part of the day's meals.

To supply one-fourth of the day's protein requirement, a main dish for a family of four must contain about 2 ounces of protein (average 1/2 ounce or 15 grams per person, more for men and teen-age boys and girls, and less for women and younger children). The following amounts of foods provide about 15 grams of protein:[17]

1/5 to 1/2 pound meat, poultry, fish (depending on bone, gristle, fat)

2½ frankfurters

Four 1-ounce slices Bologna

6 to 8 slices bacon

2¼ large eggs

1¾ cups fluid whole or skim milk

Scant ⅔ cup nonfat, dry instant milk

Less than ½ cup compact instant milk

Scant cup evaporated milk

Four 1-inch cubes or two 1-ounce slices American or Swiss cheese

½ cup creamed cottage cheese

⅓ cup dry or 1 cup canned or cooked dry beans, peas

4 tablespoons peanut butter

8 slices bread or 1⅓ cups dry crumbs

1 cup dry or 2 cups cooked macaroni, spaghetti, noodles

Best proteins (other nutrients, also) come from animal sources, such as meat, poultry, fish, eggs, cheese, and milk. It is good to include some in each meal.

Next best proteins are from soybeans and nuts, and dry beans and peas. When these or grain products are featured in main dishes, try to combine them with a little top-rating protein foods—animal proteins.

No one food is exactly like any other food and no food is complete in all nutrients, so use a variety of main dishes and wide choice of other foods to complete the meal.

WHAT ARE SOME BUYING AND MANAGEMENT POINTERS FOR LOW-COST MEALS[18]

Buying Pointers

Amount of bone, gristle and fat on a cut of meat affects cost of serving. Less tender cuts of beef as chuck, heel of round, brisket and short ribs usually provide protein for less money than some of the more tender cuts.

The less tender *Good* grade of meat (3rd grade) provides more lean meat than higher grades and costs less per pound.

Chicken and turkey are low-cost protein sources compared to some cuts and types of meats.

Larger well-fleshed birds are often better buys than smaller ones; when sold whole, price is less per pound than when halved, quartered or cut up.

Whole ready-to-cook turkey provides more meat for the money than a boned, rolled turkey roast,

Medium and small eggs are a better buy than large ones at certain seasons.

Cheaper, grade B eggs are as good as grade A for combination dishes and baked foods.

Grade B and C fishery products are as nutritious as higher grades for dishes in which appearance is unimportant.

"Light meat" tuna costs less than "white meat" tuna; flaked or grated tuna less than solid or chunk; pink or chum salmon less than red or king.

Dry beans and peas are among the least costly sources of protein.

---

[17] Ibid., p. 3.
[18] Ibid., pp. 6–10 adapted.

Buying Pointers*

Cheese wedges cost less than sliced, cubed, grated; mild natural cheese costs less than aged sharp; domestic less than imported; home-flavored cottage cheese less than similar flavored purchased products.

Nonfat dry and evaporated milk costs less than whole fluid for cooking and baking; store-bought less than home delivered; large containers ($\frac{1}{2}$ or 1 gallon) less than quart containers.

Management Pointers

Money-saving Ideas

Use *less tender cuts* of meat made tender by cooking slowly with moisture; grinding, cubing, pounding, scoring; marinating with acid ingredients; using commercial tenderizers.

Make the *most of flavor* and food value from meat, poultry, and fish by using small pieces in casseroles, sandwiches, and salads; "meaty" bones in soups and stews and for seasoning vegetables; broth in gravies, sauces, soups, stews, and other combination dishes; drippings in gravies, sauces, pan frying, and seasoning vegetables.

Extend meat, poultry, and fish by combining with mild-flavored foods such as dry beans or peas, macaroni products, rice, or potatoes in casseroles, stews, and soups; breads or cereals as stuffings in meat, poultry, fish loaves, patties, and balls.

Replace the meat in some meals with less expensive protein sources— dry beans, peas, lentils; peanut butter; eggs; American or Swiss-type cheese; cottage cheese.

Make good use of leftovers.

Time-saving Ideas

Prepare larger amounts of main dish than needed for one meal, use some, freeze rest. Freeze in meal-size packs; roasts, meat sauce; combination dishes; lunchbox sandwiches.

Use previously partly or fully prepared items for sauces and toppings for casseroles, for added flavor with little preparation time.

Prepare a major part of meal in oven. Use a pressure cooker to shorten cooking time for pot roasts, swiss steaks, meat sauces, dry beans and peas.

---

* How to Use USDA Grades in Buying Food. HG No. 196, Washington, D. C., U. S. Dept. of Agriculture, 1971.

Family Food Buying: A Guide for Calculating Amounts to Buy. Home Economics Research Report No. 37, Washington D. C., U. S. Dept. of Agriculture, 1969.

WHAT ARE SOME PATTERNS AND IDEAS FOR DAILY MEAL PLANNING?

A Breakfast Plan	One Example	More Ideas
Fruit or Juice	Grapefruit	Fruit may be fresh, canned or frozen. Suggest combining fruit with cereal sometimes: bananas and cornflakes, raisins and oatmeal. If the fruit is not citrus or tomato, urge good vitamin C sources for other meals.
Main Dish	Oatmeal with Milk	Cereal may be ready-to-eat or cooked kinds. Also suggest eggs, meat, cheese or beans as alternates or as additions for persons with higher energy needs.
Bread: Enriched or whole grain	Buttered Toast	Sometimes sweet rolls, coffee cake, pancakes, waffles, biscuits, cornbread, other hot breads, or French toast.
Milk	Milk	Adults may prefer another beverage for breakfast but should have 1 pint or more of milk a day. Hot cocoa made with milk is a good cold weather choice.
Extras: Sugar, Jam or Jelly	Sugar (on cereal) Jelly	Suggest moderation in additions of sweets.

A Lunch or Supper Plan	One Example	More Ideas
Main Dish	Egg & Celery Salad Sandwich	Hearty soups, such as cream of mushroom, chowder, bean, pea; eggs, meat or fish; macaroni and cheese; baked beans; sandwich of meat, fish, cheese or peanut butter; tacos; pizza with chesse.
Vegetable and/or Fruit	Tomato, sliced Variation: Eggs, Scrambled with Stewed Tomatoes	Urge vegetables: raw in salads—carrot-raisin, tossed green, coleslaw; or relishes—carrot, celery, green pepper rings; cooked, as part of main dish or separate. Urge fruits: raw in salads or to eat out-of-hand; cooked, in salads such as prune-cottage cheese; as dessert.
Bread	In Sandwich, or separately	May be part of main dish; also consider: rolls, cornbread, toasted biscuits, other hot breads, crackers.
Milk	Milk	Sometimes part of milk maybe in creamed soup, or as cheese, or in dessert such as custard, ice cream.
Simple Dessert sometimes	Peanut Butter Cookies	Desserts may be canned fruits plain, in gelatin or puddings; ice cream or custard; cookies, cupcakes or gingerbread; raw or cooked fruits.

A Dinner Plan	One Example	More Ideas
Main Dish	Swiss Steak with Meat Gravy	Suggest variety meats, such as liver, heart, kidney; chitterlings; frankfurters; meat extenders, such as spaghetti and meat balls, macaroni and cheese, rice and chicken; meat loaf; chops, ham hocks; meat stews or fish chowders; fish croquettes; cheese omelets; chicken pies; baked beans or chili con carne.
Potatoes or alternate	Boiled Potatoes	Suggest potatoes baked, mashed, scalloped, as salad; remember sweet potatoes; suggest rice, macaroni or dumplings as alternates to potatoes, or a starchy vegetable such as corn or lima beans.
Green or Yellow Vegetable and/or Salad	Green Beans Cucumber or Celery Slices for crispness	Urge *dark green leafy or deep yellow vegetable* rich in vitamin A *at least every other day;* raw vegetable relishes, such as carrot, green pepper, celery; salads of raw greens, such as spinach, lettuce, endive; or molded salads with shredded raw carrots, cabbage or fruit; or mixed salads, such as cabbage and pineapple. Suggest only light cooking for green vegetables.
Bread & Butter Milk Dessert	Cornbread & Butter Milk Fruit Gelatin	Suggest some desserts to add extra milk, such as custard, cheese, pudding, ice cream; fruit; bread or rice pudding with raisins; occasionally cookies, cake, pies or fruit short cakes.

Foods for Between Meals, Extra Meals and Snacks	
An extra glass of milk or fruit juice, or one saved from regular mealtime Cheese cubes and crackers Apple, banana, orange, dried apricots or other fruit	Raw vegetable sticks Sandwich—meat, cheese or peanut butter Lunch or dinner dessert, such as ice cream, saved for between-meal snack

Nutrition Source Book, Chicago, National Dairy Council, 1971, p. 18.

WHY IS IT IMPORTANT TO UNDERSTAND REGIONAL, RACIAL, AND RELIGIOUS DIETARY HABITS IN STUDYING NUTRITION AND MEAL PLANNING?

A surprisingly large number of foreign-born people are included in the population of the United States. Coming, as they do, from all parts of the world, they have brought with them, and tend to retain, habits of eating and food tastes very different from those we think of as American. These tastes and habits, some of which are poor in terms of present-day nutrition standards, have been fixed for generations and are not too easily changed.

One-sided diets have been brought from some countries where limited food production has restricted the diet to a few types of foods. Persons coming from such countries need to learn better food habits here, and how to incorporate in their native dishes the necessary nutrients for good nutrition. More adequate diets have been brought from other countries. However, foods familiar in these countries may be rare and expensive in America, and consequently they may be omitted from the diet. If a racial group does give up some of its own food habits and adopt those of the new country, it frequently chooses the poorest of the new country's nutritional habits, such as the liking for excessive sweets and breadstuffs.

If the general level of nutrition in the United States is to be improved, the education of the various racial groups in the best ways to supplement the good features of their racial diets is an important starting point in a nutrition education program. In most cases, the answer lies in the greater use of milk, fruits, and vegetables in their cheaper forms and prepared in dishes that are accepted and enjoyed. Some assistance in planning the expenditure of food money to permit the purchase of the needed supplemental foods, and also some help in combining these foods into dishes and meals that the family will eat, are also frequently needed. The problem becomes more difficult when religious restrictions are applied to the family diet.

Just as food tastes and habits differ among different racial groups, so do they differ also from region to region in the United States. From the Far West to the East Coast and New England by way of the Southwest and South or the North Central states, differences are apparent in the special regional dishes, the types of meals served, and the ways food is prepared, to say nothing of the food patterns and habits to be encountered in the metropolitan areas across the country and in less accessible areas.

HOW MAY RACIAL AND REGIONAL DIETARY PATTERNS BE EVALUATED?

A typical day's diet for any racial, regional, or religious group may be evaluated nutritionally by checking it against an acceptable diet plan such as the Daily Food guide outlined on page 29.

STUDY QUESTIONS AND ACTIVITIES

1. Explain what is meant by the following statement "Good meal planning is both a science and an art."
2. Below are shown some poor breakfasts, poor lunches, and poor dinners. How would you change each of the meals to make them more attractive and appealing and at the same time to improve nutritive value?

Poor Meals	*Good Meals*

Breakfast Orange juice
Buttered toast

Lunch   (1) Hamburger on Buttered
             Bun
           French Fried Potatoes
           Fruit Gelatin

      (2) Macaroni and Cheese
           Muffin and Butter
           Soft Drink

Lunch,   (3) Luncheon Meat Sandwich
carried   Vanilla Wafers
            Soft Drink

Dinner   (1) Meat and Vegetable Stew
            Rolls and Butter
            Frosted Layer Cake

      (2) Roast Chicken
           Parsley potato
           Rolls and Butter
           Jam
           Apple Pie

3. Using the menu form on page 134, plan menus for five days for *your* family which will include the foods in the Four Food Groups and also illustrate other important considerations in meal planning. Note that each time you use a food you indicate the food group to which it belongs.

4. Become familiar with the racial, religious, or regional diet assigned you by the instructor and summarize information about it to present to the class. Be prepared to discuss this racial diet in terms of the Four Food Groups you have studied previously. What are the good points? How could the diet be improved?
   Each student in the class will then use the chart on page 133 to record important information about each diet presented in class.

5. Students with foreign backgrounds might tell about their food customs and dietary habits and possibly demonstrate the main dishes popular in their family meals. Markets in foreign sections of a city and foreign restaurants afford good opportunity for learning about foods used by families with different racial backgrounds. The class might prepare a foreign meal for the teachers and students.

SUPPLEMENTARY READING

Bogert: Chapter 26   Mowry: Chapter 25   Robinson: Pages 146–151
Howe: Chapter 11   Peyton: Chapter 11

Family Fare—a guide to good nutrition, HG No. 1, Washington, D. C., U. S. Department of Agriculture, 1970.

Money-Saving Main Dishes. HG No. 43, Washington, D. C., U. S. Department of Agriculture, 1971.
Special references on racial diets:

Eating in Different Languages: A Handbook for Public Health Nurses. Chicago, Visiting Nurse Association, 1962.

Favorite Recipes from United Nations. Washington, D. C., U. S. Committee for the United Nations, 1960.

Foods With an International Flavor (A 4–H Food Nutrition Project), Chicago, National 4–H Service Committee, Inc., 1970.

C. H. Robinson: *Foundations of Nutrition*. New York, The Macmillan Company, 1968, Chapter 16: Cultural Food Patterns in the United States.

RACIAL DIETARY HABITS

Regional or racial diet (list foods used)	*Characteristics and main dish*	*Good nutritional features*	*Desirable nutritional improvements*

>>> SUGGESTED FAMILY MEALS FOR FIVE DAYS <<<

Basic Plan for the Three Daily Meals	MENU 1	Food Group	MENU 2	Food Group	MENU 3	Food Group	MENU 4	Food Group	MENU 5	Food Group
BREAKFAST										
Fruit or fruit juice										
Cereal in some form and/or egg										
Cereal in some form and/or meat										
Bread in some form										
Milk										
Hot beverage for adults										
DINNER										
Meat, fish, or poultry										
Potatoes										
A vegetable										
A vegetable or fruit salad or vegetable relish										
Bread and butter if extra energy food is needed										
Dessert—light or heavy depending on meal										
Milk										
Beverage for adults										
LUNCH OR SUPPER										
Hearty main dish										
Salad or relish										
Bread and butter if extra energy food is needed										
Dessert—light or heavy depending on meal										
Milk										

Form from a Cornell Extension Bulletin.

WHAT HAS HAPPENED TO YOUR FOOD HABITS AND NUTRITION ATTITUDES AS YOU HAVE STUDIED ABOUT NUTRIENTS AND FOODS FOR GOOD NUTRITION?

Now is a good time for you to check your food habits once more.

1. Keep a record of your food intake (at meals and between meals) for one week on the chart on the following page.
2. Score your diet for each day, using the Food Selection Score Card on page 25, and determine your average score for the week.
3. What is your average score for the week? How does this score compare with the score you obtained for your weekly food record when you started the course? See page 24.
4. Analyze and comment on your last food selection score in the space provided below.

Food Groups	Perfect Score	My Score	Comments
Milk Group			
Meat Group			
Vegetable-			
Fruit Group			
Bread-Cereal Group			
Water	_____		
	100		

What improvements have you made in your food selection habits thus far?

What further improvements do you think it desirable to make?

What thought have you given to the principles of meal planning as you have selected the necessary foods for your various meals?

Note to Instructor: It is suggested that each student keep and score a week's food intake at least *once more (preferably twice)* before the end of the course.

Unit Four

NUTRITION IN THE LIFE CYCLE

PART 1.   NUTRITION IN PREGNANCY AND LACTATION

PART 2.   NUTRITION OF INFANTS AND TODDLERS

PART 3.   NUTRITION IN CHILDHOOD AND
           ADOLESCENCE

PART 4.   GERIATRIC NUTRITION

Object

To help the practical nurse develop an appreciation of special nutritional needs throughout the life cycle: in pregnancy and lactation, to meet additional requirements of mother and baby; in infancy and early childhood, to lay a foundation for future health; in later childhood and adolescence, to strengthen this foundation for physical, mental, and emotional health; and in later adult life, to conserve health and postpone degenerative diseases so characteristic of this period.

PART 1.   NUTRITION IN PREGNANCY AND LACTATION

WHY ARE DIET AND NUTRITION IMPORTANT DURING PREGNANCY AND LACTATION?

Food is an important factor for good health in the young and old alike. It becomes increasingly important during pregnancy when the needs of both the developing baby and its mother need to be met adequately.

The health of expectant mothers is a subject of world-wide concern. Many studies have been made to observe the relationship between food and nutrition, the course of pregnancy, and the condition of the infant at birth. These studies indicate that women who eat nutritionally adequate diets during pregnancy are in better health themselves, have more normal pregnancies with fewer complications, are more likely to be able to nurse their babies and have better quality milk. They show further that these well-fed mothers have babies that are better developed and healthier than the babies of mothers receiving inadequate diets during pregnancy.

WHAT ARE SPECIAL NUTRITIONAL NEEDS DURING PREGNANCY?

It is advantageous for a woman to have eaten a good diet previous to pregnancy so that her body has adequate reserves of nutrients for the increased needs of pregnancy—production of new tissues, changes in metabolism and changes in endocrine secretions. The recent increase in teen-age marriages and teen-age pregnancies focuses special attention on the importance of a good prenatal diet to meet the continuing growth needs of the mother as well as those of the developing baby. Growth continues during adolescence and requires more nutrients than those needed by an adult. Studies of the diets of teen-age girls have revealed many poor food habits, and diets inadequate in calcium, vitamin C, and iron. The adolescent girl may enter pregnancy in an extremely poor nutritional state, lacking in reserves of nutrients, and the health of both mother and child may suffer as a result.

The following table compares the Recommended Daily Dietary Allowances for pregnancy and lactation with those for the moderately active, nonpregnant woman 18 to 35 years of age.

RECOMMENDED DIETARY ALLOWANCES DURING PREGNANCY AND LACTATION[1]

Nutrient	18 to 35 Years		
	Nonpregnant Women	*Pregnancy*	*Lactation*
Calories	2000	2200	3000
Protein	55 gm.	65 gm.	75 gm.
Vitamin A Activity	5000 I.U.	6000 I.U.	8000 I.U.
Vitamin D	400 I.U. (18–22)	400 I.U.	400 I.U.
Vitamin E Activity	25 I.U.	30 I.U.	30 I.U.
Ascorbic acid	55 mg.	60 mg.	60 mg.
Folacin	0.4 mg.	0.8 mg.	0.5 mg.
Niacin, mg. equivalent	13 mg.	15 mg.	20 mg
Riboflavin	1.5 mg.	1.8 mg.	2.0 mg.
Thiamine	1.0 mg.	1.1 mg.	1.5 mg.
Vitamin B6	2.0 mg.	2.5 mg.	2.5 mg.
Vitamin B12	5 μg.	8 μg.	6 μg.
Calcium	0.8 gm.	1.2 gm.	1.3 gm.
Phosphorus	0.8 gm.	1.2 gm.	1.3 gm.
Iodine (22–35)	100 μg.	125 μg.	150 μg.
Iron	18 mg.	18 mg.	18 mg.
Magnesium	(18–22) 350 mg. (22–35) 300 mg.	450 mg.	450 mg.

[1] Food and Nutrition Board, National Research Council, Revised 1968. (Consult complete table, p. 26).

WHAT ARE DAILY FOOD NEEDS DURING PREGNANCY AND LACTATION?

FOODS NEEDED EACH DAY

Food item	Before and during the first half of pregnancy	During the latter half of pregnancy	While nursing your baby
Milk, pasteurized—includes whole, nonfat, evaporated, reliquefied dry, or buttermilk	1 pint	1 quart	1½ quarts
Lean cooked meat, fish, poultry or meat alternate. Use liver or heart frequently	1 serving (2–3 ounces)	1–2 servings (5 ounces)	1–2 servings (5 ounces)
Egg	1	1	1
Dark green or deep yellow vegetable	1 serving	1 serving	1–2 servings
Fruits and vegetables rich in vitamin C Good sources: citrus fruit or juice, cantaloup, raw strawberries, broccoli, peppers	1 serving	1 serving	1 serving
Fair sources: other melons, asparagus, brussels sprouts, raw cabbage, greens, tomatoes or juice, fresh or canned chili, potatoes cooked in jackets	or 2 servings	and 1 serving	and 2 servings
Other vegetable or fruit	1 serving	2 servings	2 servings
Whole grain, restored, or enriched cereal	1 serving	1 serving	1 serving
Whole grain, restored, or enriched bread	2–3 slices	2–3 slices	3 slices
Butter or fortified margarine	Amount as caloric level permits	Amount as caloric level permits	Amount as caloric level permits
Vitamin D		Use according to physicians's instructions	Use according to physician's instructions

From *Prenatal Care*. Children's Bureau Publication No. 4. Washington, D. C., U. S. Department of Health, Education and Welfare, 1962, p. 19. (Adapted from *Nutrition During Pregnancy and Lactation*. Berkeley, California, California State Department of Public Health, revised 1960.)

Equivalents of Servings[2]

Milk. One 8-ounce cup of milk contains about the same amount of calcium as 1⅓ oz. cheddar cheese
¾ pound creamed cottage cheese
1 pound cream cheese
1 pint ice cream
(Calcium tablets are not a substitute for milk as they contain no protein or riboflavin)

Meat. A 3-ounce serving of lean, cooked meat, poultry, or fish (without bone) is roughly equal in protein to any one of the following:

½ cup of any of these diced
1 medium-sized patty

---

[2] *Prenatal Care*. Children's Bureau Publication No. 4. Washington, D. C., U. S. Department of Health, Education and Welfare, 1962, pp. 16–18.

1 slice roast meat or poultry,
$5 \times 2\frac{1}{4} \times \frac{1}{2}$ inch
1 slice round steak, $4 \times 2 \times 1$ inch
2 frankfurters
1 medium shoulder lamb chop
2 small slices liver
2 thin slices meat loaf
1 medium chicken leg (fryer)
1 medium-sized fish steak
1 cup (cooked) dry peas or beans
4 tablespoons peanut butter
Vegetable-Fruits. 4 ounces $\frac{1}{2}$ cup orange or grapefruit juice is equivalent in vitamin C to:
$1\frac{1}{4}$ cups tomato juice
$\frac{1}{2}$ medium-sized cantaloup
$\frac{1}{2}$–$\frac{3}{4}$ cups strawberries
1 cup shredded cabbage
$\frac{1}{2}$ cup broccoli
Fats, oils, and sugars may be included as ingredients in food preparation.

$\frac{3}{4}$ cup dark-green leafy vegetables such as collards or kale cooked briefly in a little water
2 tangerines
A serving of a fruit or vegetable is usually $\frac{1}{2}$ cup or an ordinary portion such as:
1 medium apple
1 medium banana
1 medium orange
1 medium potato
$\frac{1}{2}$ medium grapefruit
$\frac{1}{2}$ medium cantaloup
Breads-Cereals. One serving of cereal is equal to
$\frac{1}{2}$–$\frac{3}{4}$ cup cooked whole-grain or enriched cereal, cornmeal, grits, macaroni, noodles, rice or spaghetti or
1 ounce ready-to-eat cereal or
1 medium slice enriched bread

WHAT SAMPLE MEAL PLANS CAN BE USED AS GUIDES?[3]

Sample Meal Plans For The Second Half Of Pregnancy

For pregnant woman of normal weight

For pregnant adolescent girl of normal weight
(more calories, protein, calcium)

Breakfast: Orange slice
Shredded wheat
Scrambled egg
Toast, 1 slice
Milk, $\frac{1}{2}$ pint
Coffee

Orange juice, 8 ounces
Shredded wheat
Scrambled egg
Toast, 2 slices
Butter or margarine
Marmalade
Milk, 1/2 pint

Lunch: Meat sandwich
Carrot and green pepper sticks
Oatmeal cookies
Milk, $\frac{1}{2}$ pint

Meat sandwich on whole wheat bread
Carrot and green pepper sticks
Cheese cubes
Oatmeal cookies
Fresh fruit
Milk, $\frac{1}{2}$ pint

Midafternoon: Milk, $\frac{1}{2}$ pint

Chicken sandwich
Milk, $\frac{1}{2}$ pint

Dinner: Broiled beef liver
Steamed broccoli
Baked potato

Broiled beef liver
Steamed broccoli
Baked potato

---

[3] Ibid., p. 20.

For pregnant woman of normal weight	*For pregnant adolescent girl of normal weight*
Tomato salad with French dressing	Vegetable salad with French dressing
Baked apple	Baked apple with raisins
Bedtime: Hot milk or cocoa, ½ pint	Milk, ½ pint
	Milk or cocoa, ½ pint

Meals and Snacks. Part of the day's food may be taken in the form of snacks between meals and at bedtimes. Some doctors may recommend five small meals a day instead of three large ones (as in the above meal plans.) Smaller amounts of food at more frequent intervals help prevent hunger between meals; may also help prevent nausea, and the hot drink at night may help sleep. Avoid extras—food treats high in calories. If snack is needed between meals, milk, fruits, and raw vegetables are best.

Fluids. Physician may recommend as much as two quarts fluid daily, some of which is furnished by milk, soup, fruit juices, tea, coffee, and other beverages in addition to water.

Salt. If restricted by physician, no salt is used in cooking or at table, and the following foods omitted: bacon, ham, chipped beef, corned beef, salted and smoked fish, salted nuts, pretzels, salted crackers, popcorn, potato chips.[4]

WHY IS ATTENTION TO WEIGHT IMPORTANT DURING PREGNANCY?

Normal weight increases occur during pregnancy to the amount of 12 or more pounds. This weight gain is due to the weight of the placenta and membranes (about 1¼ pounds), enlarged uterus (about 2 pounds), increase in size of liver and volume of blood, slightly heavier breasts, and water absorbed and held in body tissues. A full term infant at birth weighs between 7 and 8 pounds. A weight gain of about 20 pounds is considered an acceptable level in most cases. Weight at beginning of pregnancy and previous history of weight gains and losses may make greater or lesser gain desirable in individual cases. Sudden gain of weight in a short period is not desirable. Extreme overweight is thought to be a factor in toxemia and complications in delivery.[5]

WHAT PROBLEMS DURING PREGNANCY REQUIRE DIETARY ADJUSTMENTS?

Overweight. Excessive weight gain, mentioned above, is undesirable for both mother and developing baby as it may predispose to delivery problems or toxemia and be detrimental to well-being of the baby. An 1800 calorie diet may be recommended.

Nausea and Vomiting. High carbohydrate foods or dry toast before arising and 5 to 6 smaller meals a day in place of the three large ones may alleviate. Fluids with meals and fats may be a common cause. Skim milk may replace whole milk.

Anemia. Liver, green vegetables, eggs, dried fruits, whole-grain and enriched cereals and breads, and molasses provide iron in the diet as a safeguard against nutritional anemia.

---

[4] *Prenatal Care.* Children's Bureau Publication No. 4. Washington, D. C., U. S. Department of Health, Education and Welfare, 1962, pp. 15, 16, 20.

[5] Ibid., pp. 21–22, adapted.

Toxemia.   Characterized by edema, albuminuria, and elevated blood pressure; may respond to a modified protein diet with restricted sodium and possible fluid restriction. Calories restricted with overweight.

Constipation.   Usually responds to the inclusion of vegetables, fruits, and whole-grain products along with adequate fluids.

Underweight.   Diet increased in calories and protein. Smaller meals of higher nutritional value, eaten more frequently, rather than fewer larger meals may enable women to consume an increased diet more easily.

STUDY QUESTIONS AND ACTIVITIES

1.   What benefits may a mother-to-be expect if she is well nourished before pregnancy and eats well during pregnancy? How will the baby benefit?
2.   Why is the health of expectant mothers of world-wide concern?
3.   Why is it important for the mother-to-be to control her weight to the figure recommended by her physician during pregnancy? What is the maximum weight gain suggested?
4.   Why are the eating habits of pregnant teen-agers of special importance?
5.   Why are protein and calcium key items in the diet during pregnancy? How are the additional demands for these nutrients met in the diet of the pregnant woman?
6.   What are other special nutritional needs during pregnancy?
7.   How and why do the foods needed daily during pregnancy and lactation differ from those of the non-pregnant woman?
8.   What problems during pregnancy may require adjustments in the diet? Why?
9.   Name several different ways for the pregnant woman to incorporate milk in her diet if she does not find it possible to drink the desirable amount?
10.   When a pregnant woman has to restrict her calories, what foods should she avoid or eat in lessened amount?
11.   Mrs. J. is told by her doctor that she is anemic. What advice can you give her about her choice of foods?
12.   Mrs. M. is bothered with constipation during pregnancy. What suggestions can you give her about foods?
13.   Although Mrs. J. does not like to drink milk, she can manage to drink 1 glass daily. Suggest ways to her for including the remainder of the 4 glasses in foods at meals and between meals.
14.   Mrs. W. wonders if she should take calcium tablets in place of some of the milk she should have in her diet. What nutrients will be lacking if she replaces milk with calcium tablets?
15.   The doctor has reduced the amounts of meat and eggs in the diet of Mrs. B. How can Mrs. B. receive adequate protein with such diet restrictions?
16.   Secure from a woman in the latter half of pregnancy who comes to the hospital's Prenatal Clinic or one suggested by a physician, a list of foods she ate at meal time and between meals during one average day. Compare this woman's diet with the foods suggested in column 3 of the table on page 139.
   What conclusions can you draw regarding the food habits of this woman?
   What suggestions could you make to her about her diet?
   Has this woman's physician prescribed any supplementary vitamins or minerals? Why?
17.   What inexpensive sources of vitamin C (ascorbic acid) can you suggest to a pregnant woman?
18.   What ways can you suggest for including raw vegetables in the diet?

SUPPLEMENTARY READING

Bogert: Chapter 21   Mowry: Pages 68–71   Robinson: Pages 126–128
Howe: Pages 137–140   Peyton: Chapter 12

Special Reference for *Unit Four; Your Age and Your Diet*. Leaflet. Chicago, American Medical Association.

Prenatal Care, Children's Bureau Publication No. 4, Washington, D. C., U. S. Department of Health, Education and Welfare, 1962.

PART 2. NUTRITION OF INFANTS AND TODDLERS

HOW DOES AN INFANT GROW AND DEVELOP?

The greatest growth and development during a lifetime takes place during the first year.

Average weight at birth: 7 pounds (boys weigh a little more than girls)

Average length at birth: 18 to 24 inches

Average weekly gain in weight: First 5 months: 5 to 8 ounces (about 1–1/2 to 2 lb. per mo.) with birth weight doubled at 5 months. Six to 12 months: 4 to 5 ounces (about 1 lb. per mo.) with birth weight trebled at 10 to 12 months. Twelve to 24 months: gain of about 1/2 pound per month

Average gain in height: 9 to 10 inches during first year with rapid growth of arms and legs (short in proportion at birth).

Stomach capacity: at birth—1 ounce (2 tablespoons); at 2 weeks—2 ounces (4 tablespoons); at 3 months—4–1/2 ounces (9 tablespoons).

Digestive ability: at birth, able to digest protein, simple carbohydrate and emulsified fat; later, digestive enzymes develop for digestion of starch and some fat.

A well-nourished infant will show steady gain in weight and height (with some fluctuations from week to week), is happy, vigorous, sleeps well, has firm muscles, will have some tooth eruption at about 5 to 6 months with about 6 to 12 teeth erupted by 12 months, has good elimination characteristic of the type of feeding—breast or formula. Each infant has his own rate of growth but all grow faster in weight than in height. A steady gain of weight is more important than a large amount gained.

A three year old child will weigh between 25 and 42 pounds and be 34 to 43 inches tall.

HOW ARE THE INFANT'S NUTRITIONAL NEEDS MET?

Infants require more calories, protein, minerals and vitamins in proportion to weight than do adults. Because of growth, more active tissues, and activity needs, fluid requirements are also high. Water is part of the formula at first; later boiled water is given between feedings.

It is generally agreed that breast feeding is desirable to get the infant off to a good start, at least for a couple of months. Mother's milk is the natural food for an infant; it agrees well, is clean, sterile, available, proper temperature, and eliminates the necessity of formula preparation. Colic, constipation, and digestive upsets are noted less frequently in breast-fed than in formula-fed infants.

The early flow of breast milk (colostrum) may provide some immunity to the infant to some infections of early life. An infant will gain satisfactorily if he receives about 2.5 ounces of breast milk per pound of body weight. Human milk also forms finer, softer, and more easily digested curds in the infant's stomach than cow's milk, containing casein, as more of the protein is in the form of lactalbumin.

Proper nutrition and hygiene habits are necessary on the part of the mother if she is to produce the right amount and quality of milk for her infant's needs.

WHAT DOES A FORMULA CONTAIN?

A formula for an infant will contain milk in some form (cow's for the most part in the United States or goat's milk in other countries), or a special form of milk or a milk substitute, some form of carbohydrate, and a liquid. Cow's milk requires special treatment to make it suitable for an infant. Water and sugar are added and it is heated to make it more digestible and free of disease bacteria.

Milks Used

Types. Pasteurized fresh, whole or skim, dried, or canned evaporated milk, any or all fortified with vitamin D. Fat is more finely divided in homogenized milk (most of which is fortified with 400 I. U. of vitamin D per quart) which forms smaller curds in the stomach.

Cow's milk generally available and easily modified to resemble human milk. Contains the same calories per ounce but has more protein than human milk.

Amount required. 1.5 ounces per pound of body weight.

Treatment. Diluted with water to dilute protein and heated or acidulated to make curd more like human milk curd. Dilution reduces proportion of sugar, so sugar is added to formula. Some pediatricians may substitute whole milk for modified milk formula at an earlier age than formerly recommended.

Special Milks

Acid milk. Made with lactic acid, lemon, or orange juice; fine soft curd so less dilution required, limits regurgitation, and acid reaction in intestine facilitates the absorption of calcium and iron.

Low-fat milk. Non-fat dry milk. Deficient in essential fatty acids and vitamins A and D unless D fortified. (Some dried milks are now being vitamin fortified.)

Protein milk. Various modified milks under different trade names, some with added minerals and vitamins. Usually in powdered or evaporated form.

Complete Commercial Formulas. (Premodified Milks) Available in powdered form or evaporated in cans or disposable feeding bottles. Usual base is cow's milk modified in one or more of the following ways: protein, lactose, fatty acids, minerals, vitamins, curd formation. Available for home delivery in certain limited areas; an expensive form. Examples are Enfamil, Modilac, Formil, Similac, and Carnilac.

Milk Substitutes

Simulate milk, particularly human milk, but contain no milk. Used for therapeutic purposes.

Soybean mixtures, for milk protein sensitivities. Examples are Pro-Sobee (Mead-Johnson); Mull-Soy (Borden).

Meat-base formulas or amino acid mixtures. For milk protein sensitivities and milk sugar-galactose intolerance. Examples are Nutramigen (Mead-Johnson); Meat Base Formula (Gerbers).

Low phenylalanine formula, used for phenylketonuria. Example: Lofenalac (Mead-Johnson).

Sugars

Granulated or brown sugar. Available, inexpensive, easy to use, but may be too sweet.

Corn syrup. Available, inexpensive, easy to use.

Dextri-Maltose (malt sugar with dextrin). Expensive, not as sweet as other sugars, fewer calories—1 tablespoon sugar equals 2 tablespoons Dextri-Maltose.

The cheapest formula is made from evaporated milk and granulated sugar.

Calculation of Infant's Formula:

Data

Fluid requirement: 2–1/2 oz. per pound of body weight.

Milk: 1–1/2 to 2 oz. per pound of body weight.

Sugar: 1/2 oz. per day for first few weeks; then 1 oz. (3 Tbsps.) per day to age of about 6 months, when sugar is omitted as other foods are added to diet.

Feedings: 5 at 4-hour intervals

Amount per feeding: 2 to 3 ounces more than age in months.

Example

Infant 4 months old

    Weight at birth—7 pounds

    Weight gain—6 oz. per week for 16 weeks: 16 × 6 or 96 oz. or 6 pounds.

Weight at 4 months—13 pounds

Size of feedings: 4 months plus 2 = 6 oz.

Number of feedings: 5; 6 oz. each = 30 oz.

Computation

Fluid: $13 \times 2\frac{1}{2} = 32\frac{1}{2}$ oz., of which milk = $13 \times 1\frac{3}{4} = 22\frac{3}{4}$ oz., therefore water required is $9\frac{3}{4}$ oz.

Formula

Quantities computed as at left are rounded off to the nearest ounce.

Milk 23 oz.   Yield:

Water 10 oz.   5 bottles

Sugar 1 oz.

Sample Formulas[6]

	First formula	Later formulas	
Evaporated milk	6 ounces	10 ounces	13 ounces
Water (boiled)	10 ounces	15 ounces	19 ounces
Sugar or corn syrup	1–1/2 tablespoons	2–1/2 tablespoons	3 tablespoons

Or

Fresh whole milk (boiled)	12 ounces	20 ounces	26 ounces
Water (boiled)	4 ounces	6 ounces	6 ounces
Sugar or corn syrup	1–1/2 tablespoons	2–1/2 tablespoons	3 tablespoons

---

[6] *Infant Care,* Children's Bureau Publication No. 8. Washington, D. C., U. S. Department of Health, Education and Welfare, 1963, p. 92.

HOW IS AN INFANT'S FORMULA PREPARED?

It is important that the baby's formula be as sterile as possible. Either of the two sterilization methods below may be used:

Method 1: Sterilizing utensils and formula together (terminal)
Prepared mixture ordered by the doctor is poured into washed and rinsed nursing bottles, then the bottles and mixture are boiled. This method eliminates possible contamination and is easy to use. It is recommended by the American Hospital Association.

Steps
1. Shake well an unopened bottle of fresh, pasteurized milk to mix in cream if not homogenized. The doctor may prescribe a modified form of fresh milk.
2. Measure exact amounts of sugar, water, and milk as ordered by doctor, in a clean quart measure (or use measuring cup and sauce pan). Stir well to dissolve and blend ingredients.
3. Pour correct amount of formula into each clean bottle.
4. Cap bottles with clean nipples (inverted if using certain types of screw tops); cover with clean discs and screw caps, or with clean nipple covers. Do not screw cap on tightly, or press down covers. They should be loose enough for steam to circulate.
5. Place bottles in rack in deep pan. Put 2 to 3 inches of hot water into pan, cover tightly, and bring water to boil. Boil 25 minutes.
6. Turn off heat and let bottles cool in covered pan until lukewarm. Tighten screw tops, or press down covers. Refrigerate bottles at once.

Method 2: Sterilizing utensils and formula separately (sterile or aseptic)
Prepared mixture is boiled for 3 minutes (counting from the time it comes to a boil), then poured into sterilized nursing bottles. This is the traditional method.

Steps
1. Sterilize utensils: Put clean nursing bottles, funnel, strainer, and tongs in rack in pan which holds 2 to 3 inches hot water. (Keep tong handles out of hot water.) Cover and boil 10 minutes. Boil clean nipples and all parts of bottle caps or nipple covers 3 minutes in small covered pan. Drain off water and keep nipples and caps in the sterile pan. Take utensils from sterilizing pan with sterile tongs. Put sterile funnel and strainer on inverted lid of bottle sterilizer. Do not let hands touch any part of sterile utensils which the formula will touch.
2. Follow steps 1 and 2 under Method 1, using enamel sauce pan.
3. Heat quickly to boiling, boil 3 minutes. Stir continuously.
4. Strain hot formula into the sterile bottles using sterilized strainer and funnel. Fill each bottle with exact amount of formula for each feeding.
5. Put on sterile nipple and cap. Do not touch nipple with hands.
6. Cool bottles at room temperature until lukewarm. Refrigerate bottles at once.

HOW IS INFANT'S FORMULA FED?

Formula temperature: Formulas at room temperature or warmed to body temperature by placing bottle in warm water.

Feeding intervals: After the first month of more frequent feedings on demand, the usual interval between feedings is 3 hours; at 2 to 3 months a gradual change to 4 hour interval feedings. Several "burpings" are desirable during a feeding period.

WHAT ADDITIONAL FOODS ARE GIVEN DURING THE FIRST YEAR?

Neither breast milk nor a milk formula will furnish adequate amounts of all the nutrients required by the infant during the first year. An important reason for introducing some solid foods into the infant's diet is to replenish the depleting body stores of iron during the early months of life. The kind of food, form, time, and sequence for adding supplemental foods vary with pediatricians; some add solid foods early in the first year while others choose to wait until nearer the middle of the year. By the end or shortly after the end of the first year, the baby will be eating the family diet. The following foods are added to the infant's diet during the first year.[7] As the baby may not be receiving enough fluid in the formula or from the breast, cool boiled water should be offered several times daily.

Vitamin C and D.   Usually started at 2 to 3 weeks, starting with orange juice for ascorbic acid. Start with 1 teaspoon strained orange juice mixed with 1 teaspoon cooled boiled water given daily. More juice is added as baby grows older; 4 tablespoons by 4 months; 6 tablespoons daily by 8 to 10 months. Doctor may suggest other juices. Source and amount of vitamin D will also be suggested by doctor.

Solid foods.   Started 2 to 3 months. Store of iron in baby's body begins to be depleted so iron foods stressed. Cereals, vegetables, or fruit started first, depending on doctor. Only one new food introduced at a time one week apart, and then just a little bit from tip of spoon. This provides a new experience of taking food from a spoon and swallowing. Foods should not be sweetened.

Cereals: enriched cream of wheat, strained oatmeal, or baby cereal food, thinned with a little of baby's formula or boiled water. Begin with 1 teaspoon, once a day, increase gradually until 2 to 5 tablespoons are given once or twice daily when baby is 6 to 7 months old.

Fruits: cooked and strained or babies' canned fruit; peaches, apricots, prunes, applesauce, mashed ripe banana.

Vegetables: cooked and strained or babies' canned vegetables; mild flavored ones such as green beans, carrots, green peas, strained dark green and deep yellow vegetables.

Egg yolk, meats, fish: about 3 to 5 months. Egg yolk, hard cooked or in custard starting with 1/4 teaspoon, adding a small amount at a time until all of yolk is fed. Some pediatricians do not advise feeding the whole egg until toward the end of the first year; meat canned for babies or scraped or finely ground before baby has teeth. Begin with a small amount and add slowly until baby receives about 2 tablespoons at a feeding; fish may be added when baby is 1 year old—steamed, poached, or tuna fish or fish prepared for babies (all bones carefully removed).

By end of first year baby will be getting mashed and chopped foods instead of strained and finely ground and will be eating, in addition to milk, many kinds of fruits, vegetables, cereals, as well as egg, meat, and fish; will be on a 3 meal a day schedule plus (midmorning and midafternoon) snacks, some, if not all, of which come from the family table. Plan to give the child some of the foods from the above list at midmorning, midafternoon, and maybe at bedtime. The day's meal plan may then be—*Breakfast:* cereal, egg, milk (orange juice). *Midmorning:* orange juice, if not given at breakfast. *Noon meal:* vegetables, meat, milk. *Midafternoon:* milk, crusty bread

---

[7] *Your Baby's First Year.* Children's Bureau Publication No. 40. Washington, D. C., U. S. Department of Health, Education and Welfare, 1962, adapted.

or crackers. *Evening meal:* cereal, fruit, milk. To help baby feed himself, some food he can eat with his fingers may be offered—pieces of banana, diced cooked carrots, chopped cooked meat. Doctor will advise kinds and amounts of other foods and time to add them as the baby grows older.

WHAT FOODS ARE NEEDED DAILY BY THE 1 TO 3-YEAR-OLD?[8]

Milk.   Two to 3 cups to drink and in dishes such as soup, custard, pudding, cheese.

Egg.   One helping each day.

Bread and Cereal.   Whole grain or enriched. Four or more helpings each day.

Butter   or fortified margarine on bread or to season vegetables. Some every day.

Vegetables.   Choose a dark-green or deep-yellow vegetable (cook vegetables and peel fruits for the 1 to 2-year-old). Two or more helpings each day.

Meat, Fish, Poultry.   One or more helpings each day. Dry beans and peas, or smooth peanut butter in place of meat, fish, or poultry at times.

Fruits.   Good source of vitamin C such as grapefruit, orange, or tomato, whole or in juice. One or more helpings each day.

Vitamin D.   Doctor will decide form to be given. Usually 400 units each day. Milk, cereals, and other foods may have had vitamin D added (stated on label). Only the amount of vitamin D suggested by doctor is to be given.

One serving for most children 1 to 3 years old amounts to 1/2 to 1 tablespoon. Some children will eat more. Some children are satisfied with three meals daily; others may want snacks—some of the foods from above list at midmorning, midafternoon, and possibly at bedtime. By now, child probably eats with family; let him feed himself. At 1 year, can handle bite-size pieces with fingers; later on can handle a spoon. He may be less hungry and more choosy and refuse certain foods. Different foods should still be offered—in time he will take them.

STUDY QUESTIONS AND ACTIVITIES

1.   What are the advantages of breast feeding for an infant?
2.   Name several reasons why breast milk is so suitable for an infant.
3.   How much breast milk per pound is required by an infant? How can it be determined if an infant is getting sufficient breast milk?
4.   What has to be done to cow's milk to make it suitable for infant feeding?
5.   Why do supplementary foods have to be given to either a breast fed or formula fed infant during the first year?
6.   What are the two first additions of food given to an infant? Why?
7.   What nutrients are supplied to the infant's diet by cereals? By fruits? By a green or yellow vegetable? By egg yolk? By meat?
8.   What is meant by the sterile technique for preparing a baby's formula? the terminal technique? Which is considered more desirable? Why?

---

[8] *Your Child from 1 to 3,* Children's Bureau Publication No. 413, Washington, D. C., U. S. Department of Health, Education and Welfare, 1964, adapted.

9. List some ways to encourage good food habits in children as soon as they begin to get foods in addition to the formula or breast feeding.

    Class activity: observe preparation of infant formulas in hospital.

    Demonstration by instructor: terminal and aseptic methods of formula sterilization.

SUPPLEMENTARY READING

Howe: Pages 140–148   Peyton: Chapter 13   Robinson: Pages 131–138
Mowry: Pages 63–66
Infant Care, Children's Bureau Publication No. 8, 1963
Your Baby's First Year, Children's Bureau Publication No. 400, 1962
Your Child from 1 to 3, Children's Bureau Publication No. 413, 1964
Available from Superintendent of Documents, Government Printing Office, Washington, D. C.

PART 3. NUTRITION IN CHILDHOOD AND ADOLESCENCE

WHAT IS THE IMPORTANCE OF NUTRITION TO HEALTHY GROWTH AND DEVELOPMENT?

"Healthy growth and development depend more on good nutrition than on any other factor. From the beginnings of growth in the prenatal period to the time when the child attains his full size as an adult, the food he eats and his ability to convert that food into energy and new body tissue will influence the state of his health not only as a child but throughout life.

"Good nutrition means more than the right kinds of foods in the right quantities. In order to be well nourished, a child must be able to digest and utilize the food he eats. His ability to do this may be affected by a great many things—the presence or absence of disease, the amount of sleep he is getting, and his emotional and mental condition. These factors must never be overlooked.

"Each period in the life of a child—infancy (birth to 1 year), preschool (1 to 6 years), school (6 to 12 years), and adolescence (12 to 18 years)—has its special needs and its special problems. But certain principles hold good for all periods. At all periods, a person's nutrition is affected, not only by the food he eats, but also his rest, his recreation, and his general mental health. At all periods, the diet must provide a number of essential food elements if the body is to function properly.

"Children like to eat. If good food is offered in a matter-of-fact way, without urging, most children will accept and enjoy it. But children, like adults, have food preferences. The best way to get children to eat is to give them some freedom in choice and not force them to eat against their will. A child will accept food one day and reject it a few days later. If children receive a lot of attention when they will not eat, refusing food may become a game with them. The wise parent will say nothing about the matter but will offer the food again some other day."[9] Steady refusal on the part of children to eat many of the foods necessary for good nutrition is a matter of real concern and may require medical advice.

WHAT IS MEANT BY GROWTH AND DEVELOPMENT?

Growth is the increase in weight and height with age, or "size" as it is popularly designated, which comes about as a result of the multiplication of cells and their differentiation for many different functions in the body. Height is the more significant factor as the type of body build and amount of fatty tissue cause weight variation. Growth is a continuous but not uniform process from conception to full maturity. During fetal life and infancy, the rate of growth is very rapid. This period is followed by one of slower growth during early and middle childhood. Another period of very rapid growth occurs during adolescence, followed by a tapering off until the growth period ends.

---

[9] *Nutrition and Healthy Growth,* Children's Bureau Publication No. 352. Washington, D. C., U. S. Department of Health, Education and Welfare, 1955 (out of print), p. ii and p. 5, adapted.

Development refers to the increasing ability of body parts to function. Factors affecting the rate of growth and development include heredity, or inborn capacity to grow, and various environmental factors, an extremely important one of which is nutrition. Better diets, which go with improved economic conditions, and advances in medical care and health services are credited for the taller stature of children and adults in the United States as compared with children and adults of similar ages some years ago. It has also been noted that in the technologically advanced countries the average height and weight of children of any given age have increased over the last 100 years. There is accumulating evidence that well nourished children reach the potential set by their heredity, not only in physical growth but also in mental development.

HOW IS THE NUTRITIONAL STATUS OF CHILDREN EVALUATED?

To accurately assess the nutritional status of a child, patterns of growth and body measurements are evaluated by using physical growth charts, as shown on pages 294 and 295, which are designed for use in schools for boys and girls 4 to 18 years of age. These charts are based on scientific studies of growth—measurements of height and weight—of white school children in Iowa City, Iowa, from 1961 to 1963. They are preferred over the formerly used height-weight tables to measure growth. In addition, extensive physical examinations and biochemical studies of the blood and urine as well as dietary studies are made. Also taken into consideration are certain environmental factors which may affect good nutrition.

WHAT ARE THE CHARACTERISTICS OF GOOD AND POOR NUTRITIONAL STATUS?[10]

"Nutritional status means state of health of the individual or group as conditioned by choice and amounts of foods, or more accurately, *nutrients,* eaten."* Positive indications of good nutrition are vitality, alertness, good muscular development and tone, body weight within 10% of desirable weight and integrity of all body tissues and organ systems. Biochemical tests, anthropometric measurements and examinations by experienced medical specialists provide the best data for evaluation of nutritional status. Records of food intake are of value in confirming the evidence and in establishing dietary needs."

The following outline lists the characteristics of good and poor nutrition.

---

[10] *Dairy Council Digest,* vol. 35, no. 1, January–February, 1964, Chicago, National Dairy Council.

* *Nutritional Status:* U. S. A., edited by A. F. Morgan, California Agricultural Experiment Station Bulletin 769, 1959.

	Good Nutrition	*Poor Nutrition*
Body	Well developed	Undersized, poorly developed, possible physical defects
Weight	Approximately average for height and age and body build	Overweight Underweight
Posture and carriage	Good with head erect, chest up, shoulders flat, abdomen in, elastic step, arms and legs straight; weight distributed evenly on balls of feet; all parts of skeleton in good alignment	Fatigue posture; shoulders rounded, wings, flat and narrow chest, protruding abdomen, head forward
Facial expression	Bright and alert and without strain	Alert but strained; drawn and worried; dull and lifeless
Spirits and disposition	Good natured and full of life; good attention span for age; gets along well with others	Irritable, apprehensive, difficult to manage; nervous; overactive and fatigues easily; or phlegmatic, listless; fails to concentrate
Activity	Active mentally and physically, good endurance, quick recovery from fatigue	Mental and physical vigor lacking, hyper active
Muscles	Well developed and firm	Small and underdeveloped; flabby
Subcutaneous fat	Good layer	Usually lacking; sometimes excessive
Hair	Smooth and glossy	Rough and lusterless
Skin and complexion	Firm skin of good color with healthy glow	Skin loose, pale, waxy, of sallow color; blemishes
Eyes	Clear and bright; no dark circles underneath	Dull; hollow or dark circles underneath
Mucous membranes	Eyelids, mouth, and tongue clear and reddish pink	Pale
Appetite	Good, relishes food	Poor, fickle, or finicky
Sleep	Sound	Difficulty getting to sleep; light or restless sleeper
Teeth	Sound, well formed in well shaped jaws without overlapping or crowding; good occlusion; firm gums pinkish	Poorly shaped jaw and poorly formed and placed teeth; caries

	Good Nutrition	*Poor Nutrition*
Body functions	Normal; good appetite and digestion; regular elimination; stable nervous system; good endurance	Disturbed digestion; subject to constipation
General health	Excellent; no physical defects; good endurance; good resistance to infections	Endurance and vigor lacking; diseased and enlarged tonsils and adenoids; susceptible to infections

WHAT ARE NUTRITIONAL REQUIREMENTS OF GROWING CHILDREN?

"The growing child needs food to supply the materials for building tissues, to regulate the functions of those tissues and to furnish energy for many activities, including basal metabolism, growth and voluntary muscular activity. The amount of energy varies widely among individuals and depends upon a number of variables such as body size, basal metabolic rate, amount of voluntary activity, efficiency of the body in using foods, and rate of growth. To permit growth to proceed normally there must be a surplus of energy over the actual energy expended by the body, as well as adequate amounts of specific nutrients, including amino acids, glucose, essential fatty acids, minerals, and vitamins. Nutrition is an important cause of the more rapid rate of growth and the increased size of abundantly fed children. Human growth, superficially seen as the increase in size of a child, is a very complex and fascinating process. It involves continuous cell multiplication as well as the differentiation of cells to perform the many different functions of the organism so that its millions of cells of many types may live as a biological unit."

"The final size a person may become is limited by heredity, but whether or not the individual realizes his full potential is determined largely by nutrition. It is well known that growth is stunted in young children receiving diets severely restricted in proteins and calories. When such children are given an adequate diet, the rate of growth is very fast at the beginning of the rehabilitation period, greatly exceeding the normal rate for the chronological age, but it slows down later on. The initial rate corresponds to the actual size of the child. However, growth ceases at the usual chronological age, and the child becomes an undersized and underdeveloped adult. Thus it is seen that the full growth potential must be used continuously if full development is to be achieved. The extent to which undernutrition influences the size of an individual depends upon the age at which it occurs—the greatest effect being at the period of maximum growth—and by its duration in relation to the total period of growth."[11]

"Growing evidence that nutrition may affect intellectual and behavioral as well as physical growth has stimulated efforts to determine the extent of malnutrition in the United States and to assess its long-term impact. The National Nutrition Survey, begun in 1968 and being carried out by the U. S. Department of Health, Education and

---

[11] *Dairy Council Digest*, vol. 36, no. 2, March–April 1965, Chicago, National Dairy Council.

Welfare, is the first comprehensive effort to assess the nutritional status of the U. S. population. The survey found an unexpectedly high prevalence of conditions associated with malnutrition. Further research is needed to give a complete answer to the question of what effect malnutrition has on intellectual development. In the meantime, however, programs are underway for improving nutritional status and eating practices of mothers and infants. Information demonstrating the benefits of good nutrition in improved health and physical growth already justifies such efforts."[12]

WHAT ARE IMPORTANT CONSIDERATIONS IN FEEDING PRESCHOOLERS?[13]

The food a child eats from his first to his sixth year has much to do with his well-being and future development. Growth continues thereafter but less rapidly. Foods must supply adequate building materials.

During early childhood, children like foods prepared in simple ways. The way food tastes and feels to a young child leads to likes and dislikes at this age which are quite different from those of adults. Warm foods are more acceptable than hot or cold ones. Foods thinner than those for adults are enjoyed. Mild flavored foods are better liked than salty, sour, or highly spiced ones. Crisp and tender vegetables are well liked. Easily identified foods are more popular than mixtures.

Gradual extension of the diet begun in infancy is continued throughout the preschool period. Plenty of water is important. The need for vitamin D continues during this period. A variety of new food is being presented at this time and lasting food habits are formed. Between-meal eating should contribute nutrients as well as satisfy appetite. Increased energy needs are provided for by larger amounts of cereals, bread, butter, or margarine, potatoes, and other foods as appetite demands. Added needs for proteins, minerals, and vitamins are met by more and larger servings of fruit, vegetables, eggs, meats, and fish.

Refer to Part 2, Daily Foods for 1 to 3 years, page 149. The preschool child needs the same basic foods but in larger amounts. The following meal plan for a child shows how little adjustment, if any, needs to be made in the family meal pattern.[13]

FAMILY MEAL PATTERN

Breakfast	*Lunch or Supper*	*Dinner*
Fruit or juice	Main dish—mainly meat, eggs, fish, poultry, dried beans or peas, cheese, or peanut butter	Meat, poultry, or fish
Cereal with milk		Vegetables
Toast		Relish or salad
Butter or margarine		Bread
Milk		Butter or margarine
	Vegetable or salad	Fruit or pudding
	Bread	Milk
	Butter or margarine	
	Dessert or fruit	
	Milk	

---

[12] *Malnutrition and Learning,* Dr. Merrill S. Read, Bethesda, Maryland, 1969, National Institutes of Health.

[13] *Your Child from 1 to 6,* Children's Bureau Publication No. 30, Washington, D. C., U. S. Department of Health, Education and Welfare, 1962, pp. 66–71, adapted.

Some small children find it difficult to eat sufficient quantities of food at one time so a snack once or twice a day may be desirable. Snacks should be part of the whole day's food plan and should make a real nutritional contribution. Nibbling of cookies, crackers, chips, bread, etc. with soft drinks spoils the appetite for the carefully planned meals. Frequent nibbling also creates mouth conditions conducive to tooth decay. The following make good snacks for between meal eating when it is thought a wise plan:

Dry cereal, with milk or out of box	Fruit sherbet or ice cream
Simple cooky, or cracker	Toast, plain or cinnamon
Raw vegetables	Fruit juice
Canned, fresh, or dried fruit	Milk
Cheese wedge	Fruit drinks made with milk and juice

"Make snacks count for more than calories"

Other considerations in addition to food values:

Foods should be easy to handle.

Serve soup in mugs to drink.

Serve meats, vegetables, and fruits as finger foods.

Provide a variety of textures in meals: soft, chewy, crisp.

Serve meats moist rather than tough or dried (liver loaf instead of broiled liver).

Color appeals to children—use colorful gelatin, bits of parsley, etc.

Temperature extremes are unpleasant to children; serve foods and beverages at room temperature.

Strong flavored vegetables are not popular with children; serve raw or mild ones.

Children do not like foods mixed together; divided plates are popular.

Desserts should be a worthwhile part of the meal so they can be eaten any time (rather than being offered as a reward).

Consider comfort and service in the way meals are served.

Provide for a short rest before meals.

Reasonable size portions (on basis of what child can handle) encourage him to complete meal and request seconds.

Children vary from time to time in how much and what they want to eat. Sometimes they want the same food over and over, another time they will refuse it. They often go on food jags, then finally settle down to an overall eating pattern.

WHAT FOODS ARE NEEDED DAILY BY CHILDREN 6 TO 12?

A DAILY GUIDE TO FOODS NEEDED BY CHILDREN AND THEIR FAMILIES[14]

Types of Foods	Daily Amounts	Special Functions in Daily Diet
Milk Group:	Children under 9: 2–3 cups	
Milk (fluid, whole, evaporated, skim dry, buttermilk)	Children 9–12: 3 or more cups	Leading source of Ca for bones and teeth. High quality protein; Ex-

---

[14] *Your Child from 6 to 12,* Children's Bureau Publication No. 324, Washington, D. C., U. S. Department of Health, Education and Welfare, 1966 revision, pp. 34–39, adapted.

Types of Foods	*Daily Amounts*	*Special functions in daily diet*
Cheddar and Cottage Cheese, Ice Cream	Sometimes in place of milk	cellent for riboflavin, other vitamins, minerals, carbohydrates, fat, and vitamin D, when fortified. Cheese and ice cream supply the same nutrients as milk but in different amounts.
Meat and Meat Substitutes	2 or more servings, including: Meat, poultry, fish, or eggs: 1 or more servings. Dried beans or peas, peanut butter, and nuts as meat substitutes. Count as serving: 2–3 ounces lean cooked meat, poultry, fish (without bone), or 2 eggs or 1 cup cooked beans or peas, etc., or 4 tablespoons peanut butter.	Amount and quality of protein for tissue building: muscle, organs, blood, skin, hair, and other living tissues. Dried beans, peas, and nuts also supply protein but of lower quality than that of meat and milk; also provide iron, thiamine, riboflavin, and niacin
Vegetable-Fruit Group	4 or more servings, including: Fruit or vegetable high in vitamin C: grapefruit, oranges, tomatoes (whole or in juice), raw cabbage, green or red sweet pepper, broccoli, fresh strawberries. 1 serving daily—1/2 cup or portion. Dark green or deep yellow fruit or vegetable high in vitamin A: broccoli, spinach, greens, cantaloup, apricots, carrots, pumpkin, sweet potatoes, winter squash. 1 serving daily—1/2 cup or portion. Other vegetables and fruits, including potatoes. 2 or more servings—1/2 cup or portion	Vitamins and minerals: Vitamin A: normal growth and development in children for normal vision, and for healthy skin condition. Ascorbic acid: essential for healthy gums and body tissues
Breads and Cereals	4 or more servings	Worthwhile amounts of

Types of Foods	*Daily Amounts*	*Special Functions in Daily Diet*
	Whole-grain, enriched, or restored bread and cereals or other grain products such as corn meal, grits, macaroni, spaghetti, and rice	thiamine, iron, niacin, protein, and food energy
	Count as serving: 1 slice bread; 1 ounce ready-to-cook cereal; 1/2–3/4 cup cooked cereal, cornmeal, grits, macaroni, noodles, rice, spaghetti.	
Plus other Foods	More of the above foods and other foods not specified—butter, margarine, other fats, oils, sugars and unenriched refined grain products—to round out meals and satisfy	appetite. "Other foods" may be part of specified foods in mixed dishes, baked goods, desserts, and other recipe dishes which are part of daily meals.

All of the foods listed in the preceding guide are obtainable from the grocery store. "Usually children will get all the vitamins and minerals they need from a good, varied diet and supplements are not necessary. Occasionally, a doctor may prescribe vitamin D in some form, if the child is not getting enough through foods like milk, margarine and cereals which often have vitamin D added to them."[15]

WHAT ARE SPECIAL CONSIDERATIONS IN FEEDING THE 6 TO 12 YEAR OLD?[16]

Appetite. "Within limits, *what* your child eats is generally more important than *how much*. Many youngsters overplay fats and sugars and underplay the other essential foods. So long as your child is healthy and not seriously under or overweight, it is a good idea not to push him to eat more or less than he naturally wants. Since each child has his own natural rate and style of growth, each will require varying amounts of food. However, if he suddenly loses his appetite, you will want to check his physical and emotional health. When a normally enthusiastic eater turns down food, it can be a sign that something ails him."[16]

Overweight. Too much food and too little exercise may cause 6 to 12 year olds to become overweight. Though children need plenty of food for energy and growth, it is easy for them to overeat, so the prevention of excessive weight or the loss of weight may become necessary. In some cases overweight may be due to children being encouraged, even as infants, to eat more than they need. Reducing the amount of between-meal snacks, and cutting down on butter, fried foods, salad dressings, and rich desserts, may help to control obesity. A continuous gain of excessive

---
[15] Ibid., p. 36
[16] Ibid., pp. 36–39, adapted

weight may indicate the desirability of examination and advice by a physician. Emotional problems may cause children to eat too much.

Underweight. Insufficient food, overactivity, lack of sleep, infectious disease, or other factors which affect appetite and total food intake may be responsible for underweight or undernourishment. A physician can determine the cause and advise methods for correcting underweight.

Mealtime conditions. A peaceful tone is important at meal times if appetites are to be keen, food good tasting, and digestion normal. Excitement of any kind is undesirable. Meals are not the time for discussing children's faults and family problems; conversation should be devoted to interesting and pleasant happenings of the day. For many families it is the only time when the whole family is together and should, therefore, be made as pleasant as possible. A table neatly prepared with adequate and good food, no matter how simple, appetizingly served, with grown-ups' table manners and conversation acceptable; meals served on time and adequate time allowed for meals, all contribute to the development of good food habits and pleasing manners for children.

Snacks and treats. "It appears that, unless parents firm up their 'No' power, our children may become a nation of unwise snackers. Not that there's anything wrong with a between-meal pick-up, but there is danger of going overboard on soft drinks and greasy foods that add pounds but not much basic nourishment. Too many sweets, moreover, are likely to damage teeth. One way to cut down on this overspending and overeating is to have snacks available at home—all kinds of fruits, simple cookies, whole grain or enriched breads, milk, cheese, and peanut butter are far better than sweets and fats."[17]

Three hearty meals a day may help to prevent "snacks unlimited." Also a definite allowance for "treats" may encourage a wiser snack choice and a greater appreciation of the "free meals" at home.

Adequate breakfast. Children who skip breakfast are less well fed (it being hard to make up the missed nutrients at other meals), do not do as good work in school as they could, and may be more irritable and emotionally unstable than if they were well fed at breakfast. Lack of time, lack of hunger on arising, dislike of "breakfast foods," and lack of a regular family breakfast time are the usual reasons given for failure to eat breakfast. A little preplanning the night before will help to overcome the time limitations.

"Breakfast menus don't have to follow a set routine. For instance, if your youngster rebels against cereal and eggs, there's nothing wrong with a frankfurter or hamburger along with fruit juice and milk. A peanut butter sandwich, a serving of custard pudding, a glass of milk and an orange in the pocket to eat on the way to school is a pretty good beginning for the day. You don't have to have the usual breakfast foods every day."[17] Milk and vitamin C foods such as oranges or grapefruit are a good idea in the morning meal; if missed then, they should be included at another meal. Breakfast should provide about one-third of the total daily food needs of the child.

Adequate lunch. A well chosen lunch, eaten at home or in school, as a carried lunch or in the cafeteria, is also important for the child's well being. The same pattern may be used for lunch at home and lunch carried to school: a hearty sandwich of meat, egg, cheese, or peanut butter; fruit, a simple cookie, a raw vegetable such as carrot sticks, and milk to drink, carried in a thermos or bought at school.

---

[17] Ibid., p. 38

A SAMPLE DAY'S MEALS FOR A 10 YEAR OLD[18]

Breakfast

Tomato juice (3/4 cup)
Hot whole wheat cereal
  (2/3 cup) with milk
  (1/2 cup)

Toast (2 slices) with butter or
  fortified margarine (2 tsp.)
Milk (1/2 pint)

Lunch
(If served at school or at home)

Creamed eggs (3/4 cup)
Green beans (1/2 cup) with butter
  or fortified margarine (1 tsp.)

Oatmeal muffins (2) with butter or
  fortified margarine (2 tsp.)
Milk (1/2 pint)

(If brought from home)

Sandwich—peanut butter and raw
  carrot on buttered whole grain
  or enriched bread

Sandwich—chopped dried fruit on
  buttered whole grain or enriched bread

Supplemented at school by—

Orange

Milk, soup (1 cup) or cocoa (1 cup)

Dinner

Meat loaf (1 serving)
Scalloped potatoes (2/3 cup)
Cole slaw with red and green
  peppers (1/2 cup)
Milk (1/2 pint)

Whole wheat bread or enriched
  bread (2 slices) with butter or
  fortified margarine (2 tsp)
Applesauce (1/2 cup)
Molasses cookies (2 thin)

WHAT IS THE IMPORTANCE OF ADEQUATE SCHOOL LUNCHES?

Adequate lunches at home, carried, or eaten in the school lunch room are important for the nutritional well-being and general health of school children. The National School Lunch Act of 1946, administered by the Agricultural Marketing Service of the U.S. Department of Agriculture in cooperation with State Education Departments, provides federal assistance and food to schools in furnishing good lunches to school children. In the 25 years since its institution, the School Lunch Program has grown in scope and emphasis. In the program's first year, a total of 6.6 million youngsters took part; in 1971 nearly 25 million were participating. Additional legislation helped expand the program. Among other provisions, the Child Nutrition Act of 1966 launched a pilot breakfast program. The improvement of all child feeding operations and their availability to needy children was provided by 1970 Public Law 91–248 amending the School Lunch and Child Nutrition Acts.[19]

---

[18] *Nutrition and Healthy Growth*, Children's Bureau Publication No. 352. Washington, D. C., Department of Health, Education and Welfare, 1955. p. 24 (out of print).

[19] Remarks of Secretary of Agriculture at 25th anniversary of School Lunch Program, June 7, 1971.

The school lunch program not only provides a way to insure adequate lunches for children, it also indirectly promotes better work in school, helps to establish good eating habits, carries over into the home and community, and helps improve the general level of nutrition in the home and community.

All lunches served in school should be palatable, attractive and suited to the children's needs. Young children should be served plate lunches with suitable combinations of foods. Lunch room food should be arranged on the counter in order of importance of the food in the meal (sweets at end of counter), and should provide a simple choice between nutritional foods.

The minimum standards for the Type A lunch served under the National School Lunch Program are as follows:

1/2 pint fluid whole milk, to drink
Main dish (protein-rich) of
  2 oz. cooked or canned lean meat, fish, or poultry; or
  2 oz. cheese; or
  1 egg; or
  1/2 cup cooked dry beans or peas; or
  4 tablespoons peanut butter; or an equivalent quantity of any combination of these; or
  in main dish, or in main dish and one other menu item.*

3/4 cup total, consisting of 2 or more servings of vegetables, fruits or both. 1 serving of full strength juice—vegetable or fruit—counts as only 1/4 of the requirement.
A vitamin C-rich food daily; a vitamin A-rich food twice weekly.

Whole-grain or enriched bread:
  1 slice; or
  1 serving of muffins, cornbread, biscuits, rolls, etc., made of whole-grain or enriched flour.
Butter or fortified margarine:
  1 teaspoon used in food preparation, seasoning, or as a spread.

A lunch including the amounts of foods above provides about 1/3 of the daily requirement for a child 10 to 12 years old.
Adolescents will require larger servings of the same foods.
The following figure shows the foods in a "Type A" school lunch.

CONFECTIONS AND SOFT DRINKS IN SCHOOLS

The Council on Foods and Nutrition of the American Medical Association has issued the following statement:

"One of the functions of a school lunch program is to provide training in sound food habits. The sale of foods, confections, and beverages in lunchrooms, recreation rooms, and other school facilities influences directly the food habits of the students. Every effort should be extended to encourage students to adopt and enjoy good food habits. The availability of confections and soft drinks on school premises may tempt children to spend lunch money for them and lead to poor food habits. Their high energy value and continual availability are likely to affect children's appetites for regular meals. Expenditures for soft drinks and most confections yield a nutritional

---

* By U.S.D.A. specifications, textured protein products (engineered foods) may be served in certain of its feeding programs for children over 12 years, applied to the 2 ounce meat or meat alternate requirements.

return greatly inferior to that from milk, fruit, and other foods included in the basic food groups. When given a choice between soft drinks and milk or between candy and fruit, a child may choose the less nutritious. In view of these considerations, the Council on Foods and Nutrition is particularly opposed to the sale and distribution of confections and soft drinks in school lunchrooms."[20]

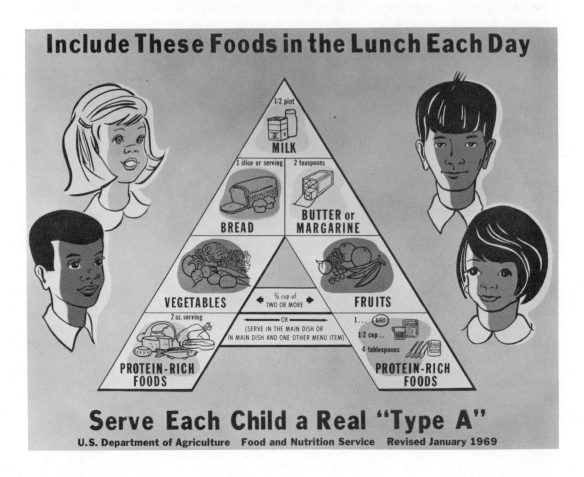

Vending Machines.   Self-service vending machines in schools which supply more of the popular, profit-making, snack-type food items (most of them providing calories only or little more) and a limited supply of nutritious foods often lead to undesirable food habits in schoolchildren. Some direction is needed to help children make desirable choices and, in some instances, to encourage a wider selection of nutritious items in the vending machines. Most desirable would be some control by schools as to what items are to be offered for sale in vending machines. Profit-making competitive food sales in schools are prohibited by School Lunch Act amendments.

Other programs, in addition to the School Lunch Program, operated through federal, state, and local governments with local activation by public officials, private organizations, and volunteer citizens to insure adequate nutrition in children include the Special Milk Program, School Breakfast Program, and the Special Food Service Program for children in day-care centers, summer camps, and summer recreation centers.

---

[20] *Journal of the American Medical Association,* vol. 180, p. 92, June 30, 1962

WHAT ARE NUTRITIONAL REQUIREMENTS OF ADOLESCENCE?

"Adolescence is a period of rapid growth and of maturation, which may occur between the ages of 10 and 20 years. On the average, girls reach this stage of development about 2 years earlier than boys. There is evidence that good nutrition, which promotes growth during childhood, is related to maturing early. At the same time that the adolescent has accelerated nutritional needs, there are many psychological and social and emotional pressures. At this age any deviation from the average in state of development may be upsetting.

"During the growth spurt the formation of muscles, of bone, and blood requires ample supplies of building materials: protein, calcium, iron. A slight rise in the basal metabolism and the constant activities of adolescents are responsible for greater food consumption than in earlier and later periods of life. Most teenagers are forever hungry.

"The 1965 Nationwide Household Food Consumption Survey showed adolescent girls (and women) represented one of the three groups of our population in need of improved diets. Past studies have shown that the percentage of young people with poor diets is likely to increase from childhood to teenage. The teenage girl is likely to be the most poorly fed member of the family. The situation is more critical than the boy's. This is partly because boys consume more food than girls so have a better chance of getting needed nutrients."[21]

Calcium, vitamin A, ascorbic acid, and in the case of girls iron are apt to be lacking in teen age diets. Some reasons include: skipping meals, especially breakfast, fad diets followed to control weight, snack eating between meals, largely of foods high in "empty calories" and low in protein, minerals, and vitamins, which make it more difficult to get the daily recommended amounts of important nutrients. Indifferent attitudes toward food also account for poor teenage food habits.

Consult Table of RDA, page 26, to compare nutritional needs of teenage boys and girls with those of their parents.

"Food habits of adolescents are the manifestations of many influences and conditions, including such factors as family eating practices, emotional environment, socioeconomic circumstances, education, and personal adjustment. Family relationships are the primary influence on eating patterns and attitudes toward food"[22]

WHAT FOODS WILL PROTECT "TEENS" IN KEY NUTRIENTS?

Daily Recommended Servings from Various Food Groups[23]

Food Group	Girls	Boys
Milk Group: Milk, Cheese, Ice Cream	At least 4 cups daily	4 or more glasses daily
Meat Group: Meat, poultry, fish, eggs or cheese, and alternates	At least 2 servings daily	2 or more servings daily

[21] *Food for Us All,* U. S. D. A. Yearbook, 1969, Washington, D. C., U. S. Department of Agriculture, pages 299, 319–320, adapted.

[22] *Factors Affecting Adolescent Food Habits,* Dairy Council Digest, vol. 36, No. 1 (Jan.—Feb.), 1965, p. 1.

[23] Adapted from: R. M. Leverton, *A Girl and Her Figure.* Chicago, National Dairy Council, 1970, pp. 7, 13. W. H. Gregg, *A Boy and His Physique.* Chicago, National Dairy Council, 1970, pp. 13, 14.

Daily Recommended Servings from Various Food Groups[23] (Cont.)

| Vegetable–Fruit Group | At least 4 servings daily | 4 or more servings daily |
| Bread–Cereals Group | At least 4 servings daily | 4 or more servings daily |

Other Foods: To round out meals and meet energy needs, almost everyone will use some foods not specified in the Four Food Groups. Sugars and unenriched, refined breads, cereals and flours are among them. Butter or other animal fats or vegetable fats and oils also belong in this category. These are the foods that are often ingredients in a recipe or added to other foods during preparation or at table. Try to use a variety of every kind of food.

WHAT CALORIE GUIDES CAN "TEENS" USE TO LEARN ENERGY NEEDS?[23]

Most girls of the same age and activity need about the same number of calories per pound of body weight per day; the same is true of boys even though no two boys are apt to grow exactly alike nor to exercise alike. To calculate how much energy you need in terms of calories, multiply the pounds you weigh by the calories you need per pound for your age (see table below). More active girls will need a few more calories per pound; less active girls a few less per pound—about 10 percent more or less than the averages on the calorie guides. For boys, about 10 percent more calories are required for a very active program such as competitive sport with daily practice and contests every week.

	Girls				*Boys*		
Age	10–12	12–14	14–16	16–18	9–12	12–15	15–18
Suggested calories/lb./day	29	24	21	19	33	31	25
For	Average-size girls of above ages who keep fairly active				Boys of above ages—average size and activity		
Average height	56 in.	61 in.	62 in.	63 in.	55 in.	61 in.	68 in.
Average weight	77 lb.	97 lb.	114 lb.	119 lb.	72 lb.	98 lb.	134 lb.
Total per day (approx.)	2250 Cal.	2300 Cal.	2400 Cal.	2300 Cal.	2400 Cal.	3000 Cal.	3400 Cal.

WHAT IS A FOUNDATION FOOD GUIDE FOR THE ADOLESCENT?[24]

The following Foundation Food Guide describes the kinds and amounts of foods to eat every day to give you the nutrients you need without using up your calorie allowance. You can have free choice in everything else you need until you have spent your total calorie allowance.

---

[24] Adapted from: R. M. Leverton, *A Girl and Her Figure*. Chicago, National Dairy Council, 1970, p. 14. W. H. Gregg, *A Boy and His Physique*. Chicago, National Dairy Council, 1970, p. 15.

Do not eat less than the amounts of foods listed every day. This guide is not a complete daily menu. It is an assortment of foods that will supply the major part of your needs for good nutrition. To this you will need to add other foods to round out your meals or to use as snacks and to satisfy your calorie need. The servings listed will supply between 1400 and 1800 calories for girls and 1600 to 2200 calories for boys (about 1/2 to 4/5 of the daily calorie allowance), depending upon the particular kinds of foods you choose.

Foods to complete daily meals and for snacks can be chosen from the Four Food Groups (they carry a wealth of nutrients) and from additional foods which frequently supply mostly calories. "Choose your calories by the company they keep."

*FOUNDATION FOOD GUIDE AND HOW IT WORKS**

Meal	Food Group	No. Servings Girls and Boys	Additional Foods for Boys	Examples of Kinds of Foods
Breakfast	Vegetables–Fruit A good source of vitamin C	1 serving		Orange juice
	Bread–Cereals	1 serving		Ready-to-eat cereals or toast
	Milk	1 serving		Milk, 1 cup ($\frac{1}{2}$ pint)
			1 serving—egg breakfast meat or other meat alternate	1 egg, 2 slices bacon, or 2 oz. other meat
Lunch or Supper	Meat	1 serving		Hamburger, hot dog, or luncheon meat
	Bread–Cereals	2 servings		Bun, buttered
	Vegetables–Fruit	1 serving		Cabbage slaw, apple, or French fries
	Milk	1 serving		Milk, 1 cup ($\frac{1}{2}$ pint or 8 oz.)
	Meat		1 serving dessert	Fruit, pudding, or ice cream; sometimes pie, cake, cookies
Dinner	Meat	1 serving		Roast beef
	Vegetable–Fruit	1 serving		Carrots–raw or cooked
	Other	1 serving		Potato, vegetable, or fruit salad
	Bread–Cereals	1 serving		Roll, buttered
	Milk	1 serving		Milk, 1 cup ($\frac{1}{2}$ pint)
			1 serving dessert	Fruit pudding, ice cream; sometimes higher calorie desserts to fit your calorie allowance and family meals.

* During the day use an additional cup of milk to drink, in milk shakes or ice cream, or in cheese or cooked. Use some butter or other animal or vegetable fats.

STUDY QUESTIONS AND ACTIVITIES

1. What do the terms "growth" and "development" mean to you?

2. List all the reasons why a good breakfast is important from early childhood throughout life.

3. Why is an adequate lunch important for everyone?

4. What suggestions can you give a mother who finds it difficult to get her young child to eat new and different foods? Who finds it difficult to get her children to eat adequate breakfasts?

5. Why might it be serious to skip breakfast repeatedly over a period of time?

6. Plan three different adequate lunches for a child to carry to school.

7. Write a short article on the importance of good nutrition for teenagers.

8. What effects later in life might be expected from foods inadequate in quantity and quality during the growing period?

SUGGESTED ACTIVITIES

1. Class observes serving of meal to preschoolers in a local nursery school.

2. Class observes food service in a school cafeteria, notes the menu for the Type A lunch and, if possible, several carried lunches and lunches chosen from the cafeteria menu. Are soft drinks, candies, and other sweets sold in the cafeteria? Are there vending machines in the school building? What foods or products are offered for sale?

SUPPLEMENTARY READING

Bogert: Chapter 22.   Mowry: Pages 66–67.   Robinson: Pages 138–143
Howe: Pages 149–151   Peyton: Chapter 14.

R. M. Leverton, *Food Becomes You.* 3rd edition, Ames, Iowa, Iowa State University Press, 1965, Chapters 13–14.

Your Child from 1 to 6, Children's Bureau Publication No. 30, Washington, D. C., U. S. Department of Health, Education and Welfare, 1962 (slight revision 1967).

Food Before Six, National Dairy Council, Chicago, 1969

Your Child from 6 to 12, Children's Bureau Publication No. 324, Washington, D. C., U. S. Department of Health, Education and Welfare, 1966.

Can Food Make the Difference?, American Medical Association, Chicago, 1964.

Food Choices: the Teen-Age Girl, New York, The Nutrition Foundation, 1966.

Your Food—Chance or Choice?, Chicago, National Dairy Council, 1967.

Give Yourself a Break, Teenage Leaflet. Chicago, American Dietetic Association.

Can Food Make the Difference? Chicago, American Medical Association, 1964

R.M. Leverton, *A Girl and her Figure.* Chicago, National Dairy Council, 1970

W.H. Gregg, *A Boy and his Physique.* Chicago, National Dairy Council, 1970.

PART 4. GERIATRIC NUTRITION[25]

WHAT IS MEANT BY GERONTOLOGY AND GERIATRICS?

Gerontology is the scientific study of the various aspects of aging and its problems (including social problems), with special emphasis on health in the later years. Geriatrics, a comparatively recent phase of the medical sciences, is concerned with the prevention and treatment of diseases in aging persons.

Scientific advances in the field of medicine and health have increased life expectancy in the United States from the 1850 average of 40 years to today's average of 70 years. In our population, about 20 million persons (over 11 million of them women, mainly widows and many living alone) are over 65 years of age, the mandatory retirement age for many, regardless of their physical health and remaining abilities.[26] Most of the men are married, with about 90 per cent living as heads of households. Since these added years extend the so-called "prime of life" or useful years, the maintenance of health and vigor for this group becomes an important consideration in any health and nutrition program—the aim of geriatric nutrition being to conserve health and delay the onset of chronic degenerative disease. "Longer life is both a major achievement and a major challenge of our time."

Our society is assuming greater responsibility for its older citizens. A Task Force on Problems of Aging was appointed in 1969 to assist with ideas and recommendations. By Presidential proclamation, a White House Conference on Aging was held in late 1971. Beginning with the Older Americans Act of 1965, which established the Administration on Aging in the U. S. Department of Health, Education and Welfare (supports research and programs for improving nutrition of older persons), legislation has been passed to benefit the aging.[27]

WHY IS GOOD NUTRITION IMPORTANT?[28]

Aging is a normal but continuous process from birth (or even before) to death. It progresses at various rates, being more rapid during the growing years and less in later years. The changes in appearance, mental outlook, and body functions that occur as one passes from youth into middle age and then into older age are well recognized by most persons. Less obvious than these outer changes are those which occur in the body and its workings as one grows older.

Long life is commonplace but many older persons are not as healthy and happy as they might be if they made a strong ally of food, letting it help in every possible way. Being badly nourished is often responsible for complaints that prevent the

---

[25] The material in this Part is largely adapted from *Food Guide for Older Folks,* Home and Garden Bulletin no. 17. Washington, D. C., U. S. Department of Agriculture, 1969, and *Helping Older Persons Meet Their Nutritional Needs,* I. H. Wolgamot, Washington, D. C., Nutrition Program News, U. S. D. A., January–February, 1970.

[26] I. H. Wolgamot, *Helping Older Persons Meet Their Nutritional Needs,* Washington, D. C. Nutrition Program News, January–February, 1970.

[27] Ibid.

[28] Ibid. and *Food,* U. S. D. A. Yearbook 1959, p. 311.

feeling of well-being. The right food helps the body to be at its best and, in the event of illness, a well-nourished body responds better to treatment than one in a run-down condition.

"Good nutrition plays an important role in the health of older persons. Problems of health and nutrition may be related to other aspects of their living—housing, clothing, transportation and recreation. They are influenced by income and social situations—family ties, social relations with friends and neighbors, and community involvement."

Nutrition is one of the factors affecting the rate of aging. Premature aging is believed to be related to poor nutrition. Along with other desirable health practices, good nutrition may even help to delay the progress of aging. "Many persons who work with the elderly are convinced that a better diet brings about marked improvement in both physical and mental health." Adverse changes in aging may be caused by impaired nutrition preventing the body cells from performing their functions rather than by the process of aging as such.

HOW WELL DO OLDER PERSONS EAT?[29]

The last U. S. D. A. Nationwide Food Consumption Study (1965) showed that older persons in families had poorer diets than the younger family members and that the women's diets were not as good as those of the men. The diets of women 65 years and over averaged more than 30 per cent below recommended allowances for calcium and were below amounts recommended for thiamin, riboflavin, iron and vitamin A value. The diets of men 75 years and over averaged 24 per cent below recommended allowances for calcium, 16 per cent below those for riboflavin, and about 10 per cent below those for vitamin A and ascorbic acid values. The women used the equivalent of less than one cup of milk daily and the men used slightly more.

A survey in Iowa of women's diets found that as these women grew older, the amount of protein and calcium in their diets decreased along with energy value; ascorbic acid and vitamin A values also declined. The food groups most neglected were the milk and meat groups. Although sufficient amounts of fruits and vegetables were chosen, the selection did not include enough of those high in ascorbic acid and vitamin A. Survey findings suggested that diets would be improved by replacing some of the sweets and fatty foods with those higher in needed nutrients.

Poor food habits carried over from earlier years and illness are responsible for poor nutritional states of older persons. They may be a contributing factor in the high incidence of chronic disease in the aging. Low incomes coupled with high living costs may result in inadequate diets. Indifference or lack of knowledge in choosing an adequate diet, waste of money on food fads and special, unneeded, diet products, lack of proper food preparation facilities which leads to "snacks" rather than regular meals, and loneliness and alienation are other causes of inadequate diets.

WHAT ARE NUTRITIONAL REQUIREMENTS?

A diet adequate in all the essential nutrients but slightly decreased in calories is the basis for good nutrition in later years. Reduction of 10 to 15 per cent in total calories is called for due to gradual reduction in the basal metabolic rate as well as lessened activity. RDA for calories decline in the "reference" man from 2800 at age

---

[29] Ibid.

22 to 2400 at age 65; for the "reference" woman, from 2000 at age 22 to 1700 at age 65. Weight should be maintained as near as possible to the ideal figure.

Requirement for protein remains the same—1 gram per kilogram of body weight or 65 gm. for men and 55 gm. for women—and should be met largely through the use of milk, eggs, cheese, fish, and meat. Illness and prolonged diet inadequacy raise requirements.

Larger amounts of foods high in minerals and vitamins are desirable. Liver should be served frequently to prevent anemia in the older person; generous amounts of fruits and vegetables high in vitamin A and ascorbic acid.

Requirement for calcium may be greater—milk and milk products are important in the diet.

The increasing prevalence of osteoporosis with aging may be due to a long-term diet low in calcium.

WHAT DAILY FOOD GUIDE WILL HELP THE OLDER PERSON SELECT THE RIGHT KINDS OF FOOD?

The following food guide,[30] which is the same as that for the young adult, will help the older person select the right kinds of food whether he or she eats at home or out. All the kinds of foods that make up well-balanced meals will be included by following this guide. Foods within a group are similar enough to replace one another and to give ample choice for variety. The minimum number of servings in each group should be included.

Daily Food Guide

Milk, cheese, ice cream
    Fresh fluid—whole or skim
    Evaporated; dry
    Buttermilk; or in cheese and ice
      cream
	2 or more cups of their equivalent daily.

Meat, poultry, fish; eggs; dry beans and peas; nuts (2 or more servings from these groups daily)	1 serving of any kind of meat, poultry or fish every day. Include heart, liver, and other variety meats. 4 or more eggs every week. 1 serving of dry beans and peas, nuts, occasionally as alternate for meat, fish, poultry, or eggs.
Grain products (baked products and bread; cereals to cook; ready-to-eat cereals; rice, grits, noodles, etc.)	4 or more servings daily of whole-grain, enriched, or restored products.

Vegetables and fruits	At least 4 servings vegetables and fruits daily.
	    (at least 1 serving daily of citrus fruits, tomatoes)
	    (a serving at least every other day of dark green or deep yellow vegetables)

---

[30] *Food Guide for Older Folks*. Home and Garden Bulletin No. 17, Washington, D. C., U. S. Department of Agriculture, 1969.

Daily Food Guide

	Potatoes every day, if desired
	1 to 3, or more, servings other fruits and vegetables.
Fats and oils	Use some butter or fortified margarine every day.
	Use fats sparingly in cooking.
Sugars and sweets	Use sparingly to add flavor to meals and for cooking.

WHAT FOOD PLANS CAN HELP IN PLANNING FOR ADEQUATE NUTRITION?

"One of the three food plans below[31] can serve as a shopping guide as it stands.

"Amounts in each food group are for a man and woman of about 60 years of age—somewhat less active than in younger years. For those regularly working or exercising in strenuous fashion, the quantities need to be stepped up to take care of extra energy needs. Potatoes, bread, and cereals will provide the extra calories and additional nutrients at low cost.

"Any one of the plans will provide for nutritional needs. The main difference is that meals will be less varied with the low-cost plan. The moderate-cost and liberal plans provide larger amounts of meat, eggs, fruits, and vegetables. Also more expensive items within the groups, such as foods out of season and more highly processed foods, can be used. Regardless of whether more or less is spent for food, the

THREE FOOD PLANS—low-cost, moderate-cost, and liberal
(Quantities for a couple for a week)

KIND OF FOOD	LOW-COST PLAN		MODERATE-COST		LIBERAL PLAN	
	MAN	WOMAN	MAN	WOMAN	MAN	WOMAN
Milk, cheese, ice cream (milk equivalent)	3½ qt.	3½ qt.	3½ qt.	3½ qt.	4 qt.	4 qt.
Meat, poultry, fish	3¼ lb.	2½ lb.	5 lb.	4¼ lb.	5¼ lb.	4¾ lb.
Eggs	6	5	7	6	7	6
Dry beans and peas, nuts	4 oz.	4 oz.	2 oz.	2 oz.	2 oz.	1 oz.
Grain products—whole-grain, enriched, or restored (flour equivalent)	3½ lb.	2¼ lb.	3¼ lb.	1¾ lb.	3¼ lb.	1½ lb.
Citrus fruits, tomatoes	2¼ lb.	2 lb.	2¾ lb.	2¼ lb.	3 lb.	3 lb.
Dark-green and deep-yellow vegetables	¾ lb.	¾ lb.	¾ lb.	¾ lb.	¾ lb.	¾ lb.
Potatoes	2½ lb.	1¼ lb.	2¼ lb.	1¼ lb.	2 lb.	1 lb.
Other vegetables and fruits	4¾ lb.	3½ lb.	5½ lb.	4¼ lb.	6 lb.	4½ lb.
Fats and oils	⅔ lb.	¼ lb.	¾ lb.	⅜ lb.	¾ lb.	⅜ lb.
Sugars, sweets	⅔ lb.	⅜ lb.	⅞ lb.	½ lb.	1⅛ lb.	¾ lb.

Count 1 lb. bread or other baked goods as ⅔ lb. flour or cereal.

If choices within the group are such that the amounts specified are not sufficient to provide the suggested number of servings, increase the amounts and use less from the "other vegetables and fruits" group.

---

[31] Ibid.

quantities suggested for milk and milk products, dark-green and deep yellow vegetables, and tomatoes and citrus fruits should not be changed very much."[32]

Sample menus for a week are shown below. The same food might be divided into four or five meals. See Table on page 122 for weekly cost of food plans for men and women 55 to 70 and older.

Sample Menus for a Week

Butter or margarine would be served with these meals, a glass of milk at least once a day, tea or coffee as desired

SUNDAY	MONDAY	TUESDAY	WEDNESDAY	THURSDAY	FRIDAY	SATURDAY
Orange juice Scrambled egg Toast	Orange juice Oatmeal Milk Toast	Prunes French toast Sirup	Orange slices Soft-cooked egg Toasted rolls	Prunes Ready-to-eat cereal Milk Peanut butter biscuits	Tomato juice Milk toast Jelly	Orange juice Oatmeal Milk Toasted corn muffins
Swiss steak Mashed potatoes Broccoli Bread Chocolate pudding	Frankfurters stuffed with mashed potatoes and cheese Scalloped tomatoes Hot rolls Apple brown betty	Lamb stew Beets Tossed green salad Bread Rice and raisin pudding	Meat loaf Scalloped potatoes Steamed cabbage Peanut butter biscuits Fruit in season	Cream of tomato soup Egg salad-shredded lettuce sandwich Gingerbread	Creamed egg and mushrooms on noodles Cabbage, carrot, raisin salad	Braised liver Potatoes boiled in jackets Green peas Grated carrot salad Bread Orange-milk sherbet
Welsh rarebit Crisp bacon strip Apple-raisin salad Ice cream Cookies	Lamb stew with potatoes Snap beans Bread Chocolate pudding	Spaghetti, tomato, chopped meat casserole Broccoli Bread Grapefruit segments	Cheese fondue Snap beans Bread Peaches Gingerbread	Meat loaf— tomato sauce Creamed potatoes Spinach Bread Tapioca pudding	Baked fish Baked potato slices Green peas Corn muffins Tapioca pudding	Vegetable-bean soup Toasted cheese sandwich Fruit in season

WHAT ARE SPECIAL FOOD PROBLEMS WITH OLDER FOLKS?

The following may prove to be special problems for an oldster planning his food:

Cooking for only two— or one
Limited cooking equipment
Eating out
Living with others

Need to watch weight
Lack of appetite
Easy-to-chew foods
Living and eating alone

"Indigestion"
Constipation
Chronic disorders
"Special" diets
Coping with food fads

CLASS ACTIVITIES

1. The problems noted above are discussed in *Food Guide for Older Folks* (Home and Garden Bulletin No. 17. Washington, D.C., U.S. Department of Agriculture, 1959). Each of the problems may be assigned to one or two students to review and present as a report to the class, to focus their attention on food problems of oldsters.

2. Class will observe facilities and meal service in a local home for elderly people, if possible. If a "Meals on wheels" project is being carried on locally, students might also observe this food service to oldsters.

---

[32] *Food Guide for Older Folks,* Home and Garden Bulletin No. 17. Washington, D. C., U. S. Department of Agriculture, p. 6.

SUPPLEMENTARY READING

Bogert: Chapter 23   Mowry: pages 71–73   Robinson: Pages 123–126
Howe: Pages 151–152   Peyton: Chapter 15

Lower Cost Meals That Please—in Senior Years. Chicago, National Dairy Council, 1965.
Eating is Fun for Older People, Too. Chicago, American Dietetic Association, 1961.
Food Guide for Older Folks. Home and Garden Bulletin No. 17, Washington, D. C., U. S. Department of Agriculture, 1969.
Your Retirement Food Guide, California, American Association of Retired Persons, 1970.
Food Hints for Mature People. C. G. Kind and G. Britt, New York, New York, Public Affairs Pamphlet No. 336, 1962.
Better Health in Later Years, New York, Public Affairs Pamphlet No. 446, 1970.
Cooking for One, Ithaca, New-York, Cornell Miscellaneous Bulletin 93, New York State College of Human Ecology, Cornell University, 1968.

Unit Five

PUBLIC HEALTH AND COMMUNITY NUTRITION

Object

To acquaint the practical nurse with aspects of public health as they are related to food and nutrition, nutrition education programs of public health organizations, and community nutrition programs for the improvement of nutrition and health.

The right kinds and amounts of food in the daily diet for optimal health have been discussed in the previous units. The care with which these foods are handled from production through preservation, refrigeration, storage, distribution, and handling in the market and in the home will determine the final nutritive value and safety of these foods when they appear on the table. At many points along the line government agencies help to safeguard the food supply; at other points, the responsibility lies with the individual handling the food.

HOW IS FOOD RELATED TO PUBLIC HEALTH?

"The matters which concern the health of the community and require cooperative effort, such as water supply, food inspection [sanitation and safety], and the control of epidemics, are generally regarded as appertaining to the questions of public health. Three goals of public health are: (1) the prevention of disease, (2) the development of healthy bodies and minds, and (3) extension of longevity."[1]

Public health as it is related to food is concerned with bacterial food poisoning, food and water-borne and utensil-borne infections, food poisons of natural origin, pesticides, and radioactive foods, food sanitation and safety in food handling and processing in the home, public eating places, and the processing establishments; food spoilage; food for survival under atomic or hydrogen bomb attack; food preservation; food quality control; food laws; food additives; or, in short, safeguarding the food supply and protection of public health.

The United States Public Health Service, which is the principal health agency of the federal government, concerns itself with all factors affecting the health of people, including nutrition. Other agencies at the national level—official, voluntary, professional, and industry-sponsored—and agencies of the same type at state and local levels are also concerned with factors affecting health and nutrition.

---

[1] M. V. Krause, *Food, Nutrition, and Diet Therapy*, 4th edition, Philadelphia, W. B. Saunders Company, 1966, p. 168.

HOW IS THE CONSUMER PROTECTED IN BUYING FOODS?[2]

Federal, state, and municipal laws and regulations protect the consumer's right to buy safe, wholesome food, to be adequately informed about what she is buying and to safeguard her health and pocketbook. "Foods that pass across state lines in commercial trade are under the jurisdiction of such federal agencies as the U. S. Department of Agriculture and the Food and Drug Administration, U. S. Department of Health, Education and Welfare. Foods produced and sold within a state are under the jurisdiction of the State Department of Agriculture and Markets. Food protection services are cooperative efforts of the city, state and federal governments."

"All foods are subject to mandatory inspection for adulteration, sanitary quality and wholesomeness in all establishments where food is prepared, manufactured, processed, stored or sold—eating places, bakeries, dairies, canning, freezing and other processing plants, slaughtering plants, beverage plants, stores and markets, and vending machine operations. Some voluntary federal–state inspection services are also provided for some foods and many producers and processors use this service. Dependable and uniform quality is assured by the grading of foods, mandatory for some and on a voluntary basis for others. Federal and state laws require that labels on foods and food advertisements must not be false or misleading in any manner and that foods must measure up to the label information; also, that no harmful or dangerous substance be added to food."[2]

The following table indicates some federal and other laws and regulations which safeguard food supply and health and nutrition.

Law or Regulation	*Provision*
Federal, Food, Drug and Cosmetic Act of 1938 ("Pure Food and Drug Law") and amendments enforced by Food and Drug Administration	Safe, effective drugs and cosmetics; pure (unadulterated), wholesome foods; honest labeling and packaging (no misbranding).
1954 Pesticides Amendment	Safe limits for chemical residues on fresh fruits and vegetables.
1958 Food Additives Amendment	Safe limits for intentional and accidental food additives.
1960 Color Additives Amendment	Approves all colors used in foods and safe limits of permitted colors.
1967 Fair Packaging and Labeling Act	More complete provisions and prominent labeling information to help shopper with best buys.
Federal Meat Inspection Act of 1906, enforced by Meat Inspection Service, U. S. D. A. (See inspection stamp, page 105.)	Regulations regarding all meat and meat products shipped across state lines and imported meat and products for wholesomeness.
Federal Wholesome Meat Act of 1967	Inspection equal to federal for plants selling meat solely in the state.
Poultry Products Inspection Act of 1957	Similar to Meat Inspection Act regarding poultry inspection for all poultry crossing state lines.
1968 Amendment—Wholesome Poultry Products Act	Inspection equal to federal for all poultry regardless of movement only in or across state lines.

---

[2] *Food in the Light of the Law.* Gail Harrison, Consumer Education Leaflet 16, New York State Colleges of Human Ecology and Agriculture and Life Sciences, Cornell University, 1968, adapted.

Law or Regulation	Provision
1970 Amendment	Tighter controls on moisture picked up during poultry processing.
Food Standards—adopted by F. and D. A.	Definitions of food content and quality for 200 basic foods for (1) identity (2) quality (3) fill of container (4) enrichments.
Grade standards for processed foods, adopted by U. S. D. A. Marketing Service. Some industries and producers as well as federal and state agencies have established grades based on above food standards.	Foods in interstate commerce failing to meet standards (above) must be labeled "below standard" or "substandard."
Advertising of foods, drugs, cosmetics, enforced by Federal Trade Commission.	Controls false, misleading information on package labels.
Nutritional labeling of foods with therapeutic claims	Current work in progress on such foods as special diet foods, diet supplements, etc., with baby foods, frozen foods and foods generally eaten by low-income groups on priority list.

HOW IS NUTRITION RELATED TO PUBLIC HEALTH?

Food sanitation and safety and disease control have always been the responsibility of health departments—national, state, and local. With the growth of the science of food technology and the science of nutrition and the more effective use of our better knowledge in preventive medicine, nutrition and nutrition education have become the added responsibility of health departments and other agencies interested in the health of people.

Although deficiency diseases are either eliminated or better controlled in our country by improved agricultural procedures, improved economic conditions, enrichment programs and increased attention to nutrition needs, nutrition education continues a never-ending process both to maintain what is good and to improve where needed, to promote a longer healthier life by the application of the principles of good nutrition.

The health and well-being of infants and their mothers were probably the first angles of nutrition to be included in public health and nutrition programs. Prenatal and well-baby clinics were established to help improve the health of these two groups and to provide continuing education for them.

Nutrition services have expanded over the years to give attention to health and nutrition needs of various age groups in the United States and other types of groups in the total population—schoolchildren, teenagers, senior citizens, industrial workers, and special population groups throughout the country. Also increased attention is given to persons living in situations where group feeding is involved—orphanages, nursery and other schools, homes for the handicapped, nursing homes, homes for the aged, summer camps, public institutions, and the like.

Some types of the many agencies and organizations which include nutrition services in their programs are shown on the following page.

Governmental

National Level	State and Local Levels
U. S. Department of Agriculture	Departments of Agriculture
Agricultural Research Service	State extension services
Interagency Committee on Nutrition Education	State experiment stations
Food and Nutrition Service	State universities
National School Lunch Program	Departments of Welfare
Special milk Program	Departments of Health
Consumer and Marketing Service	Department of Education
Extension Service	

U. S. Department of Health, Education and Welfare
  Children's Bureau
  Food and Drug Administration
  Office of Education
  Public Health Service
    Bureaus of Various Health Services
    National Institutes of Health

Non-Governmental

National Level

American Medical Association
  Council on Foods
National Academy of Sciences, National Research Council, Food and Nutrition Board
American Red Cross
Professional Organizations
  American Medical Association
  American Dietetic Association
  American Home Economics Association
  American Dental Association
  American Public Health Association
  American Heart Association
  American Nurses' Association
  American Institute of Nutrition
Funds and Foundations
  Milbank Memorial Fund
  Nutrition Foundation
  Ford and Rockefeller Foundations
Metropolitan Life Insurance Company

National Level

Industry-sponsored
  American Dry Milk Institute
  National Dairy Council
  Cereal Institute
  National Livestock and Meat Board

State and Local Levels

Educational agencies
Social agencies
Civic groups
United Community Services
Industry sponsored
American Red Cross
Infant Welfare Organizations
Church groups

International

See page 19.

WHAT ARE THE AIMS OF COMMUNITY NUTRITION PROGRAMS?

"Nutritional problems are to be found in all age and socioeconomic groups but the most vulnerable groups include children and mothers, low-income groups, children and other groups living in various types of institutions where group feeding is provided, persons with chronic illnesses and individuals handicapped in one or more ways. Many problems are best solved by group action, whether at the community or state level. The term 'community' is used here to designate any group of people, large or small; it might be a relatively homogeneous and small group . . . or it might refer to a people of a given geographic area with divergent cultural patterns.

"Nutrition is an integral part of many community services in health and welfare. The opportunities for nutritionists, dietitians and home economists and for subprofessional personnel in these areas are unlimited in public and voluntary agencies of health, welfare and education. A cooperative extensive survey by all community agencies concerned regarding all facets of the nutrition problem—age groupings, income level, health facilities, working mothers, food consumption with correlation of nutrient intakes with nutritional status—is needed to determine special needs and types of programs."[3]

"Community programs of nutrition seek to improve nutrition through research, education, improvement of food supply and feeding. The individual reaps the reward through legislation such as protects the food supply; methods for preserving the food supply; the development of new and better foods through food technology; research concerning the preventive and therapeutic aspects with respect to disease; education concerning an adequate diet. Many community programs at the local and county level also provide direct services, such as those given by a public health nurse, a visiting dietitian, a homemaker from a social agency, or a volunteer who delivers meals to an aged person. The several members of the health team also provide direct services under coordinated home-care programs."[4]

WHAT ARE THE TYPES OF COMMUNITY NUTRITION PROGRAMS[5]

Nutrition Division of State Department of Health. Representative activities (1) provide materials on nutrition information; (2) provide consultant services to institutions with group feeding; (3) work with schools of all types and at all levels; (4) cooperate with health groups in rehabilitation and chronic disease programs; (5) work with patients (through clinics and nurses); (6) work with other groups such as social and welfare agencies; (6) assist in programs of research in universities, departments of health, federal, and private agencies.

Nutritional Services to Families. (1) *Adult Education*—nutrition education in a nutrition clinic, in home, one's place of work, day care centers for older people, maternal and child health centers, home economics extension centers, hospital

[3] C. H. Robinson, *Fundamentals of Normal Nutrition*. New York, The Macmillan Company, 1968, pp. 481–482.

[4] Ibid, p. 487.

[5] C. H. Robinson, *Fundamentals of Normal Nutrition*. New York, The Macmillan Company, 1968, pp. 473–474; 485–487; 491; 493–495; 496–497, adapted. Courtesy of publisher and author.

nutrition clinics, public high school evening programs. (2) *"Dial-a-Dietitian"* program of telephone answering service for persons with food and nutrition questions (initiated by Detroit Dietetic Association and adopted by 16 or more regional associations). (3) *Project Head Start* (an Office of Economic Opportunity program), includes feeding of children and nutrition education for them and mothers. Especially for low-income families are nutritional services included in (1) *Program Aides Services* by trained non-professional home economics aides in a joint federal and state extension program, (2) *Food Stamp Program* with available simplified leaflets showing how to improve low-cost foods.

Nutritional Services to Patients. (1) *Homemaker Services* sponsored by public or voluntary health and welfare agencies; (2) *training* in food preparation, feeding, and kitchen adaptation for *"Handicapped Individuals"* in home or rehabilitation center; (3) "home-delivered" meals—*Meals-on-Wheels*—providing two daily meals to older citizens living alone and sponsored by various community organizations under guidance of trained home economists.

Legislation Related to Nutrition Programs. "The major programs in public health, including nutrition, are authorized and financed through laws enacted by Congress and the state legislatures. Of great social significance and of major assistance toward better health care and nutrition are: '(1) *Medicare* provided by 1965 amendments to Social Security Act (2) *Maternal and Child Health Welfare* provided by 1935 Social Security Act and 1963 and 1965 amendments (3) *Commodity Distribution*—laws providing donations and food stocks to various feeding programs and (4) *Child Nutrition Act of 1966.*' "

WHAT IS THE IMPORTANCE OF THE SCHOOL LUNCH PROGRAM IN COMMUNITY NUTRITION EDUCATION?

The school lunch furnishes a large share of the child's daily nutrition needs if eaten regularly and completely. It is supplemented by the home diet. In addition to being an important factor in improving nutrition of children and their performance in school, it provides an educational experience for forming good habits and can have far-reaching effects on nutrition in the family and community.

In 1946 the United States Congress passed the National School Lunch Act which provided, on a permanent basis, federal aid to state and community lunch programs in the form of financial assistance by cash reimbursement (matched in amount with funds from state sources), and also foods suitable for the school lunch program purchased and distributed by the U. S. Department of Agriculture. A local sponsor or sponsoring agency is required for a school operating under this act and lunches must meet certain nutritional standards. Operation on a non-profit basis and availability of lunches to all children regardless of ability to pay and without discrimination are also requisites. The total amount of money and food a school may receive depend on the type of lunch served (highest rate of reimbursement going for the complete lunch), the amount spent for food, the need for aid, and the number of lunches served to the children. Over the years the school lunch has become an essential part of the whole educational program. See pages 160–162 regarding school lunch.

WHY IS FOOD AND NUTRITION MISINFORMATION A PROBLEM IN COMMUNITY EDUCATION AND HOW CAN IT BE COMBATED?

Food fads and nutritional quackery have multiplied as the science of nutrition has grown. It is probably not too far from the truth to say that every scientific finding in nutrition has been converted into misinformation by the food faddist or nutritional quack for his own ends. A trained person can easily differentiate between the accurate and the unsound. Unfortunately, the lay person is not always able to do this. In addition, the dramatic (but misleading) manner in which fads and fallacies (sometimes with a grain of truth in them) are propounded, with zip and emotional appeal, shrouds the falseness. As many as 200 fallacies regarding food and nutrition were listed in one report, from very simple, harmless ones to those of dangerous proportions.

Anything which is out of line with current scientific evidence is considered misinformation. Some fallacies are furthered by the nutritional or food quack who pretends to be a specialist in the field of food, nutrition or medicine, or by the food faddist who follows and advocates with great enthusiasm certain food customs and habits. No single food is essential to health, but some 60 nutrients now recognized by nutrition scientists are essential. These nutrients may be obtained by eating a varied diet. The food faddist would have one believe otherwise. He either makes exaggerated claims for the value of certain foods or advocates the omission of other foods from the diet because of the harmful properties he believes they possess. Another type of food faddist emphasizes "natural" foods and wishes them to be consumed in place of others. Special devices of one kind or another, either with or without an accompanying food fad, are another stock-in-trade of the faddist.

The food quack of today has been likened to the patent medicine man of yesterday except that he uses a lot of scientific jargon (important sounding to the untrained ear) to sell his product, be it a "special food," "special food preparation," "special diet," "special regime," or a book, magazine, or reducing gadget. It is well to be suspicious of any writer or lecturer who makes claims contrary to accepted information, claims wholesome food to be harmful or undesirable in some way, uses a scare technique in regard to health, claims to be a scientist or authority, claims association with an unheard-of organization, makes extravagant or unscrupulous claims, or who attacks the Food and Drug Administration or medical, public health or nutrition authority. One should also be suspicious of any material which comes from an anonymous source.

Nutrition authorities agree that the more widespread and more effective dissemination of sound scientific information on nutrition is necessary to combat food and nutrition misinformation. The references listed at the end of this unit discuss many food fads, how they can be recognized and how they can be scientifically refuted.

The Food and Drug Administration of the U. S. Department of Health, Education and Welfare has long been concerned about the promotion of food supplements as cure-alls for conditions which require medical attention. Misleading promotion of food supplements violates Federal Law. It is carried on in the following ways:

1. So-called 'health food lecturers' who claim, directly or indirectly by inference, that the products they are promoting are of value in preventing and curing disease, when in fact they are ineffective for such purposes.

2. Door-to-door sales agents posing as nutrition experts.

3. Pseudo-scientific books and journals frequently recommending some particular food or combination and often written by persons with little nutrition background or training. These may include advertisements for various products in which the publisher has a commercial interest.

False ideas about food are the stock in trade of the food faddist and the following four ideas are used by practically all operators in the field:

1. Myth that all diseases are due to faulty diet.
2. Myth that soil depletion causes malnutrition.
3. Myth that overprocessing of foods is causing malnutrition.
4. Myth of subclinical deficiencies.

Nutrition authorities agree that the best way to buy vitamins and minerals is in the packages provided by nature—vegetables, fruits, milk, eggs, meat, fish, and whole-grain and enriched bread and cereals. The normal American diet now includes such a variety of foods that most persons can hardly fail to have an ample supply of the essential food constituents. The public should distrust any suggestion of self-medication with vitamins and minerals to cure diseases of the nerves, bones, blood, liver, kidneys, heart or digestive system.

QUESTIONS AND ACTIVITIES

1. List all the reasons you can think of why persons take up food fads.

2. What are the signs of a food faddist?

3. Why is self-medication dangerous?

4. Become familiar with the food fad or fad diet assigned you by the instructor so you may report about it to the class. Be sure you can refute the fad or fad diet.

5. What laws in your state safeguard food and health?

Visit the health department in your city. Learn about any nutrition activities which are carried on by the department.

Are there other organizations in your city which carry on nutrition programs?

What are they and what do their nutrition programs cover?

SUPPLEMENTARY READING

Bogert: Chapter 28
Howe: Chapters 2 and 29

Mowry: Chapter 13
Peyton: Chapter 16
Robinson: Pages 15–17

Food Fads Talk Back; Food Information—Fallacies and Facts. Chicago, American Dietetic Association, 1957.

The Role of Nutrition Education in Combatting Food Fads. New York, The Nutrition Foundation, Inc.

Fact, Fad and Fraud About Food. East Lansing, Mich., Michigan State University Cooperative Extension Service.

R. L. Huenemann. Combatting Food Misinformation and Quackery. *Journal of the American Dietetic Association,* vol. 32, p. 627, 1956.

A. M. Beeuwkes, Characteristics of Self-styled Scientists. *Journal of the American Dietetic Association,* Vol. 32, P. 627, 1956.

Food Fact or Fad. Brookings, South Dakota, South Dakota State College, 1959

R. M. Deutsch, *The Nuts Among the Berries.* New York, Ballantine Books, 1961

Food Facts and Fallacies. Chicago, Department of Foods and Nutrition, American Medical Association. (Mimeographed article.)

J. N. Bell, Let 'em Eat Hay. *Today's Health,* September, 1958. Reprint available.

The Merchants of Menace. Leaflet. Chicago, American Medical Association, 1964.

Fads, Myths, Quacks—and Your Health. J. Seaver, New York, Public Affairs Pamphlet No. 415, Public Affairs Committee, 1968.

Don't Be Fooled by Fads. U. S. D. A. Yearbook, 1959, U. S. Department of Agriculture, pp. 660–668.

Nutrition Nonsense—and Sense, FDA Fact Sheet CSS-F4, 1971, Food and Drug Administration, Rockville, Md. 20852.

Quackery, FDA Fact Sheet CSS-g7, Food and Drug Administration, Rockville, Md. 20852.

Food Labeling, FDA Fact Sheet CSS-F6, Food and Drug Administration, Rockville, Md. 20852.

Some Questions and Answers About Dietary Supplements. FDA Fact Sheet CSS-Fll, Food and Drug Administration, Rockville, Md. 20825.

Facts About Nutrition, Public Health Service Publication 917, 1968, Washington, D. C., U. S. Department of Health, Education and Welfare.

Section Two

THERAPEUTIC NUTRITION

Object

To help the practical nurse understand the role food plays in the treatment of disease; how the normal basic diet is modified for nutritive therapy of a corrective or curative nature; the interpretation of a diet order in terms of daily foods and meals; and the psychological factors in feeding the sick.

Introduction

Unit

1. BASIC HOSPITAL DIETS AND THERAPEUTIC MODIFICATIONS

2. DIETS IN OVERWEIGHT AND UNDERWEIGHT AND THYROID DISTURBANCES

3. DIET IN DIABETES MELLITUS

4. DIET IN CARDIOVASCULAR AND RENAL DISEASES

5. DIET IN DISEASES OF THE GASTROINTESTINAL TRACT

6. DIET IN MISCELLANEOUS DISEASES AND CONDITIONS

Introduction

Object

To define terms, discuss important considerations in feeding patients and discuss topics for consideration in a clinical conference on patients on a therapeutic diet.

In the previous section on normal nutrition, the following topics were discussed:

The relation of good nutrition to health;

The nutrients required for good nutrition: their functions, recommended dietary allowances, food sources, and use by the body;

Foods to supply the necessary nutrients: nutritional contributions, selection and care, daily requirements, principles of preparation, and daily food plans;

Application of basic nutrition principles to family feeding;

Special nutritional needs in the life cycle;

Public health nutrition and community nutrition.

This section on therapeutic nutrition will consider the application of the basic principles of nutrition to the treatment of disease.

HOW ARE DIET PRINCIPLES RELATED TO TREATMENT OF DISEASE?

Evidence has accumulated rapidly over the years to show the value of food as a therapeutic agent. Corresponding changes and developments have occurred in medical practice. More is known regarding the maintenance of good nutrition during acute illness, convalescence, and rehabilitation. Better understood also is the manner in which certain illnesses increase requirements for nutrients beyond the usual recommended dietary allowances.

WHAT IS THERAPEUTIC NUTRITION?

Therapeutic nutrition is simply the role of food and nutrition in the treatment of various diseases and disorders. Also referred to as Diet Therapy, Nutritive Therapy, or Diet in Disease, it involves the modification or adaptation of the normal diet in one or more ways to meet the physiologic needs of an ill or injured person.

The normal diet may be modified in

consistency—to make it semisolid, soft, or fluid

flavor—to omit strong flavors

types of foods—to omit hard-to-digest, fried, or rich foods
preparation methods—to mash, chop, or puree
feeding techniques—to feed by tube
amounts of specific foods—increased or decreased amounts
amounts of specific nutrients—increased or decreased amounts
Or, in a combination of any of these modifications.

All therapeutic diets start with a basic normal adequate diet which is then modified in the manner required by the individual patient. See nutritional evaluation of Foundation Diet on page 117.

WHAT ARE IMPORTANT CONSIDERATIONS IN FEEDING PATIENTS?

Meals served the patient in the hospital make an important contribution to his total nursing care and his recovery from illness. Good nutritional condition needs to be maintained and poor nutritional condition improved as he is treated for and recovers from an illness or injury. The diet order of the physician is no less important than his order for any special treatment or medication. It is important also that the patient actually eat the diet ordered by the physician. While the correct diet is important for all patients, it carries special importance in diseases of long duration and for the chronically ill patient.

"Diet is an integral part of total patient care. In her care of the patient, the nurse accepts certain responsibilities related to ensuring comfort and providing therapy according to the physician's order. Included in these aspects of the patient's care are the daily meals and plans for dietary instruction.

"The feeding of the patient involves the coordinated activities of the nursing, medical, and dietary staff, but the nurse is a central figure in a number of ways since she has the closest and most constant association with the patient.

1. She assists the patient at mealtimes as the situation may require.
2. She serves as a liaison between the physician and patient or the dietitian and patient by:
   a. Helping the patient to select his menu when a selective menu is available;
   b. Interpreting the patient's attitudes and problems to the nursing, medical and dietary staff;
   c. Observing the patient's acceptance or rejection of food, noting the response on the patient's record, and assuming responsibility for calling problems to the attention of the physician, dietitian, or both, as may be needed;
   d. Interpreting the prescribed diet to the patient, and developing understanding and acceptance.
3. She assists in or assumes responsibility for dietary instruction of the patient under supervision of the dietitian.[1] (Practical nurse will probably observe in this case and, when asked questions she can not answer, either find out the correct answer or ask professional nurse or dietitian to talk to patient.)

No therapeutic diet will be effective if the meals are not eaten. Therefore, thought must be given to the cultural or regional food patterns of the patient and his family, as well as to his already developed food tastes and habits which can not

---

[1] Robinson, C. H., Proudfit-Robinson *Normal and Therapeutic Nutrition,* 13th edition, New York, The Macmillan Company, 1967, p. 419.

be changed overnight. Patients' meals must also be planned around foods which the patient can afford to buy when he leaves the hospital, if he is to follow the diet successfully after he returns home. There must also be some understanding of the psychological significance food may hold for the individual patient.

The patient's own acceptance of the therapeutic diet is as important, or more important in some cases, than medication or physical treatment as a factor in his recovery. Some attention to his food preferences, insofar as is possible with the necessary diet restrictions and limited hospital and personnel facilities, as well as attention to the appearance and service of his food and the attitude of the nurse who serves his food, all contribute to the acceptance of the diet and the success of therapeutic treatment.

The illness itself and the different conditions imposed on eating when a patient goes from home to hospital, diet restrictions and changes imposed by a therapeutic diet (possibly with different foods and different forms of foods), all accompanied by patient's fears, also affect food acceptance. Part of diet care in patient nursing is educating the patient in new food habits which he will take home with him and which will require some adjustment in his home environment and family group.

HOW DOES FOOD SERVICE CONTRIBUTE TO FOOD ACCEPTANCE AND ENJOYMENT?

Importance of Attractive Food Service

Plays important role in stimulating the appetite and the enjoyment of food.

Especially important for ill persons where meals may be the major events of the day. Patient's room and patient himself should be properly readied to receive meal.

Attitude of patient toward food may reflect his general attitude towards his illness.

General Considerations in Food Service

Table should be appropriately and properly set for the meal being served.

Use clean linen (or good quality paper products for hospital tray service) attractive china, glassware, and silver.

Place silver in order of use (from outside in).

Food portions should be neither too large nor too small and placed on plate attractively.

Hot foods should be served *hot;* cold foods served *cold.*

Mealtime conversation should be pleasant without discussion of disagreeable subjects or "shop," and no disparaging remarks about the food or mention of likes and dislikes.

Food Service on a Tray.   Characteristics of a good tray service are:

Tray lightweight and sufficiently large to hold all necessary articles and foods and permit convenient and neat arrangement, without overcrowding. If possible, dessert may be served on a separate small tray to avoid overcrowding.

Fresh linen or paper tray cover and napkin for each meal.

Small sized sugar bowl, cream pitcher, salt and pepper shakers and a low flower vase all in scale with size of tray.

Lightweight china, glassware, silverware of attractive design and scrupulously clean and shining.

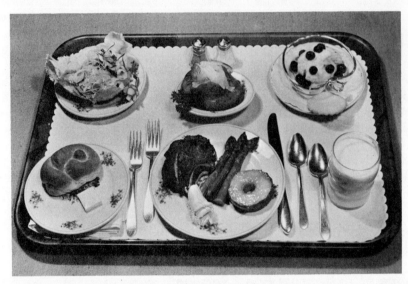

A tray adequate in size and correctly set for dinner for a patient. (From M. V. Krause, *Food, Nutrition and Diet Therapy,* 4th ed. Philadelphia, W. B. Saunders Co., 1966.)

Same placement of foods on tray from day to day.

Food portions of appropriate size, attractively arranged on dishes and garnished.

No spilled foods or liquids.

Tray served on time with a smile with only good remarks about the food.

Tray solidly placed in view of patient and foods within easy reach with patient in a comfortable position.

Plenty of time allowed for eating, with assistance given as needed.

Tray removed without any appearance of hurry.

WHAT INFORMATION IS DESIRABLE IN DISCUSSION OF A PATIENT'S THERAPEUTIC DIET REGIMEN?

RECORD FORM FOR CLINICAL CONFERENCE ON PATIENTS ON THERAPEUTIC DIETS

Participation by Nursing School Clinical Instructor, Therapeutic Dietitian, and Nutrition Instructor.

Patient: Name_____ Age_____ Nationality_____

Symptoms	Laboratory findings	Diagnosis	Medications important in disease

DIET ORDER

Diet prescription	Relation of diet to disorder	Nutritional adequacy	Place of diet in total nursing care

Dietary problems	Adjustments in diet and reasons	Social, economic, and psychological problems	Response of patient to food, physically and emotionally

Instructions about diet	Progress report on patient during stay in hospital and changes effected in diet

SUGGESTED ACTIVITIES

1. For an overall picture of good food service, set up a table properly for breakfast, luncheon, and dinner.

2. Sample trays from hospital dietary department set up for breakfast, noon, and night meals, and nourishment service. Discuss trays: size, cover, napkins, china, glassware, silver, etc. If trays not available from hospital, set up a series of tray service for hospital patients.

3. Comment on the dinner setting on a tray, page 188.

4. Observe a clinical conference on a patient receiving a therapeutic diet. See Form for Clinical Conference on page 188.

5. Write a short paper on the important considerations in feeding a patient.

6. List factors which might affect a patient's nutrition during illness.

SUPPLEMENTARY READING

Howe: Pages 155–157
Peyton: Chapter 18

Robinson: Chapter 18

Unit One

BASIC HOSPITAL DIETS AND THERAPEUTIC MODIFICATIONS

PART 1.   BASIC PROGRESSIVE HOSPITAL DIETS

PART 2.   THERAPEUTIC DIETS

PART 3.   DIET IN FEVERS AND INFECTIONS

Object

To discuss basic routine hospital diets, planned to expedite food service uniformly and conveniently to patients who do not require therapeutic diets; the modifications of the basic normal diet for therapeutic purposes; and diet modifications imposed by fevers and infections.

PART 1.   BASIC PROGRESSIVE HOSPITAL DIETS

WHAT IS MEANT BY A BASIC HOSPITAL DIET?

A basic routine diet is a necessity in the many hospitals and other types of institutions that care for the sick, for reasons of economy, efficiency, convenience, and uniformity of service. Such a routine diet must be nutritionally adequate to maintain good nutrition or to improve nutritive status. It is based on the same foundation diet pattern for normal nutrition stressed throughout this book: certain numbers of servings daily from each of the Four Food Groups which in total meet the recommended dietary allowances for all the essential nutrients, combined into attractive and palatable meals. Refer to pages 29 and 118.

The basic routine diet, variously referred to from hospital to hospital as House, General, Regular, Standard, or Full Diet, is served to ambulatory patients and those patients who do not require nutritive therapy (therapeutic diet). Many factors affect the choice of foods within each group to be served on this General or House Diet: type of hospital (private, state, etc.); budget; socioeconomic level of patients; adaptability to large quantity preparation, etc. It may contain any or all foods that any healthy person may eat, but possibly with fewer calories. There will be a minimum of rich foods and foods requiring a long time for digestion, because hospital patients are less active than average people. This basic normal nutritionally adequate diet is the foundation for planning any or all adaptations or modifications needed by any patient to meet his particular needs due to illness of one kind or another, accident or injury.

PROGRESSIVE BASIC HOSPITAL DIETS

	Clear Liquid Diet	Full Liquid Diet	Soft Diet	Regular-house General-Full
Characteristics	Temporary diet of clear liquids without residue. Nonstimulating, nongas-forming, nonirritating.	Foods liquid at room temperature or liquefying at body temperature.	Normal diet modified in consistency to have no roughage. Liquids and semisolid food; easily digested.	Practically all foods. Simple, easy-to-digest foods, simply prepared, palatably seasoned.
Adequacy	Inadequate: deficient in protein, minerals, vitamins, and calories.	Can be adequate with careful planning: adequacy depends on liquids used.	Entirely adequate liberal diet.	Adequate and well balanced.
Use	Acute illness and infections. Postoperatively. Temporary food intolerance. To relieve thirst. Reduce colonic fecal matter. 1 to 2 hour feeding intervals.	Transition between clear liquid and soft diets. Postoperatively. Acute gastritis and infections. Febrile conditions. Intolerance for solid food. 2 to 4 hour feeding intervals.	Between full liquid and light or regular diet. Between acute illness and convalescence. Acute infections. Chewing difficulties. Gastrointestinal disorders. 3 meals with or without between-meal feedings.	For uniformity and convenience in serving hospital patients. Ambulatory patients. Bed patients not requiring therapeutic diets.
Foods	Water, tea, coffee, coffee substitutes. Fat-free broth. Carbonated beverages. Synthetic fruit juices. Ginger ale. Plain gelatin. Sugar No milk or fats Orange juice may cause distention	All liquids on clear liquid diet plus: All forms milk. Soups, strained. Fruit and vegetable juices. Eggnogs. Plain ice cream and sherbets Junket and plain gelatin dishes. Soft custard. Cereal gruels.	All liquids. Fine and strained cereals. Cooked tender or pureed vegetables. Cooked fruits without skins and seeds. Ripe bananas. Ground or minced meat, fish, poultry. Eggs and mild cheeses. Plain cake and puddings. Moderately seasoned foods.	All basic foods. No foods that may cause digestive distress or take long to digest; rich foods
Modification	Liberal clear liquid diet includes: fruit juices, egg white, whole egg, thin gruels.	Consistency for tube feedings: foods that will pass through tube easily.	Low residue—no fiber or tough connective tissue. Bland—no chemical, thermal, physical stimulants. Cold soft—tonsillectomy. Mechanical or "Dental" soft—requiring no mastication—diced, chopped, mashed foods in place of pureed. Light or convalescent diet—intermediate between soft and regular.	For a light or convalescent diet, fried foods, rich pastries, fat-rich foods, coarse vegetables, possibly raw fruits and vegetables and gas-forming vegetables may be omitted.

Note: Because of trend toward more liberal interpretation of diets and foods, soft diet may be combined with light diet in some hospitals with cooked low-fiber vegetables allowed in place of purees.

When the General Diet is modified in consistency to become a Soft Diet or a Liquid Diet, these three diets are known as Basic Hospital Diets and represent the progressive steps through which a regular hospital patient, requiring no therapeutic food prescription, is carried. In some hospitals, a Light Diet is included in the list as a transitional convalescent diet between a Soft Diet and a General Diet for minor illnesses or if the patient is not ready for a Full Diet. See fourth column in the table on page 192. Semisolid foods and liquid foods are allowed on the soft diet. The Fluid Diet comprises a Full Fluid Diet and a Clear Liquid Diet.

WHAT TYPES OF FOODS ARE ALLOWED ON BASIC HOSPITAL DIETS?

The chart on page 192 lists information about each of the routine hospital diets. There are some differences from hospital to hospital, in the foods allowed in each category, as well as in the number of kinds of diets. When a patient is admitted to the hospital, the type of diet he is to receive will be ordered by his physician. This order will be changed if and when the patient's condition makes it desirable. Or, if the patient requires a modified basic diet, such as listed below and on page 197, such a therapeutic diet order will be written. Note that on page 196, the nurse is asked to attach a list of diets in her hospital and become familiar with them.

IN WHAT WAYS IS THE BASIC GENERAL DIET MODIFIED?

Modifications in consistency of the diet are discussed above. Other modifications include the following:

1. Type of foods—omission of fried, hard-to-digest, rich, and possibly gas-forming, foods.
2. Preparation—mashing, pureeing, homogenization, blending.
3. Flavor—omission of foods with extractives and strong flavors (stimulating), spices and condiments.
4. Exclusion of foods—allergens for persons with allergies.
5. Feeding techniques—tube and intravenous feedings.
6. Intervals of feeding—every hour or two or 6 times daily instead of 3 meals.

Modifications in amounts—increases or decreases—of calories, one or more of various nutrients and roughage, or proportions of various nutrients follow in Part 2.

ACTIVITIES

1. Class makes a tour of the Dietary Department with the dietitian explaining the various units and their relation to each other.

2. List your own hospital's routine Hospital Diets. A copy should be available for each student to attach to the following page indicated for this purpose. Compare the foods on your hospital's diets with those on the chart on the preceding page.

3. Sketch below tray setting used in your hospital for breakfast and dinner service.

Comments.

Linen	Silver	Extras
China	Glassware	Convenience
Attractiveness	Other points	Ways to improve

4. Class observes at every meal time for one day the tray set-ups for the regular diet, soft diet, full liquid diet, and clear liquid diet, in their own or other hospital and writes menus below. If hospital has printed menus, student may attach a copy to this page and use it for checking foods allowed on each type diet.

Typical Hospital Diets Served from One Menu   Date

Menu	Regular Diet	Soft Diet	Full Liquid Diet	Clear Liquid
Breakfast				
Midmorning				
Dinner				
Midafternoon				
Supper				
Night				

SUPPLEMENTARY READING

Howe: Chapter 14   Mowry: Chapter 14   Peyton: Chapter 19
Robinson: Chapters 18–19

BASIC ROUTINE HOSPITAL DIETS

(attach copy of *your* hospital's diets)

PART 2. THERAPEUTIC DIETS

WHAT ARE THE OBJECTIVES AND INDICATIONS FOR THERAPEUTIC DIETS?

Therapeutic diets are ordered by the physician for one or more of the following reasons:

1. To maintain or improve nutritive status.
2. To improve nutritional deficiencies—clinical or sub-clinical.
3. To maintain, decrease, or increase body weight.
4. To rest certain organs or the whole body.
5. To eliminate particular food constituents to which patient may be allergic.
6. To adjust the composition of the diet to meet the ability of the body to digest, metabolize, and excrete certain nutrients and other substances.

HOW ARE HOSPITAL DIETS MODIFIED FOR THERAPEUTIC PURPOSES?

In addition to the ways hospital diets are modified as listed on page 193, the foundation basic normal diet may be modified as follows:

1. Energy value (calories)—increased or decreased
2. Fiber (bulk, roughage)—increased or decreased
3. Specific nutrients (one or more)—increased or decreased
4. Specific foods—included or excluded
5. Any of the above modified diets may be further modified to become a soft or liquid diet

HOW ARE THERAPEUTIC DIETS NAMED?

Therapeutic diets (no longer called "special diets") are named in terms of the diet modification without reference to the name of the disease (except in the case of the diabetic diet) or symptoms, or to the names of persons who may have originated or modified the diet. This makes possible the universal understanding of terms and also reduces the number of therapeutic diets. Adaptations are sometimes classified as *qualitative* where the adaptations are in types of foods or consistency, and *quantitative* where the modifications are increases or decreases of certain nutrients or calories. It is desirable that every therapeutic diet be planned for the particular patient for whom such a diet is ordered.

The modified diets discussed in this unit include, in addition to usual hospital diets (Part 1), further modifications in the soft diet; caloric, protein, fat, sodium, purine, and allergen modifications, and the diabetic diet.

WHAT STEPS DOES THE PHYSICIAN FOLLOW IN WRITING A PRESCRIPTION FOR A THERAPEUTIC DIET?

Before a prescription for a therapeutic diet (which may serve the same purpose for certain disorders as the drug prescription does for others) is formulated, it is desirable to know something about the customary food intake of the patient. This can be accomplished by taking a nutritional history. From a record of food eaten during the past 24 hours or a more detailed record of food consumed during a given period, an estimate of the nutritive content of the home diet may be made. This information can then be correlated with clinical and laboratory findings. The diet prescription is written in terms of caloric requirements based on the individual's weight and activity, and requirements for protein, fat, carbohydrate, minerals, vitamins, and fiber, with due regard for increased or decreased needs for each because of the patient's illness. This prescription is translated into foods and meals by the dietitian who, in turn, instructs the patient regarding the diet, its importance as a single therapeutic measure or as a supplement to medication, and how to prepare and serve it when he returns to his home.

WHAT ARE EXAMPLES OF THERAPEUTIC DIETS AND INDICATIONS FOR USE?

Therapeutic Diet	*Uses*
Low-Calorie Diet	Obesity, diabetes mellitus, cardiovascular and renal diseases, hypertension, gallbladder disease, gout, severely ill patient with low food tolerance, hypothyroidism
High-Calorie Diet	Fevers, hyperthyroidism, following prolonged and severe illness, underweight-malnutrition
Restricted Carbohydrate Diet	Diabetes mellitus, hyperinsulinism, obesity, celiac disease, epilepsy with high fat diet, dumping syndrome
High-Carbohydrate Diet	Toxemias of pregnancy, liver disturbances, uremia, febrile conditions, Addison's disease, preoperative, hyperthyroidism
Moderate to Low-Fat Diet	Gallbladder disturbances, obesity, celiac disease, sprue, pancreatic disease, cardiovascular disease, certain intestinal diseases
Modified-Fat Diet (fat restricted or fat controlled)	Atherosclerosis
High-Fat	Underweight, malnutrition, convalescence, epilepsy
Protein-Free Diet	Hepatic coma, acute anuria
Protein-Restricted Diet	Hepatic coma, chronic uremia, acute glomerulonephritis, certain other kidney diseases

Therapeutic Diet	*Uses*
High-Protein Diet	Any protein inadequacy, preoperative and postoperative, high fevers, burns, injuries, increased metabolism, nephrosis (children), chronic nephritis unless with nitrogen retention, pernicious anemia, ulcerative colitis, hepatitis, celiac and cystic fibrosis, tuberculosis and other wasting diseases, wounds, anemia (nutritional)
Potassium-Restricted Diet	Oliguria, anuria
Increased Sodium Diet	Addison's disease
Sodium-Restricted Diet	Edema, cardiac diseases, kidney disorders, liver cirrhosis, toxemias of pregnancy, hypertension, ACTH therapy
Iron-High Diet	Nutritional and hemorrhagic anemias
High Calcium and Phosphorus Diet	Rickets, osteomalacia, tetany, dental caries, acute lead poisoning
Restricted Calcium and Phosphorus Diet	Urinary calculi (kidney stones)
Low-Purine Diet	Gout
Low-Cholesterol Diet	Atherosclerosis
High Vitamin Diet	Vitamin A—night blindness and xerophthalmia; D—rickets and osteomalacia; K—liver and gallbladder disease where vitamin not stored; thiamine—beriberi and polyneuritis; niacin—pellagra; ascorbic acid—wound healing and scurvy
Gluten-free Diet (wheat-, oatmeal-, rye-free)	Celiac disease, nontropical sprue
Galactose-free Diet	Galactosemia
Low Phenylalanine Diet	Phenylketonuria
Low Residue Diet	Severe diarrhea, ulcerative colitis, partial intestinal obstruction, after G. I. surgery, typhoid fever
High Residue Diet	Atonic constipation (intestinal stasis)
Bland Diet	Gastric and duodenal ulcers, gastritis, diarrhea, ulcerative colitis
Tube feeding (consistency modification)	Esophageal obstruction, anorexia nervosa, severe burns, gastric surgery, inability to chew or swallow
"Elimination Diet"	Allergies; offending allergen is omitted
Acid-ash or Alkaline-ash diet	Certain kidney stones, depending on solubility in either one

SUGGESTED ACTIVITIES

1. Instructor will provide a list of therapeutic diets currently being prepared and served in the hospital with name of disorder or disease for which each has been prescribed. Any pertinent details regarding the patient and his care might be discussed incidentally. Student will list these therapeutic diets below. Student should become acquainted with any diet manual prepared by the hospital's dietary department.

SUPPLEMENTARY READING

See References under Part 1, page 195.

PART 3. DIET IN FEVERS AND INFECTIONS

(Diet Modification: *High-Protein, High-Calorie Diet;* fluid, soft, or regular consistency.)

WHAT ARE THE MEANING AND SIGNIFICANCE OF FEVERS AND INFECTIONS?

Fever is an elevation of body temperature above normal. It indicates infection in the body and increased metabolic processes (all of which are aggravated by malnutrition).

Protein metabolism is increased (end products excreted in the urine along with other toxic products). Stored fat and body protein are utilized for energy if food intake is inadequate, with loss of protein from the tissues. Stored carbohydrate (glycogen) is depleted. With loss of body fluids, sodium chloride and potassium levels are lowered. Disturbances of appetite, digestion, and absorption may occur.

WHAT ARE THE TYPES OF FEVERS?

Fevers of Short Duration (Acute). Tonsillitis, colds, grippe, influenza, children's diseases (measles, chicken pox, scarlet fever), typhoid and certain pneumonias, when treated with antibiotics, rheumatic fever when treated with hormones, poliomyelitis (short but destructive).

Fevers of Long Duration (Chronic). Tuberculosis, malaria (recurrent).

WHAT IS THE DIETARY TREATMENT FOR FEVERS AND INFECTIONS?

Increased calories: 50 per cent or more above normal requirement (3000–4000 calories) with high carbohydrate to replenish glycogen stores and high fat in emulsified form for easy digestion.

High protein: 100–150 grams daily.

Increased vitamins: especially vitamin A, ascorbic acid and B Complex vitamins. Vitamin supplements may be ordered.

Sufficient Sodium chloride and potassium; increased fluids— 3–4 quarts daily.

Frequent small feedings—tube feedings if appetite is poor, then full liquid as soon as possible with protein supplements added to milk, fruit juices and soups as needed.

Some Commonly Used Supplements[1]	*Low in Sodium		*How to Use*
Alacta	*Kralex	*Protinal	1. Include in meat, egg, and cheese dishes.
Aminoids	*Lonalac	Protenum	2. Add to gravies, sauces, and salad dressings.

---

[1] M. V. Krause, *Food, Nutrition and Diet Therapy,* 4th edition, Philadelphia, W. B. Saunders Company, 1966, pages 588–589, adapted.

Some Commonly Used Supplements[1]			How to Use
Brewer's yeast	Meritene	Provimal	3. Stir in cooked cereals, and mashed potatoes or squash.
Casec	Powdered egg	Sobee	4. Mix with milk, eggs, flavorings in hot or cold beverages.
Dryco	Powdered milk	Soy flour	
Klim	Dried egg	Peanut flour	5. Incorporate in custards and other simple desserts. See page 203 also.

Additional Dietary Considerations

Typhoid fever: Large quantities of milk is basis of diet.

Low-fiber diet to prevent intestinal irritation.

3–6 eggs daily, if tolerated.

Frequent, small feedings.

High-Calorie, High-Protein, Low-Fiber Diet.

Fruit juices may cause distress.

Poliomyelitis: Liquid to soft diet during acute stage. Then High-Calorie, High-Protein, High-Vitamin Diet to compensate for rapid tissue destruction.

Protein supplements may be better tolerated than milk.

Vitamin supplements may be indicated.

Tube feeding may be necessary in early stages.

Rheumatic Fever: High-Calorie, High Protein liquid diet in early stages.

Diet gradually increased to one high in iron, vitamin A, protein and calories to maintain normal weight.

Restricted sweets to avoid appetite reduction for other foods.

Possible sodium chloride restriction with ACTH therapy.

Tuberculosis: 2500–3500–5000 calories; 100–150 grams protein.

Optimum minerals and vitamins with special attention to calcium and iron, vitamins A and D, and ascorbic acid.

Easily digested, simple food, attractively served; "forced feeding" undesirable.

WHAT IS A DIET PATTERN FOR A HIGH-PROTEIN, HIGH-CALORIE DIET?

HIGH-PROTEIN, HIGH-CALORIE DIET[2]
Approximately 130 gm. protein, 3500 calories

Breakfast	Luncheon or Supper	Dinner
Citrus fruit or juice	Cream soup	Clear soup or fruit juice
Cereal, 2/3 cup	Meat, fish, poultry, eggs, or cheese; 2 ounces	Meat, poultry, or fish; 3 ounces
Cream, light, 1/2 cup	Potato or substitute	Potato
Eggs, 2	Green leafy or yellow vegetable	Cooked vegetable
Toast or roll, 1–2 slices	Salad and salad dressing	Bread or roll, 1–2 slices
Butter or fortified margarine, 2 teaspoons	Bread or roll, 1–2 slices	Butter or fortified margarine, 2 teaspoons
Jelly, 1 tablespoon		

---

[2] F. T. Proudfit and C. H. Robinson, *Normal and Therapeutic Nutrition*, 12th ed. New York, The Macmillan Company, 1961, p. 395.

Breakfast	*Luncheon or Supper*	*Dinner*
Milk, 1 cup	Butter or fortified mar-	Dessert
Sugar, 3 teaspoons	garine, 2 teaspoons	Milk beverage
Hot beverage	Milk, 1 cup	
	Fruit	

Midmorning	*Midafternoon*	*Evening*
Milk beverage	Citrus fruit juice	Milk beverage
	Crackers or plain cookies	Sandwiches, plain dessert,
		cookies, or crackers

WHAT ARE CHARACTERISTICS OF FLUID AND TUBE FEEDINGS?

Fluid feedings

Forms of Milk Used

Plain, malted, acidulated.

Reinforced with egg, glucose, lactose, gelatin, yeast, dried milk.

Flavored with chocolate, coffee, fruit extracts.

Milk beverages used in high protein diets.

Fruits added to milk beverages with blender.

An example of an adequate 85 gm. protein, 2150 calorie *full liquid diet* given in 6 or more feedings daily includes:[3]
6 cups milk
2 eggs
1–2 ounces strained meat
1/2 cup strained cooked cereal for gruel
1/4 cup vegetable puree for cream soup
1 cup citrus fruit juice
1/2 cup tomato or vegetable juice
1 tablespoon cocoa
3 tablespoons sugar
1 tablespoon butter
2 servings plain gelatin dessert. Junket, custard, ices and plain ice cream
Broth or bouillon

Ways of Increasing Food Value

Calories: replace or supplement sugar with lactose (less sweet so more can be used).

Substitute cream or evaporated milk for all or part of milk.

Butter added to cereal waters and gruels.

Ice cream added to beverages: fruit, milk, carbonated.

Protein: Add egg white to fruit juices.

Add dried milk solids to beverages.

Add protein hydrolysates.

Add whole egg or increase eggs.

Add gelatin to fruit juices, soups, broth.

Add commercial protein supplements.

Tube feedings

Indications

Inability to eat or refusal of food

Considerations

Tube feedings must be adequate for all

---

[3] C. H. Robinson, Proudfit and Robinson's *Normal and Therapeutic Nutrition*, 13th edition. New York, The Macmillan Company, 1967, page 446.

Indications	*Consideration*
following operation, accident, unconsciousness, resection in digestive tract.	nutritional needs if used for a long time.
Obstruction or surgery in upper gastrointestinal tract.	High in protein and low in fat usually.
Inability to chew and swallow.	Heated over hot water to body temperature for serving and strained.
Intolerance for food by mouth.	Food introduced directly into stomach by nasogastric tube from mouth, nose, or artificial opening.
	Food must be partially predigested if introduced directly into jejunum.
	Tube feeding should be served as any meal on a tray.
	Commercially prepared tube feedings (expensive):
	Sustagen Lipoprotein

EXAMPLES OF TUBE FEEDINGS[4]

Standard Tube Feeding

Protein, 100 gm.; fat, 110 gm.; carbohydrate, 190 gm.; calories, 2140; Na 155 mEq; K 100 mEq; fluid, 1500 ml. May be inadequate in iron for men and women.

$3\frac{1}{3}$ cups whole milk

2/3 cup eggnog powder

3/4 cup powdered skim milk

$2\frac{1}{2}$ cups half and half

1 teaspoon salt

$1\frac{1}{4}$ teaspoons vitamin preparation (2 mg. thiamine; 3 mg. riboflavin; 30 mg. niacin; 100 mg. ascorbic acid)

Milk-base tube feeding to which eggnog powder and vitamin preparation have been added.

150 to 200 ml. given at a time, diluted if not tolerated at this concentration.

Modifications made when variations in one or more nutrients necessary.

Blenderized Tube Feeding

Protein, 150 gm.; fat, 60 gm.; carbohydrate, 230 gm.; calories 2050; Na 100 mEq; K 143 mEq; fluid 1500 ml.

1 cup meat, strained

2 cup eggnog powder

$\frac{1}{2}$ cup vegetable, strained

1 cup fruit juice

3 cups whole milk

2 cups powdered skim milk

5/8 cup half and half

Water to make 1500 ml.

Variety of basic foods used in preparation; these foods are mixed in a blender and strained. Foods from the general diet such as meat, fruits, vegetables, eggnog powder and milk products are used.

Amount of feeding at any one time may vary from 150–200 ml.

STUDY QUESTIONS AND ACTIVITIES

1. Discuss the old saying "Feed a cold and starve a fever."

---

[4] Mayo Clinic Diet Manual, Committee on Dietetics of the Mayo Clinic, Philadelphia, W. B. Saunders Company, 1971, pages 94–95.

2.   Why is a High-Carbohydrate, High-Protein, High-Calorie, High-Vitamin Diet given in fevers and infections?

Demonstration.   Preparation of tube feedings with and without blender: High protein beverages: milk, fruit, vegetable juices, soups. Scraped beef; minced meat; sieved foods.

SUPPLEMENTARY READING

Howe: Chapter 18; pages 422–423   Peyton: Chapter 21   Robinson: Pages 203–205

Unit Two

DIET IN OVERWEIGHT AND UNDERWEIGHT
DIET IN THYROID DISTURBANCES

Object

To discuss the use of the Low-calorie *and the* High-calorie
Diets *as modifications of the normal basic diet in weight control
and thyroid disturbances, and how to adapt family menus for
overweight or underweight family members.*

OVERWEIGHT AND UNDERWEIGHT
(Diet Modification: *Calorie-Controlled Diets*)

WHY IS WEIGHT CONTROL DESIRABLE FOR HEALTH?

Overweight, once considered a sign of success and prosperity, is now considered
a form of malnutrition and a major problem in preventive medicine. Excess weight
places undue strain on the body, lowering resistance to infection and increasing the
susceptibility to certain diseases: diabetes, cardiovascular and renal disorders, and
other degenerative diseases. Changes in some body functions may also occur. It also
reduces life expectancy. Surgery is a greater risk for an obese person, and overweight
during pregnancy predisposes to complications during pregnancy and at childbirth.
Statistics also show that very obese persons are accident-prone. Obesity handicaps
a person physically in many ways and may cause emotional and psychological
problems.

Considerable overweight is considered an indication for reduction. It is always
wise for any person to check with his physician before starting a reducing program,
to learn if the body is in condition to lose weight, the rate and extent of loss desirable,
the correct types of foods and number of calories to be eaten, and the type and extent,
if any, of exercise. A reduction program may be a preliminary requirement to the
treatment of a disorder by surgery, drugs, and/or diet.

Underweight associated with undernutrition can be a health problem because of
lowered resistance to disease, accompanied by fatigue and impaired efficiency. It may
be a symptom or a predisposing factor in disease. It is especially serious in younger
individuals as underweight persons are more subject to tuberculosis. In children,
it may result in retarded growth. Additional calories over and above those needed
for basal metabolism and activity are required to meet growth needs during infancy,
childhood and pregnancy. A physician's examination and advice is essential before
starting a program for gaining weight.

WHAT IS DESIRABLE WEIGHT AND HOW IS IT DETERMINED?

Revised Height-Weight Tables (Appendix, page 293) indicate "desirable" weights, those associated with lowest mortality rates, based on the weights of individuals approximately 25 years of age. They take into consideration differences in body frame—small, medium, large—and height. Unlike older tables, they do not consider increases of weight with age to be ideal. Rather, the proper weight for one's height and body build at age 25 is recognized to be the ideal one to be maintained for the remainder of life. These tables are published by the Metropolitan Life Insurance Company following extensive research on their insurance policyholders, relating weight to health and longevity.

Because height-weight tables cannot determine the degree of body fatness—an important factor in proper weight evaluation—current studies are concerned with thickness of subcutaneous tissues in certain parts of the body, anthropometric measurements (by calipers) and other detailed procedures.

HOW IS THE NORMAL DIET MODIFIED IN ENERGY (CALORIES)?

The energy value of the normal diet may be modified for therapeutic purposes by decreasing the caloric value below the allowance recommended for maintenance, so that some of the body fat will be utilized for energy. Conversely, the calorie value may be increased above the maintenance requirement to allow fat to be stored. In either case, the protein, minerals and vitamins must meet or exceed the recommended dietary allowances. A further modification may be made in the consistency of either diet as needed.

WHAT ARE THE MEANING, CAUSE, AND DIET TREATMENT OF OVERWEIGHT?

Meaning.   Slight overweight—10% above desirable weight.

Excessive—10–20% above desirable weight.

Obesity—20% and more above desirable weight: Excessive deposit of fatty (adipose) tissue.

Causes.   Excessive food intake because of family food customs, social eating, excessive appetite, or emotional problems; changes in living patterns; too little exercise; sedentary occupations and leisure-time activities; nibbling, skipping meals and overeating at other times. See also page 56.

Very small percentage of overweight due to glandular disturbances.

Calories eaten exceed energy needs of body.

Lessening of activity.

Adult obesity may have started in childhood and adolescence; prevention of early obesity is desirable.

Principles of Diet.   Calorie intake must be reduced to less than output so body will draw on reserve fat for some of needed calories; otherwise diet should be completely adequate.

Calories reduced to about basal requirement or roughly 500 to 1000 calories less than actual requirement. Theoretically, this should bring about the recommended maximum daily weight loss of two pounds.

Emphasis on low calorie foods, regular eating and no nibbling.

Diet adapted to eating habits and easily obtainable.

WHAT ARE THE PURPOSE, INDICATIONS, CHARACTERISTICS, FOODS ALLOWED AND TO BE AVOIDED ON LOW-CALORIE DIETS?

Purpose.   To maintain or restore good nutrition.
To bring about a gradual loss in body weight by depletion of body fat.

Indications

Overweight	Obesity	Arthritis
Gout	Diabetes	Cardiac insufficiency
Gallbladder disease with obesity		Circulatory problems

Characteristics.   Normal diet about 500 calories lower than actual requirement—or 12–15 calories per pound for sedentary man or woman; adequate in other nutrients and satiety value.

Approximate daily calories: women—1000–1500; men—1500–2000

Protein, minerals and vitamins at recommended allowance.

Some low-calorie diets have slightly higher calories and higher fat and protein than others for better satiety value. See page 210.

Possible iron and vitamin supplementation on doctor's orders for diets of 1000 calories or less.

Foods allowed	*Foods to be avoided*
Milk—whole, skim, buttermilk, cottage cheese	Salad dressings
Lean meats	Gravies Fat meat Bacon
Bulky low-calorie fruits and vegetables	Sauces
Small amounts of whole-grain and enriched cereal products	Creamed dishes
Seasonings	Rich and sweet desserts
Tea and coffee without cream or sugar	Fried foods
Low calorie dark green and yellow vegetables and fruits high in vitamin C	Bottled beverages
Broth—fat free	High carbohydrate vegetables
	Sweets—jams, jellies, candies
	Sweetened fruits
	Concentrated sweets and fats
	Alcoholic beverages
	"Snack" foods

WHAT FOODS ARE INCLUDED IN A 1200 CALORIE DIET AND HOW ARE THEY COMBINED INTO MEALS?

Foods for the Day	*Notes*
1 pint whole milk	Vitamin supplements may be ordered by the physician.
1 egg	
5 oz. meat, poultry, fish, or cheese	Diets furnishing less than 1000–1200

Foods for the Day
(divided between 2 meals)
1 serving green or yellow vegetable from List 2A
1 other vegetable from List 2A
1 serving vegetable from List 2B
1 serving citrus fruit
2 other servings fruit
1 small potato
2 slices whole wheat or enriched bread
2 teaspoons butter or fortified margarine

Notes
calories should be used only under supervision of physician.
Accompanying diet may be increased to 1500 calories by adding

2 slices bread	140
2 teaspoons butter	90
1 oz. American cheese	75
	305

Nutritive Values of Foods for the Day[1]
Carbohydrate, gm. 106
Protein, gm. 66
Fat, gm. 55
Calories, 1200

MEAL PATTERN FOR 1200 CALORIE DIET[2]
(Moderate Carbohydrate, Normal Protein, Low Fat)

Breakfast
1 serving citrus fruit or juice
1 egg (cooked without fat)
1 slice bread or small serving of cereal
1 level teaspoon butter
1/2 glass (4 oz.) whole milk
Clear coffee or tea

Lunch or Supper
1/2 cup cottage cheese, or 2 oz. meat, or
1 oz. cheese and 1 oz. meat
1/2 cup green or yellow vegetable (List 2A)
1/2 cup of another vegetable (List 2B)
1 serving fruit—no sugar
1 glass (8 oz.) whole milk
Tea

Dinner
3 oz. lean meat, fish, or poultry (not fried; liver once a week)
1 small potato
1/2 cup vegetable (List 2A)
1 serving fruit—no sugar
1/2 glass (4 oz.) whole milk

MEAL PATTERN FOR 1400 CALORIE DIET

A *1400 Calorie Diet* containing *high protein* (90 grams), *moderate fat* (80 grams), and *low carbohydrate* (80 grams), developed first at Michigan State University and later adapted by the School of Nutrition, Cornell University, has proved satisfactory for weight loss in different age groups. This diet is easy to follow. The higher amount of protein and fat provides greater satiety value than the usual 1200–1400 calorie diet. The foods and their distribution among the meals of the day are shown below with some adaptations by the author.

Foods for the Day
3 glasses (6 oz. each) whole milk to drink and to use in tea and coffee, on cereal, in cooked foods, etc.
1 egg
2 servings (4 oz. each, cooked weight)

Meal Pattern
Breakfast
1 serving citrus fruit   1 egg
1 thin slice enriched or whole wheat bread
or

---

[1] Calculated from Exchange Lists on pages 221–224.
[2] See Exchange Lists on pages 221–224 for choices and amounts among various forms of milk, vegetables, fruits, breads, meats and fats.

Foods for the Day

of meat (beef, veal, lamb, pork); poultry (chicken, turkey); fish, eggs, or cheese, or any combination of these. (4 oz. cooked meat, fish, or poultry equals a large serving [piece about 4 × 3 × 1 inches]; about 1/3 pound uncooked.)

2 servings (1/2 cup each) vegetables
   1 serving green or yellow vegetable
   1 serving of another vegetable

2 servings of fruit without sugar
   1 serving of citrus fruit
   1 serving of another fruit

1 thin slice enriched or whole wheat bread,
   or 1/2 cup cooked cereal,
   or 1/2 to 3/4 cup flaked or puffed unfrosted cereal

1 level teaspoon butter

Note:

Large-framed men may add an extra egg at breakfast and use 3 thin slices of bread daily and 1 extra level teaspoon of butter.

Meal Pattern

1/2 cup cooked cereal
     or
1/2 to 3/4 cup flaked or puffed dry cereal
1 level teaspoon butter
3/4 cup (6 oz.) whole milk
Coffee or tea

Noon

4 oz. meat, cooked weight
1/2 cup vegetable
Small wedge lettuce, or 2 to 3 strips carrot, celery, green pepper, cucumber, or 1 or 2 thin slices tomatoes, or small tossed salad with lemon or vinegar and seasonings
3/4 cup whole milk (6 oz.)
Tea or coffee

Night

Occasionally 1/2 cup tomato juice or 1 cup fat-free bouillon
4 oz. meat, cooked weight
1/2 cup vegetable
1 serving fruit
3/4 cup (6 oz.) whole milk
Tea or coffee

Suggestions for a Person Following a Low-Calorie Diet

Be satisfied to lose not more than 2 pounds a week: large weekly weight losses are not desirable.

Follow diet exactly and stay on it until desired weight loss has been achieved. Then add foods (200 to 500 calories per day) gradually to learn the amount that will hold desirable weight. This is your maintenance diet.

Eat slowly and stretch out eating time.

Discover, if possible, why you overeat and replace food craving with another activity.

Eat the full breakfast as it will make it easier to stick to the diet. You will not become hungry during the morning and be inclined to nibble.

Learn to be satisfied with smaller amounts of food.

Keep your mind on the rewards of reducing: feel better, more vigor, less tired, wear smaller clothes, live longer, etc.

Serve meals as attractively as possible: don't cut on niceties of meal.

Learn seasonings, flavorings, and garnishes to make low calorie food interesting.

Learn to like a variety of low-calorie foods.

If you like to eat before going to bed, save a glass of milk or serving of fruit from your day's allowance to eat then.

If you are going to a party where food will be served, eat less at home that day.

When you eat in a restaurant, choose plain foods, salads without dressings, fruit for dessert, broiled or roasted meats.

Don't skip meals.

Learn to enjoy foods without added sugar or fat.

"Concentrate on what you can have, not what you have to forego."

A cup of tea sweetened with artificial sweetener, or a cup of fatfree bouillon helps hungry feeling between meals.

Avoid mineral oil dressings as the oil absorbs and interferes with absorption of some of the nutrients. French dressings made with tomato juice, lemon or vinegar, grated onion, herbs, are good additions to salads or heated overcooked vegetables.

Reducing "Fads" and "Diets"

Dangers and Reasons for Failure. Fad diets *are* fast and may take off weight easily but they *do not* keep it off.

Fad diets do nothing to change eating habits permanently, which is basic for a reducing regime.

Many are so limited in types of foods allowed that they become monotonous and cannot be adhered to.

Drastic short term dieting is hard on the body.

Many fad diets do not follow "Basic Four Food Plan," are low in protein and other important nutrients, and as such are a serious menace to health of everyone, but especially of teenagers, convalescents, people with low disease resistance and certain ailments, and women during childbearing years.

Fad Diets

"Fabulous" formula diet

Elimination diet

Banana and skim milk diet

Egg and leafy vegetable diet

Various 7-day, 9-day, and other "wonder diets"

The "low protein" diet and the "high protein" diets

Reducing pills, candies, etc.

"Eat all you want" diet

"Air Force" diet (no connection with Air Force)

Grapefruit diet

Grapejuice diet

"Starvation diet"

"Mayo Diet" (no connection with Mayo Clinic)

HOW CAN ONE FAMILY MEMBER DIET WHILE OTHERS EAT NORMALLY?

The following menus show how a normal 3000 calorie diet may be modified to give one family member a 1200 calorie diet without preparing separate meals. Some items are omitted, some served in smaller portions, and some served in modified form —skim milk instead of whole milk; black coffee instead of coffee with cream and sugar.

FIRST DAY[3]

1,200 Calories

3,000 Calories

BREAKFAST

Grapefruit......... ½ medium.
Wheat flakes....... 1 ounce.
Skim milk......... 1½ cups.
Coffee (black), if desired.

Grapefruit......... ½ medium.
Wheat flakes....... 1 ounce.
Banana........... 1 medium.
Whole milk........ 1½ cups.
Toast, enriched..... 2 slices.
Butter or margarine.. 1½ teaspoons.
Coffee............ 1 cup.
   Cream.......... 1 tablespoon.
   Sugar........... 1 teaspoon.

LUNCH

Chef's salad:
   Julienne chicken.. 1 ounce.
   Cheddar cheese.. ½ ounce.
   Hard-cooked egg. ½ egg.
   Tomato........ 1 large.
   Cucumber...... 6 slices.
   Endive........ ½ ounce.
   Lettuce........ ⅛ head.
   French dressing... 2 tablespoons.
Rye wafers....... 4 wafers.
Skim milk........ 1 cup.

Chef's salad:
   Julienne chicken.. 2 ounces.
   Cheddar cheese.. 1 ounce.
   Hard-cooked egg. ½ egg.
   Tomato........ 1 large.
   Cucumber...... 6 slices.
   Endive........ ½ ounce.
   Lettuce........ ⅛ head.
   French dressing... 2 tablespoons.
Rye wafers........ 4 wafers.
Gingerbread....... 2-inch square
                    piece.
   Lemon sauce..... ¼ cup.
Whole milk........ 1 cup.

DINNER

Beef pot roast...... 3 ounces.
Mashed potatoes... ⅓ cup.
Green peas........ ½ cup.
Whole-wheat bread. 1 slice.
Butter or margarine.. ½ teaspoon.
Fruit cup:
   Orange......... ½ small.
   Apple.......... ½ small.
   Banana........ ½ medium.

Beef pot roast...... 3 ounces.
Gravy............ ¼ cup.
Mashed potatoes... ⅔ cup.
Green peas, but-
   tered.
Rolls, enriched..... 2 small.
Butter or margarine.. 1 teaspoon.
Fruit cup:
   Orange......... ½ small.
   Apple.......... ½ small.
   Banana......... ½ medium.
Plain cooky....... 1 medium.

BETWEEN-MEAL SNACK

Sandwich:
   Enriched bread... 2 slices.
   Beef pot roast.... 2 ounces.
   Mayonnaise..... 2 teaspoons.
   Lettuce........ 1 large leaf.
Whole milk........ 1 cup.

---

[3] From *Food and Your Weight*, Home and Garden Bulletin no. 74. Washington, D. C., U. S. Department of Agriculture, 1969, p. 10.

SECOND DAY[4]

1,200 Calories

3,000 Calories

BREAKFAST

Orange juice...... ½ cup.
Soft-cooked egg.... 1 egg.
Whole-wheat toast.. 1 slice.
Butter or margarine.. 1 teaspoon.
Skim milk......... 1 cup.
Coffee (black), if desired.

Orange juice...... ½ cup.
Soft-cooked egg.... 1 egg.
Bacon............ 2 strips.
Whole-wheat toast.. 2 slices.
Butter or margarine.. 2 teaspoons.
Whole milk........ 1 cup.
Coffee............ 1 cup.
   Cream.......... 1 tablespoon.
   Sugar.......... 1 teaspoon.

LUNCH

Sandwich:
   Enriched bread... 2 slices.
   Boiled ham...... 1½ ounces.
   Mayonnaise..... 2 teaspoons.
   Mustard
   Lettuce........ 1 large leaf.
Celery.......... 1 small stalk.
Radishes......... 4 radishes.
Dill pickle........ ½ large.
Skim milk........ 1 cup.

Tomato soup...... 1 cup.
Sandwich:
   Enriched bread... 3 slices.
   Boiled ham...... 3 ounces.
   Mayonnaise..... 2½ teaspoons.
   Mustard
   Lettuce........ 2 large leaves.
Celery.......... 1 small stalk.
Radishes......... 4 radishes.
Dill pickle........ ½ large.
Apple........... 1 medium.
Whole milk........ 1 cup.

DINNER

Roast lamb....... 3 ounces.
Rice, converted..... ½ cup.
Spinach.......... ¾ cup.
Lemon........... ¼ medium.
Salad:
   Peaches, canned 1 half peach.
   Cottage cheese... ⅓ cup.
   Lettuce........ 1 large leaf.

Roast lamb....... 4 ounces.
Rice, converted..... ⅔ cup.
Spinach, buttered... ⅔ cup.
Lemon........... ¼ medium.
Salad:
   Peaches, canned.. 2 halves.
   Cottage cheese... ⅓ cup.
   Lettuce........ 1 large leaf.
Rolls, enriched..... 2 small.
Butter or margarine.. 1 teaspoon.
Plain cake, iced.... 2-inch piece
              layer cake.

BETWEEN-MEAL SNACK

Apple........... 1 medium.

Soda crackers..... 4 crackers.
Peanut butter...... 2 tablespoons.
Whole milk........ 1 cup.

---

[4] From *Food and Your Weight,* Home and Garden Bulletin no. 74. Washington, D. C., U. S. Department of Agriculture, 1969, p. 11.

WHAT ARE THE MEANING, CAUSE AND DIET TREATMENT OF UNDERWEIGHT?

Meaning. 10–15% or more below desirable weight. Serious if 20% and more below desirable weight.

Causes. Food insufficient for needs in quality or quantity; most frequently the wrong kinds of foods are eaten.

Poor absorption and utilization of food.

Wasting disease.

Increased metabolic rate.

Mental strain and worry.

Excessive activity.

Calories less than energy expended by body.

Principles of Diet Treatment. Stimulate appetite.

Allow plenty of time for meals. Serve meals at regular intervals.

Encourage relaxation at meals.

Increase calorie intake to 500–1000 or more over need, to allow weekly gain of 1 to 2 pounds.

Use vitamin supplements to allow storage and improve appetite.

Well-balanced diet with emphasis on high calorie foods, large meals, and well chosen in-between snacks.

WHAT ARE THE PURPOSE AND INDICATIONS, CHARACTERISTICS, AND FOODS ALLOWED AND TO BE AVOIDED ON THE HIGH-CALORIE DIET?

Purpose. To maintain or restore normal nutrition.

To bring about a weight gain by the storage of fatty tissue.

Indications. Underweight

Malnutrition	Hyperthyroidism
Infections	Typhoid fever
Fevers	Tuberculosis

Characteristics. Normal adequate diet with suggested number of servings from "Basic Four Food Groups" plus additions to provide more calories than actual requirement.

About 1200 calories above requirement to allow an approximate weekly gain of 2 lbs or more.

Higher protein—90–100 grams per day.

High thiamine and other B-complex vitamins.

Minerals and vitamins to exceed Recommended Allowances.

3 large meals or 3 average meals and 2 to 3 between meal feedings.

For some patients: Smaller volume meals and more concentrated food value.

Easily digested foods.

Foods Allowed. Almost any foods liked by patients at meals, between meals and at night.

Skim milk powder added to milk, cottage cheese, macaroni, cereals, mashed potatoes, for extra protein and calories.

High calorie desserts.

Jams and jellies.

Cream added to foods and on foods, if tolerated.

Concentrated foods with more calories but less bulk

Foods to be Avoided.   Concentrated fats and sweets when poor appetite is a problem.

HOW IS THE HIGH-CALORIE DIET PLANNED?

As with all other therapeutic diets, the basis of a high-calorie diet is the normal adequate diet. Additional amounts of the basic foods, particularly those with high energy value, may be added to each meal or in an extra evening small meal; or the energy value of between meal foods may be stepped up. Two slices of bread generously spread with butter or fortified margarine or peanut butter or cheese, and 2 glasses of milk added during the day easily add about 500 calories. With further increases in servings of bread and spread, cereals, cream, egg, and glucose or lactose in fruit juices, an additional 1000 calories may be obtained. The addition of dry skim milk powder to milk used for drinking, and also to cottage cheese, cereals, macaroni dishes, and mashed potatoes, adds energy value and also additional nutrients. High calorie milk beverages, high calorie sandwiches with extra meat, cheese, and mayonnaise, additional desserts and sweets, and additional butter may also be used.

HYPOTHYROIDISM AND HYPERTHYROIDISM

(Diet Modification: *Calorie-Controlled Diets*)

WHAT ARE CHARACTERISTICS AND DIET TREATMENT FOR HYPOTHYROIDISM AND HYPERTHYROIDISM?

Hypothyroidism.   Deficient secretion of thyroid gland.

Low metabolic rate—15 to 30% below normal.

Rapid gain in weight.

Personality changes.

May be related to iodine deficiency.

Obesity may be a problem.

Diet.   Low Calorie Diet: Refer to page 210.

Hyperthyroidism.   Excessive secretion of thyroid gland which regulates energy metabolism.

High metabolic rate—15 to 75% above normal.

Loss of weight.

Fatigue and weakness.

Rapid pulse.

Rapid breakdown of tissue.

Enlarged thyroid.

Increased appetite.

Diet.   High calories—up to 5000 per day.

Liberal diet.

High protein—100 to 125 grams.

Increased vitamins—possibly supplements.

Limited stimulants.

High Calorie Diet—Refer to page 215.

SUGGESTED ACTIVITIES

Exhibits: Reducing Fads and Diets

Snack Foods—What they do to the day's calories.

Each student might collect information about a single fad reducing regime and report to the class its characteristics, nutritional deficiencies, dangers, printed materials, etc. This material could then be assembled in the form of a permanent exhibit.

SUPPLEMENTARY READING

Howe: Chapter 15   Mowry: Chapters 22–23   Peyton: Chapter 20

Robinson: Chapters 20–21

Food and Your Weight. Home and Garden Bulletin No. 74, Washington, D. C., U. S. Department of Agriculture, 1969.

Four Steps to Weight Control. New York, Metropolitan Life Insurance Company, 1969.

The Healthy Way to Weigh Less. New York, Metropolitan Life Insurance Company, 1966.

G. Christakis and R. K. Plumb, *Obesity.* New York, The Nutrition Foundation, 1966.

P. Weyden, *The Overweight Society.* New York, William Morrow and Company, 1965.

Unit Three

DIET IN DIABETES MELLITUS

Object

To understand how the normal basic diet is modified for the therapeutic treatment of diabetes mellitus.

(Diet Modification: *Modifications for Carbohydrate, Protein, and Fat*)

WHAT ARE BASIC FACTS ABOUT DIABETES MELLITUS?

Characteristics. Diabetes is a metabolic disorder (inborn error of metabolism) in which the body is unable to metabolize carbohydrates. This in turn prevents complete oxidation of fats and interferes with protein metabolism.

Causes	*Symptoms and Clinical Findings*
Direct: Inability of pancreas to produce insulin (secreted by special cells in the pancreas) which metabolizes carbohydrates.	High blood sugar (hyperglycemia).
	Glucose in urine (glycosuria).
	Increased thirst (polydipsia).
	Increased appetite (polyphagia).
Indirect: May be an hereditary tendency.	Increased urination (polyuria).
Overweight is a predisposing factor.	Ketone bodies in urine (ketonuria).
Vascular disease may be an associated factor.	Loss of weight and strength.
	Fatigue and loss of strength.
Occurs at all ages; greater incidence in middle and later years.	Dehydration.

WHAT TYPES OF DIETARY TREATMENT ARE USED IN DIABETES?

Diet is a very important part of treatment for a patient with diabetes mellitus to control high blood sugar, keep the urine sugar-free, and help allay the appearance of undesirable conditions of vascular disease. It alone may suffice for a few diabetic patients with early detected and early treated mild diabetes but, for the more severe cases, complete control requires supplemental therapy with insulin or other hypoglycemic agents.

Opinion differs as to the extent of diet restriction and insulin therapy needed. At one extreme is the carefully controlled so-called *chemical regulation* of blood sugar. The diet and insulin are so balanced that all carbohydrates are metabolized, the blood sugar is kept within normal limits and the urine is sugar free. The diet is carefully calculated for prescribed amounts of carbohydrate, protein, and fat, and all foods are weighed. Patients frequently find it difficult to adhere to the severe diet restrictions.

At the other extreme is the more liberal, "free" *clinical regulation* of blood sugar. The diet is practically unrestricted (except for sugar and foods high in sugar) as long as there are no diabetic symptoms, no ketonuria, no more than a mild glycosuria, and correct weight is maintained. Insulin is prescribed to metabolize most of the carbohydrate in the diet.

The usual diet is liberal compared with early diets for diabetics but it is not completely "free." This diet is planned easily with *Exchange Lists* shown on pages 221–224; it allows a wider choice of foods, is easier for the patient to follow, being based on household measures, and blood and urine sugar levels are moderately controlled.

HOW IS THE NORMAL DIET MODIFIED FOR THE DIABETIC PATIENT?

The diet for a diabetic patient represents the normal nutritionally adequate diet modified in protein, fat, and carbohydrate.

The calorie and protein content of the diabetic diet approximates the recommended normal dietary allowances with any adjustment in calories necessary to meet either overweight or underweight. The carbohydrate content is restricted, ranging from 100 to 300 grams. The protein content is figured on the basis of 1 to 1–1/2 grams per kilogram of body weight. The fat content is sufficient to meet the total calorie allowance, but restricted to prevent ketosis. The exact proportion between protein, carbohydrate, and fat is an individual problem and is adjusted by the physician according to the needs of his patient. The diet must be adequate in all other nutrients—minerals and vitamins.

WHAT ARE THE FOODS ALLOWED AND TO BE AVOIDED ON THE DIABETIC DIET?

Foods Allowed

All forms of milk, cheese, fats, meats, fish, poultry.

Eggs.

Clear soups and broths.

All vegetables: fresh, frozen, canned, raw, cooked, including potatoes.

All breads and cereals (except sugar-coated).

All fruits except those with added sugar.

Clear tea and coffee.

Unsweetened gelatin.

Pepper, spices, vinegar, lemons.

Unsweetened desserts or desserts sweetened with artificial sweeteners.

Foods to be Avoided

(or used, if at all, in very small amounts)

All forms of sugar (honey included).

Dried fruits (except those on Exchange List) and those prepared with sugar.

All sweetened desserts.

Dried vegetables and legumes (except those on Exchange List).

Soft drinks and alcoholic beverages.

Special "diabetic" foods.

Food mixtures unless composition is known.

HOW IS THE DIABETIC DIET PRESCRIPTION CALCULATED?

The diabetic diet prescription is calculated by the physician on the basis of the patient's nutritional requirements, sex, age, height and weight, activity, the severity of his diabetic condition, and the type and amount of insulin required. The physician will also determine the way the carbohydrate is to be distributed among the feedings of the day, depending upon the type of insulin, whether regular, crystalline, protamine zinc, globin, or Lente. With certain types of insulin, a feeding at bedtime may be required; with other types an additional afternoon feeding may be desirable. An example of the doctor's final diet prescription might be: protein 80 gm.; carbohydrate 180 gm.; fat 80 gm. The dietitian then translates the diet prescription into foods and meals.

HOW IS THE DIET PRESCRIPTION TRANSLATED INTO FOODS AND THE THREE MEALS OF THE DAY?

Early diets for diabetes were very carefully calculated, all foods weighed, and very little choice among foods was allowed. Today dietary treatment may start with weighed foods so the patient will become familiar with the size of food portions, but in most cases, the food for the diabetic patient is no longer exactly weighed. Instead, it is carefully measured and patients are taught to measure their diets. Detailed calculation of diets requires the use of extensive food value tables and lists of foods, particularly fruits and vegetables, classified according to carbohydrate content.

A simplified but moderately accurate method for calculating diets and planning meals for the diabetic patient was published in 1950, a joint project of the American Dietetic Association, American Diabetes Association, and the Diabetes Section of the U.S. Public Health Service. This method is based on the following six Food Exchange Lists. Foods in each list are grouped in terms of similarity in composition, and supply approximately the same amount of protein, fat, and carbohydrate. One serving of any food may be exchanged for another on the same list.[1] These Food Exchange Lists may also be used in the calculation of a diet in which one, two, or three of the nutrients—protein, fat, and carbohydrate—need to be controlled.

FOOD EXCHANGE LISTS

List 1. Milk Exchanges

One exchange of milk contains:
Carbohydrate—12 gm., Protein—8 gm.,
　　Fat—10 gm., Calories—170
*Milk, whole—plain or
　　homogenized　　　　　　　　1 cup

Milk, evaporated	1/2 cup
*Milk, powdered, whole	1/4 cup
*Buttermilk (whole milk)	1 cup
*Milk, skim	1 cup
*Add 2 fat exchanges if fat free	

---

[1] The Exchange Lists and the Composition of Food Exchanges are based on material in *Meal Planning with Exchange Lists* prepared by Committees of the American Diabetes Association, Inc., and The American Dietetic Association in cooperation with the Chronic Disease Program, Public Health Service, Department of Health, Education and Welfare. Food Exchange Lists and Meal Plan reprinted by permission.

FOOD EXCHANGE LISTS

List 2. Vegetable Exchanges A
These vegetables may be used as desired in ordinary amounts. Carbohydrate, protein and fat negligible. Servings: raw unlimited; cooked 1/2–1 cup.

Asparagus	*Greens:	Mushrooms
*Broccoli	Beets	Okra
*Brussels	Chard	*Pepper
Sprouts	Collard	Radishes
Cabbage	Dandelion	Sauerkraut
Cauliflower	Kale	String Beans,
Celery	Mustard	young
*Chicory	Spinach	Summer Squash
Cucumbers	Turnip	*Tomatoes
*Escarole		*Watercress
Eggplant		
Lettuce		

Vegetable Exchanges B
1 Serving = 1/2 cup = 100 grams.
Carbohydrate—7 gm., Protein—2 gm.,
Calories—35

Beets	Peas, green	*Squash, winter
*Carrots	*Pumpkin	Turnip
Onions	Rutabaga	

*High Vitamin A value. Use one daily.

List 3. Fruit Exchanges
One exchange of fruit contains:
Carbohydrate—10 gm., Calories—40
Fresh, dried, cooked, canned, frozen
   without sugar

Apple	1 sm. 2″ diam.
Applesauce	1/2 cup
Apricots, fresh	2 medium
Apricots, dried	4 halves
Banana	1/2 small
Berries; *Strawberries, Raspberries,	
Blackberries	1 cup
Raspberries	2/3 cup
Blueberries	2/3 cup
*Canteloup	1/4 (6″ diam.)
Cherries	10 large
Dates	2
Figs, fresh	2 large
Figs, dried	1 small
*Grapefruit	1/2 small
*Grapefruit Juice	1/2 cup
Grapes	12
Grape Juice	1/4 cup
Honeydew Melon	1/8 (7″ diam.)
Mango	1/2 small
*Orange	1 small
*Orange Juice	1/2 cup
Papaya	1/3 medium
Peach	1 medium
Pear	1 small
Pineapple	1/2 cup
Pineapple Juice	1/3 cup
Plums	2 medium
Prunes, dried	2 medium
Raisins	2 tbsp.
*Tangerine	1 large
Watermelon	1 cup

*High Vitamin C value.

List 4. Bread Exchanges
One bread exchange contains: Carbohydrate—15 gm.,
Protein—2 gm., Calories—70

	Meas.		Meas.
Bread	1 slice	Vegetables	
Biscuit, Roll (2″ diam.)	1	Beans and Peas, dried,	
Muffin (2″ diam.)	1	cooked (lima, navy,	1/2 cup
Cornbread (1½″ cube)	1	split pea, cowpeas, etc.)	
Flour	2½ tbsp.	Baked Beans, no pork	1/4 cup
Cereal, cooked	1/2 cup	Corn	1/3 cup
Cereal, dry (flake, puffed)	3/4 cup	Popcorn	1 cup
Rice, Grits, cooked	1/2 cup	Parsnips	2/3 cup
Spaghetti, Noodles, etc.		Potatoes, white,	
cooked	1/2 cup	baked, boiled	1 (2″ diam.)

FOOD EXCHANGE LISTS

Crackers,

Graham (2½″ sq.)	2
Oyster	20 (1/2 cup)
Saltines (2″ sq.)	5
Soda (2½″ sq.)	3
Round, thin (1½″ diam.)	6 to 8

Potatoes, white, mashed	1/2 cup
Potatoes, sweet, or Yams	1/4 cup
Sponge Cake, plain (1 ½″ cube)	1
Ice Cream (Omit 2 fat exchanges)	1/2 cup

List 5. Meat Exchanges

One meat exchange contains:
Protein—7 gm., Fat—5 gm., Calories—75

Meat and Poultry (med. fat) (beef, lamb, pork, liver, chicken, etc.)	1 oz.
Cold Cuts (4 ½″ × ⅛″ thick)	1 slice
Frankfurter (8 to 9/lb.)	1
Fish: Cod, Mackerel, etc.	1 oz.
Salmon, Tuna, Crab	1/4 cup
Oysters, Shrimp, Clams	5 small
Sardines	3 med.
Cheese, cheddar, American	1 oz.
Cottage	1/4 cup
Egg	1
Peanut Butter*	2 tbsp.

* Limit use or adjust carbohydrate.

List 6. Fat Exchanges

One fat exchange equals:
Fat—5 gm., Calories—45

Butter or Margarine	1 tsp.
Bacon, crisp	1 slice
Cream, light, 20%	2 tbsp.
Cream, heavy, 40%	1 tbsp.
Cream Cheese	1 tbsp.
French Dressing	1 tbsp.
Mayonnaise	1 tsp.
Oil or Cooking Fat	1 tsp.
Nuts	6 small
Olives	5 small
Avocado	1/8 (4″ diam.)

Composition of Food Exchanges

List	Food	Meas.	gm.	C	P	F	Cal.
1	Milk Exchanges	1/2 pint	240	12	8	10	170
2a	Vegetable Exchange	as desired					
2b	Vegetable Exch.	1/2 cup	100	7	2	—	35
3	Fruit Exch.	varies	—	10	-	—	40
4	Bread Exch.	varies	—	152	—		70
5	Meat Exchanges	1 oz.	30	—	7	5	75
6	Fat Exchanges	1 tsp.	5	—	-	5	45

Foods Allowed as Desired

Negligible Carbohydrate, Protein and Fat

Vegetables, List 2A

Coffee	Rhubarb (unsweetened)
Tea	Mustard
Clear Broth	Pickle, sour
Bouillon (fat free)	Pickle, dill— unsweetened
Gelatin, unsweetened	Saccharine
Rennet Tablets	Pepper
Cranberries (no sugar)	Spices
Lemon	Vinegar

With the use of the preceding Food Exchange Lists the dietitian converts a diet prescription into the foods for the day and then into three meals. An example of a diet prescription with its foods for the day follows.

FOOD EXCHANGE LISTS

Diet Prescription			*Foods for the Day*	
Carbohydrate	180 grams	1 pint	Milk	List 1
Protein	80 grams	any amount	Vegetable Exchanges	List 2A
Fat	80 grams	1	Vegetable Exchanges	List 2B
Calories	1800	3	Fruit Exchanges	List 3
		8	Bread Exchanges	List 4
		7	Meat Exchanges	List 5
		5	Fat Exchanges	List 6

HOW IS THE TOTAL AMOUNT OF FOOD FOR THE DAY DIVIDED INTO MEALS?

In distributing the food for the day among the various meals for the diabetic it is necessary to take into consideration his usual meal patterns, the particular conditions associated with the disease, and also the type of insulin which the physician has prescribed for him. For this reason, it is well for the dietitian to work out a food plan *with* the patient. The carbohydrate will be distributed among the day's meals (and snacks, if any) according to the type of insulin prescribed—fast or slow-acting insulin by hypodermic injections or oral hypoglycemic agents, in another manner for the diet of the patient who requires no insulin—and urine sugar tests. Some good source of protein will be included in each meal. The fat will be fairly evenly distributed among the meals. The distribution of the foods for the diabetic diet prescription above, and menus (from "Meal Planning with Exchange Lists")[2] follow. This plan is one of nine meal plans for diabetic diets at varying levels of calories, carbohydrate, protein, and fat developed by the American Dietetic Association and the American Diabetes Association. Plans are also available for diabetic patients who require a sodium-restricted diet or a fat-controlled diet or a bland, low-fiber diabetic diet.

Plan No. 3

Meal Plan[2]	*Sample Menu*
Break- 1 Fruit Exchange from List 3	This menu shows one of the ways Ex-
fast: 1 Meat Exchange from List 5	change Lists can be used in plan-
2 Bread Exchanges from List 4	ning the day's meals.
2 Fat Exchanges from List 6	Breakfast:
Coffee or Tea (any amount)	Orange Juice—1/2 cup
Lunch 2 Meat Exchanges from List 5	Egg—1
or 2 Bread Exchanges from List 4	Toast—2 slices
Supper: Vegetable from List 2A	Butter—2 teaspoons
(any amount)	Coffee—2 tablespoons Evaporated
1 Fruit Exchange from List 3	Milk**
1 cup Milk from List 1*	Lunch or Supper:

---

[2] From *Meal Planning with Exchange Lists*, Chicago, American Dietetic Association. Reprinted by permission.

* Part of milk may be used for coffee, tea or for cereal.

** 2 tablespoons evaporated milk equal 1/4 cup whole milk. Part of the milk is taken from bedtime to use at breakfast.

Meal Plan	Sample Menu
1 Fat Exchange from List 6	Ham and Cheese Sandwich
Coffee or Tea (any amount)	(Cheese—1 ounce,
Dinner 3 Meat Exchanges from List 5	Ham—1 ounce,
or 2 Bread Exchanges from List 4	Bread—2 slices,
Main Vegetable from List 2A	Butter—1 teaspoon)

Dinner
or
Main
Meal:

1 Fat Exchange from List 6
Coffee or Tea (any amount)
3 Meat Exchanges from List 5
2 Bread Exchanges from List 4
Vegetable from List 2A
    (any amount)
1 Vegetable Exchange from
    List 2B
1 Fruit Exchange from List 3
2 Fat Exchanges from List 6
Coffee or Tea (any amount)

Bedtime: 1 cup Milk from List 1*
    2 Bread Exchanges from List 4
    1 Meat Exchange from List 5

Ham and Cheese Sandwich
  (Cheese—1 ounce,
  Ham—1 ounce,
  Bread—2 slices,
  Butter—1 teaspoon)
Lettuce and Tomato Salad, Salad
  Dressing (zero)***
Apple—1 small
Milk—1 cup (8 ounces)
Coffee or Tea
Dinner:
  Hamburger Patties—3 ounces
  Mashed Potato—1/2 cup
  Carrots—1/2 cup Spinach
  Bread—1 slice   Butter—2
  Banana—1/2 small teaspoons
  Coffee or Tea
Bedtime:
  Milk—3/4 cup (6 ounces)**
  Peanut Butter Sandwich
  (Peanut Butter—2 tablespoons
  Bread—2 slices)

CONSIDERATIONS IN PLANNING THE DIABETIC DIET AND INSTRUCTING THE PATIENT REGARDING IT

Planning

Diabetic diet and meals must be adapted to patient's way of living.

Diet must fit in with family menus and cultural preferences.

Diet must take into account:
Age
Patient's religious, social and cultural customs.
Economic status.
Food habits of family.
Occupation and whether a lunch is carried.
Idiosyncrasies, likes and dislikes.
Any other pathological condition present.
Ability of patient to interpret the diet.
Diet must satisfy appetite and be appealing as well as meet nutritional demands.

"Diabetic Foods"

Expensive and composition is variable.

Question whether they add anything in the way of palatability and interest not obtainable with good food well prepared.

Undesirable psychologically as they make the diabetic patient "different."

Diabetic should eat the same foods as the family except food mixtures of unknown compositions.

Flavor usually disappointing.

Diabetic diet should not be considered a "special" diet.

Artificial sweetening agents allowable.

Packaging may be misleading.

Important Points in Teaching Patient About Diet

Cooperation of patient is essential.

*** Made with 1/2 cup tomato juice, 2 tablespoons lemon juice or vinegar, 1 tablespoon chopped onion salt and pepper. Use in any amount.

Instruction and methods must be adapted to patient's intelligence and background.

Patient needs to know: reasons for diet; size of servings; what substitutions he can make in diet.

Instruction must be simple but carefully given.

Importance of watching weight and not overeating.

Adjust diet instruction to whether or not patient can and will use recipes.

Good understanding of foods patient may eat and those he may not eat.

Modifications of Diabetic Diet

Caloric modification.

Bland, low-residue diabetic diet.

Semi-liquid diabetic diet preoperatively and postoperatively.

Sodium-restricted diabetic diet.

Fat controlled diabetic diet.

MATERIALS FOR TEACHING DIABETICS

Prepared by Committees of the American Dietetic Association and the American Diabetes Association, Inc. in cooperation with Diabetes Branch, U.S. Public Health Service. Available from the American Dietetic Association, Chicago.

Meal Planning with Exchange Lists
Diabetic Diet Card for Physicians
A.D.A. Meal Plans 1 through 9 (Meal Plan No. 3 shown on page 224)
Diabetes Guide Book for the Physician
Sodium-restricted Diabetic Diet Modification
Bland, Low-Fiber Diabetic Diet Modification
Fat-Controlled Diabetic Diet Modification

Available from the Diabetes Branch, U. S. Public Health Service: Film strip on the use of Exchange Lists and the teaching of the diabetic.

Diabetic Recipes

General References, page 291: Cooper, Krause, Robinson (Proudfit-Robinson)

Behrman, Des. M., *A Cookbook for Diabetics,* Chicago, The American Dietetic Association.

ACTIVITIES

Have individual class members or the class as a whole observe the meals served a diabetic patient for one day and learn about the insulin given: type, dosage, etc.

Have class members observe instruction to diabetic patient about his diet given by the nurse or dietitian.

SUPPLEMENTARY READING

Howe: Pages 205–206; 406–411   Mowry: Chapter 21   Peyton: Chapter 24
Robinson: Chapter 22

Unit Four

DIET IN CARDIOVASCULAR AND RENAL DISEASES

PART 1. DIET IN ATHEROSCLEROSIS

PART 2. DIET IN CARDIAC DISORDERS AND HYPERTENSION

PART 3. DIET IN KIDNEY DISORDERS

Object

To understand the relation of diet to atherosclerosis, cardiac disorders and kidney disorders and how the basic normal diet is modified for therapeutic treatment.

PART 1. DIET IN ATHEROSCLEROSIS

(Diet Modification: *Fat-Controlled Diet*)

WHAT ARE THE MEANING, CHARACTERISTICS, AND FACTORS IN DEVELOPMENT OF ATHEROSCLEROSIS?

Meaning. Atherosclerosis is a complex disease of the arteries—a form of arteriosclerosis or hardening of the arteries.

Atherosclerosis is thought to be cause of heart attack (coronary thrombosis or myocardial infarction, or plain "coronary").

Characteristics. Passageway through arteries becomes roughened and narrowed by fatty deposits so blood can not flow freely.

Factors In Development[1]

The American Heart Association lists the following factors associated with the increase in atherosclerosis:[1]

1. A familial history of coronary heart disease; the presence of diabetes mellitus, hyperlipidemia, gout, hypertension, obesity, and certain personality characteristics.

2. Sex and age: Men are generally more susceptible than women; both become increasingly susceptible with advancing years.

---

[1] Diet and Heart Disease, Statement, New York, American Heart Association, 1968, pp. 1–2.

3. Environmental factors such as a diet rich in saturated fat and cholesterol, cigarette smoking, and habitual physical inactivity.

It has become increasingly evident that the early identification and correction of the above risk factors may favorably influence the course of the disease. Repeated documentation shows a lower frequency of coronary disease in populations with lower cholesterol concentrations in their serum. Evidence now indicates that avoidance of prolonged elevations of serum cholesterol can decrease the hazard of developing premature coronary disease.

"It has already been shown that in most (but not all) persons, elevated concentrations of cholesterol in the serum can be decreased significantly and can be maintained at a lower level by conscientious adherence to a nutritionally sound, modified fat diet. It has been suggested, but it has not been proven, that this type of diet will minimize the progressive rise in serum cholesterol concentration that generally occurs in most adults."

WHAT DIETARY MEASURES DOES THE HEART ASSOCIATION SUGGEST TO REDUCE RISK OF HEART ATTACK?[2]

"In general, a diet designed to decrease the risk of coronary disease involves the following recommendations:

1. A calorie intake adjusted to achieve and maintain proper weight. Obesity is statistically associated with both hypertension and diabetes, and secondarily, with coronary heart disease. Correction of obesity may also reduce serum lipid concentration.

2. A decrease in the intake of saturated fats which studies show elevate serum cholesterol and an increase in the intake of polyunsaturated fats which studies show lower serum cholesterol. This will lower increased serum cholesterol concentration in most people. The ideal quantity of dietary fat is not known, but an intake of less than 40% of calories is considered desirable with polyunsaturated fats probably comprising twice the quantity of saturated fats (2:1) ratio.

3. A substantial reduction of cholesterol in the diet to less than 300 gm. daily being recommended, for hypercholesteremic individuals. A sharp reduction has been found to lower serum cholesterol in most people. The average daily diet in the United States contains approximately 600 gm. of cholesterol. Cholesterol is abundant in many protein foods of high biological quality, so careful planning is necessary to lower cholesterol intake without impairing intake of high protein foods.

4. Possible role of other dietary factors: simple sugars versus complex carbohydrates, alcohol, coffee, artificial sweeteners (cyclamates and saccharin), all under study but evidence incomplete. Dependence on foods as vegetables, cereals and fruits to supply dietary carbohydrates is preferable to excessive use of sugar, including candy, soft drinks, and other sweets."

HOW CAN DIET INTAKE OF CHOLESTEROL-RICH FOODS AND AMOUNT AND TYPE OF FAT BE CONTROLLED?[3]

1. Eat no more than three egg yolks a week, including eggs in cooking.
2. Limit your use of shellfish and organ meats.

---

[2] Ibid., pp. 2–3
[3] *The Way to a Man's Heart*, New York, American Heart Association, 1971. pp. 4–5.

3. In most of your meals for the week, use fish, chicken, turkey and veal; and limit beef, lamb, pork and ham to five moderate-sized portions a week.

4. Avoid deep fat frying; use cooking methods that help remove fat—baking, broiling, roasting, stewing.

5. Restrict your use of fatty "luncheon" and variety meats like sausages and salami.

6. Instead of butter and other cooking fats that are solid or completely hydrogenated, use liquid vegetable oils and margarines that are rich in polyunsaturated fats.

7. Instead of whole milk and cheese made from whole milk, use skimmed milk and skimmed milk cheeses. Margarines high in polyunsaturates usually can be identified by the listing of a "liquid oil" first among the ingredients. Margarines and shortenings that are heavily saturated or contain coconut oil, which is quite saturated, are ineffective in lowering serum cholesterol; they may also raise serum cholesterol.

Remember also: (1) To meet your daily needs for protein, vitamins, minerals and other nutrients (2) To control calories and maintain a desirable weight (3) To avoid eating excessive amounts of foods containing saturated fat and cholesterol, by lowering your total intake of such foods (4) To see that more of the fat you eat is polyunsaturated, and less of it saturated."

WHAT IS A FAT-CONTROLLED, LOW-CHOLESTEROL MEAL PLAN?[4]

> Every day, select foods from each of the basic food groups in lists 1–5, and follow the recommendations for number and size of servings.

1 MEAT POULTRY FISH DRIED BEANS and PEAS NUTS - EGGS

1 serving...
    3-4 ounces of cooked meat or fish (not including bone or fat) or 3-4 ounces of a vegetable listed here

Use 2 or more servings (a total of 6-8 ounces) daily

RECOMMENDED

Chicken • turkey • veal • fish • in most of your meat meals for the week.

Shellfish: clams • crab • lobster • oysters • scallops • shrimp • are low in fat but high in cholesterol. Use a 4-ounce serving in a meat meal no more than twice a week.

Beef • lamb • pork • ham • in no more than 5 meals per week.

Choose lean ground meat and lean cuts of meat • trim all visible fat before cooking • bake, broil, roast, or stew so that you can discard the fat which cooks out of the meat.

Nuts and dried beans and peas:

Kidney beans • lima beans • baked beans • lentils • chick peas (garbanzos) • split peas • are high in vegetable protein and may be used in place of meat occasionally.

Egg whites as desired.

AVOID OR USE SPARINGLY

Duck • goose

Heavily marbled and fatty meats • spare ribs • mutton • frankfurters • sausages • fatty hamburgers • bacon • luncheon meats.

Organ meats: liver • kidney • heart • sweetbreads • are very high in cholesterol. Since liver is very rich in vitamins and iron, it should not be eliminated from the diet completely. Use a 4-ounce serving in a meat meal no more than once a week.

Egg yolks: limit to 3 per week including eggs used in cooking.

Cakes, batters, sauces, and other foods containing egg yolks.

[4] *The Way to a Man's Heart,* New York, American Heart Association, 1971.

2 VEGETABLES and FRUIT

(Fresh, frozen, or canned)

1 serving ... ½ cup
Use at least 4 servings daily

RECOMMENDED

One serving should be a source of Vitamin C:
Broccoli • cabbage (raw) • tomatoes.
Berries • cantaloupe • grapefruit (or juice) • mango • melon • orange (or juice) • papaya • strawberries • tangerines.

One serving should be a source of Vitamin A—dark green leafy or yellow vegetables, or yellow fruits:
Broccoli • carrots • chard • chicory • escarole • greens (beet, collard, dandelion, mustard, turnip) • kale • peas • rutabagas • spinach • string beans • sweet potatoes and yams • watercress • winter squash • yellow corn.
Apricots • cantaloupe • mango • papaya.

Other vegetables and fruits are also very nutritious; they should be eaten in salads, main dishes, snacks, and desserts, *in addition* to the recommended daily allowances of high vitamin A and C vegetables and fruits. If you must limit your calories, use a serving of potatoes, yellow corn, or fresh or frozen cooked lima beans in place of a bread serving.

AVOID OR USE SPARINGLY

Olives and avocados are very high in fat calories and should be used in moderation.

If you must limit your calories, use vegetables such as potatoes, corn, or lima beans sparingly. To add variety to your diet, one serving (½ cup) of any one of these may be substituted for one serving of bread or cereals.

3 BREAD and CEREALS

(Whole grain, enriched, or restored)

1 serving of bread ... 1 slice
1 serving of cereal ...
   ½ cup, cooked
   1 cup, cold,
   with skimmed milk
Use at least 4 servings daily

RECOMMENDED

Breads made with a minimum of saturated fat:
White enriched (including raisin bread) • whole wheat • English muffins • French bread • Italian bread • oatmeal bread • pumpernickel • rye bread.

Biscuits, muffins, and griddle cakes made at home, using an allowed liquid oil as shortening.

Cereal (hot and cold) • rice • melba toast • matzo • pretzels.

Pasta: macaroni • noodles (except egg noodles) • spaghetti.

AVOID OR USE SPARINGLY

Butter rolls • commercial biscuits, muffins, donuts, sweet rolls, cakes, crackers • egg bread, cheese bread commercial mixes containing dried eggs and whole milk.

4 MILK PRODUCTS

1 serving ... 8 ounces (1 cup)
Buy only skimmed milk that has been fortified with Vitamins A and D.
Daily servings:
Children up to 12 ...
   3 or more cups
Teenagers ...
   4 or more cups
Adults ...
   2 or more cups

RECOMMENDED

Milk products that are low in dairy fats:

Fortified skimmed (non-fat) milk and fortified skimmed milk powder • low-fat milk. The label on the container should show that the milk is fortified with Vitamins A and D. The word "fortified" alone is not enough.

Buttermilk made from skimmed milk • yogurt made from skimmed milk • canned evaporated skimmed milk • cocoa made with low-fat milk.

Cheeses made from skimmed or partially skimmed milk, such as cottage cheese, creamed or uncreamed (uncreamed, preferably) • farmer's, baker's, or hoop cheese • mozarella and sapsago cheeses made with partially skimmed milk.

AVOID OR USE SPARINGLY

Whole milk and whole milk products:

Chocolate milk • canned whole milk • ice cream • all creams including sour, half and half, whipped • whole milk yogurt.

Non-dairy cream substitutes (usually contain coconut oil which is very high in saturated fat).

Cheeses made from cream or whole milk.

Butter.

5 FATS and OILS
(Polyunsaturated)

An individual allowance should include about 2-4 tablespoons daily (depending on how many calories you can afford) in the form of margarine, salad dressing, and shortening.

RECOMMENDED

Margarines, liquid oil shortenings, salad dressings and mayonnaise containing any of these polyunsaturated vegetable oils:

Corn oil • cottonseed oil • safflower oil • sesame seed oil • soybean oil • sunflower seed oil.

Margarines and other products high in polyunsaturates can usually be identified by their label which lists a recommended *liquid* vegetable oil as the *first* ingredient, and one or more partially hydrogenated vegetable oils as additional ingredients.

Diet margarines are low in calories because they are low in fat. Therefore it takes twice as much diet margarine to supply the polyunsaturates contained in a recommended margarine.

AVOID OR USE SPARINGLY

Solid fats and shortenings:

Butter • lard • salt pork fat • meat fat • completely hydrogenated margarines and vegetable shortenings • products containing coconut oil.

Peanut oil and olive oil may be used occasionally for flavor, but they are low in polyunsaturates and do not take the place of the recommended oils.

6 DESSERTS BEVERAGES SNACKS CONDIMENTS

The foods on this list are acceptable because they are low in saturated fat and cholesterol. If you have eaten your daily allowance from the first five lists, however, these foods will be in excess of your nutritional needs, and many of them also may exceed your calorie limits for maintaining a desirable weight. If you must limit your calories, limit your portions of the foods on this list as well.

Moderation should be observed especially in the use of alcoholic drinks, ice milk, sherbet, sweets, and bottled drinks.

ACCEPTABLE

Low in calories or no calories

Fresh fruit and fruit canned without sugar • tea, coffee (no cream), cocoa powder • water ices • gelatin • fruit whip • puddings made with non-fat milk • sweets and bottled drinks made with artificial sweeteners • vinegar, mustard, ketchup, herbs, spices.

High in calories

Frozen or canned fruit with sugar added • jelly, jam, marmalade, honey • pure sugar candy such as gum drops, hard candy, mint patties (not chocolate) • imitation ice cream made with safflower oil • cakes, pies, cookies, and puddings made with polyunsaturated fat in place of solid shortening • angel food cake • nuts, especially walnuts • non-hydrogenated peanut butter • bottled drinks • fruit drinks • ice milk • sherbet • wine, beer, whiskey.

AVOID OR USE SPARINGLY

Coconut and coconut oil • commercial cakes, pies, cookies, and mixes • frozen cream pies • commercially fried foods such as potato chips and other deep fried snacks • whole milk puddings • chocolate pudding (high in cocoa butter and therefore high in saturated fat) • ice cream.

The American Heart Association, 44 East 23rd Street, New York, New York 10010, has prepared and published two booklets on the planning of fat-controlled, low cholesterol diets (available to patients, on doctor's prescription only): (1) *Planning Fat-Controlled Meals for 1200 and 1800 Calories,* revised 1970; and (2) *Planning Fat-Controlled Meals for Approximately 2000-2600 Calories,* 1970. Also available for the general public, no prescription required, are the following leaflets: (1) The Way to a Man's Heart—a fat-controlled, low-cholesterol meal plan to reduce the risk of heart attack, 1971; (2) Diet and Heart Disease Statement 1968; (3) Eat Well But Wisely—to reduce your risk of heart attack, 1970; and (4) Recipes for Fat-controlled, Low-cholesterol Meals 1969.

WHAT ARE DIET PLANS FOR 1200 AND 1800 CALORIE FAT-CONTROLLED MEALS?[5]

Foods you should have each day on 1200-calorie diet[5]	Foods you should have each day on 1800-calorie diet[5]	In following your diet . . .
1 pint of *Skim Milk*	1 pint of *Skim Milk*	Use skim milk, nonfat dry milk powder, or buttermilk made from skim milk.
3 or more servings of *Vegetables*	3 or more servings of *Vegetables*	Use any vegetables or vegetable juices you wish, since they contain little or no fat. At least 1 serving a day should be a yellow or a leafy green vegetable. (A few vegetables—dried peas and beans, corn, and potatoes—have many more calories than other vegetables. For this reason they are grouped with breads and cereals and should not be counted as part of your vegetable servings.)
3 servings of *Fruit*	3 servings of *Fruit*	Use medium size servings of any kind of fresh or canned unsweetened fruit or fruit juice you wish. The only exception is avocado, which contains fat. At least one serving a day should be a citrus fruit or juice—orange, grapefruit, tangerine.
4 servings of *Breads and Cereals*	7 servings of *Breads and Cereals*	Use breads, cereals, and the high-calorie vegetables from the *Breads and Cereals List.*
6 ounces (cooked) of *Meat, Fish, or Poultry*	6 ounces (cooked) of *Meat, Fish, or Poultry*	Use the kinds and amounts of meat, fish, poultry, and meat substitutes specified on the *Meat, Fish and Poultry List.*
Use no more than 3 egg yolks each week (or less, depending on advice from doctor)	Use no more than 3 egg yolks each week (or less, depending on advice from doctor)	Count the egg yolks used in cooking as well as those you eat at the table. Egg whites need not be counted or limited.
2 level tablespoons of *Fat* (1 teaspoon of this may be special margarine or shortening)	4 level tablespoons of *Fat* (1 tablespoon of this may be special margarine or shortening)	Use only the oils and fats given on the *Fat List.* Be sure to use your full allowance each day.
1 serving of *Sugars or Sweets* allowed only if substitute for one serving Breads and Cereals	2 servings of *Sugars and sweets*	Use sugars, sweets, and desserts from the *Sugars and Sweets List.*

[5] *Planning Fat-Controlled Meals for 1200 and 1800 Calories.* New York, New York, The American Heart Association, 1970, pages 8–9, adapted.

WHAT FOODS ARE ALLOWED ON THE LOW-CALORIE FAT-CONTROLLED DIETS?[6]

Foods are selected from the following lists. The number of servings allowed daily and sample menus for each diet are given on pages 235–237. Avoid foods not on this list.

Breads and Cereals List

Any one of the following is a serving:

Breads, Rolls, Cereals, etc.:

1 slice bread (white, whole wheat, rye, pumpernickel, French, Italian or Boston brown bread)

1 roll (2 to 3 inches across)

1 home-made biscuit or muffin (2 to 3 inches across)

1 square of home-made cornbread (1½ inches)

1 griddlecake (4 inches across), made with skim milk and with allowed fat or oil from day's allowance

1/2 cup cooked cereal

3/4 cup dry cereal

1/2 cup cooked rice, grits, or hominy, barley or buckwheat groats

1/2 cup cooked spaghetti, noodles, or macaroni

1/4 cup dry bread crumbs

3 tablespoons flour

2½ tablespoons corn meal

4 pieces Melba toast (3½ × 1½ ×1/8″)

1 piece matzo (5 × 5″)

3/4 oz. bread sticks, rye wafers, pretzels

1½ cups popcorn (popped at home with fat or oil from day's allowance)

Use biscuits, muffins, griddle cakes, cornbread, corn muffins only if made at home from daily allowed fat or oil, counting the amount as part of daily fat allowance.

Vegetables:

1/2 cup cooked dried peas, or beans, lentils, chick peas

1/3 cup corn, kernels or cream style

1 ear corn on the cob (4 inches long)

1 small white potato

1/4 cup sweet potato, cooked

Meat, Fish, and Poultry List

Choose only lean cuts of meat and trim off all visible fat.

Make selections from this list for 11 of the 14 *main meals* each week:

Poultry (without skin)—chicken, turkey, cornish hen, squab

Fish—any kind (not shellfish)

Veal—any lean cut

Or you may choose any of these:

Cottage cheese, preferably uncreamed

Yogurt, from partially skimmed milk

Dried peas, beans, etc.

Peanut butter

Nuts, especially walnuts

Make selections from this list for the other 3 meals. (Limit servings to 3 ounces.)

Beef:

Hamburger—ground round or chuck

Roasts, pot roasts, stew meats—sirloin tip, round, rump, chuck, arm

Steaks—flank, sirloin, T-bone, porterhouse, tenderloin, round, cube

Soup meats—shank or shin

Other—dried chipped beef

Lamb:

Roasts or steak—leg

Chops—loin, rib, shoulder

Pork:

Roast—loin, center cut ham

Chops—loin

Tenderloin

Ham:

Baked, center cut steaks, picnic, butt, Canadian bacon

---

[6] Ibid., pages 10–13.

Fats and Oils

You may use any of the following poly-unsaturated vegetable oils and salad dressings on your diet:

>Corn oil
>Cottonseed oil
>Peanut oil (in place of special margarine or shortening only)
>Safflower oil
>Sesame seed oil
>Soybean oil
>Sunflower seed oil
>Mayonnaise (1 teaspoon of mayonnaise equals 1 teaspoon of oil)
>French dressing made with allowed oil (1 ½ teaspoons of dressing equals 1 teaspoon of oil)

You may also use a limited amount of special margarine or shortening as part of the fats and oils allowance.

Sugars and Sweets List

The following sugars, other sweeteners, and desserts are allowed. A serving is 1 tablespoon of sugar or other sweetener, or the amount given for each dessert listed.

Sugars and Other Sweeteners:
White, brown, or maple sugar
Corn syrup or maple syrup
Honey
Molasses
Jelly, Jam, or marmalade

Desserts:
(Each serving listed contains about the same number of calories as 1 tablespoon of sugar—about 50 calories.
All desserts except the one marked *are fat-free.)

>1/4 cup tapioca or cornstarch pudding made with fruit and fruit juice (such as apple, cherry, pineapple) or with skim milk from milk allowance
>1/4 cup fruit whip (such as prune or apricot)
>1/3 cup gelatin dessert
>1/4 cup sherbet (preferably water ice)
>1/3 cup sweetened canned or frozen fruit (sweetened fruit equals 1 portion of fruit and 1 tablespoon of sugar)
>1 small slice angel food cake
>*2 sugar cookies
>3 cornflake and nut meringues
>3/4 cup (6 ounces) sweetened carbonated beverage
>2/3 cup cocoa (not chocolate) made with skim milk from milk allowance
>Candies: 3 medium or 14 small gum drops; 3 marshmallows; 4 hard fruit drops; 2 mint patties (no chocolate)

*Count the fat as part of your daily allowance.

FOODS TO AVOID[7]

These are the foods that are not allowed on your diet—because they contain too much fat, the wrong kind of fat, or too much cholesterol.

Do Not Use

Meats

Beef high in fat or "marbled"
Lamb high in fat

Pork high in fat
Bacon, salt pork, spareribs

---

[7] Ibid., p.14.

Meats

Frankfurters, sausage, cold cuts

Canned meats

Organ meats such as kidney, brain, sweetbread,* liver*

Any visible fat from meat

Poultry and Fish

Skin of chicken or turkey

Duck and goose

Fish roe (including caviar)

Fish canned in olive oil

Shellfish (shrimp, crab, lobster, clams, etc.)*

Dairy Foods

Whole milk, homogenized milk canned milk

Sweet cream, powdered cream

Ice cream unless homemade with nonfat dry milk powder

Sour cream

Whole milk buttermilk and whole milk yogurt

Butter

Cheese made from whole milk

Fat and Oils

Butter

Ordinary margarines

Ordinary solid shortenings

Lard

Salt pork

Chicken fat

Coconut oil

Olive oil

Chocolate

Breads and Bakery Goods

Commercial biscuits, muffins, cornbreads, griddlecakes, waffles, cookies, crackers

Mixes for biscuits, muffins, and cakes (except angel food)

Coffee cakes, cakes (except angel food), pies, sweet rolls, doughnuts, and pastries

Desserts

Puddings, custards, and ice creams unless homemade with skim milk or nonfat dry milk powder

Whipped cream desserts

Cookies unless homemade with allowed fat or oil

Miscellaneous

Sauces and gravies unless made with allowed fat or oil or made from skimmed stock

Commercially fried foods such as potato chips, French fried potatoes, fried fish

Cream soups and other creamed dishes

Frozen or packaged dinners

Olives

Macadamia nuts

Avocado

Chocolate

Candies made with chocolate, butter, cream, or coconut

Coconut

Foods made with egg yolk unless counted as part of your allowance

Fudge, chocolate

Commercial popcorn

Substitutes for coffee cream (usually contain saturated fats or hydrogenated vegetable oils)

* Except as a substitute for eggs.

SAMPLE MENUS FOR FAT-CONTROLLED DIETS[8]

1200 Calories	
Sample Menu # 1	*Sample Menu # 2*
Breakfast	*Breakfast*
Chilled half grapefruit	1/2 cup orange juice
3/4 cup dry cereal	2 plain muffins (special recipe)
1 cup skim milk	Coffee or tea

[8] Ibid., pp. 19–20.

1800 Calories

Sample Menu # 1	*Sample Menu # 2*

Breakfast

1 soft-boiled egg (optional)
1 slice toast
1 teaspoon special margarine
Coffee or tea

Breakfast

Lunch

Tomato stuffed with chicken (use 1 tomato; 1/2 cup diced chicken; 2 teaspoons mayonnaise; capers; parsley; celery; lettuce)
1 small hard roll
1 cup skim milk
1 small banana, sliced
Coffee or tea

Lunch

Open roast beef sandwich (use 2 very thin slices—2 ounces—lean roast beef; 1 slice bread)
1/2 cup cole slaw with 2 teaspoons mayonnaise
Sliced sour pickles
Melon or other fresh fruit in season
1 cup skim milk
Coffee or tea

Dinner

Baked fish fillet (3 ounces) with 1 teaspoon oil
Broccoli with 1 $\frac{1}{2}$ teaspoons. Hollandaise sauce (special recipe)
Scalloped tomatoes (use 1/2 cup canned tomatoes; 1 slice diced bread; 1 teaspoon oil; salt; pepper; basil)
1 fresh or canned pear (unsweetened)
Coffee or tea

Dinner

1/4 barbecued chicken—3 ounces—with 2 teaspoons oil (special recipe)
1 small ear corn
1/2 cup mixed carrots and peas
1/2 cup fresh fruit cup
1 cup skim milk
Coffee or tea

You may use these as desired: coffee, tea, coffee substitutes, unsweetened carbonated beverages, lemons and lemon juice, unsweetened gelatin, artificial sweeteners, fat-free consomme or bouillon, pickles, relishes, vinegar, mustard, catsup, and seasonings.

1800 Calories

Sample Menu #1	*Sample Menu #2*

Breakfast

Chilled half grapefruit
3/4 cup dry cereal
1 cup skim milk
1 soft-boiled egg (optional)
1 slice toast
1 teaspoon special margarine
1 tablespoon marmalade
1 tablespoon sugar for cereal, fruit, or beverage
Coffee or tea

Breakfast

1/2 cup orange juice
2 plain muffins (special recipe)
1 teaspoon special margarine
1 cup skim milk
Coffee or tea

Lunch

Tomato stuffed with chicken (use 1 tomato; 1/2 cup diced chicken; 2 tablespoons mayonnaise; capers; parsley; celery; lettuce)

1 large or 2 small hard rolls

2 teaspoons special margarine

1 cup skim milk

1 small banana, sliced

Coffee or tea

Dinner

Baked fish fillet (4 ounces) (use 1 teaspoon oil and 1/4 cup bread crumbs)

Broccoli with 1 $\frac{1}{2}$ teaspoons Hollandaise scace (special recipe)

Scalloped tomatoes (use $\frac{1}{2}$ cup canned tomatoes; 1 slice diced bread; 1 teaspoon oil; salt; pepper; basil)

1 baked potato

1 teaspoon special margarine

1 canned pear, sweetened, with syrup

Coffee or tea

Lunch

Roast beef sandwich (use 2 very thin slices—2 ounces—lean roast beef; 2 slices bread)

$\frac{1}{2}$ cup cole slaw with 2 teaspoons mayonnaise

Sliced sour pickles

Melon or other fresh fruit in season

1 cup skim milk

Cofffee or tea

Dinner

1/2 cup chilled fruit juice

1/3 barbecued chicken—3 ounces—with 2 teaspoons oil (special recipe)

2 small ears corn, or 1 large ear, with 2 teaspoons special margarine

$\frac{1}{2}$ cup mixed carrots and peas

Mixed green salad

1 tablespoon French dressing (special recipe)

1 slice French bread

$\frac{1}{2}$ cup sherbet

1 cup skim milk

Coffee or tea

SUPPLEMENTARY READING

Robinson: Pages 251–257

Howe: Pages 42–45

PART 2. DIET IN CARDIAC DISORDERS AND HYPERTENSION

(Diet Modification: *Sodium-Restricted Diet*)

WHAT ARE THE TYPES AND CAUSES OF CARDIAC DISORDERS?

Types. Acute or chronic. Extent of heart damage determines whether condition is *compensated*, with mild or slight damage, or *decompensated* (cardiac insufficiency) where there is severe damage. In diseases of the heart, one or several parts may be damaged:

muscle (myocardium)   blood vessels
outer covering (pericardium)   valves
lining (endocardium)

Causes

Organic	*Functional*
Congenital	Infections
Rheumatic fever	Inflammation
Arteriosclerosis with hypertension	Fatigue
Atherosclerosis	

WHAT ARE PRINCIPLES OF DIETARY TREATMENT FOR CARDIAC DISORDERS?

Acute. (Coronary Occlusion) Minimum nutritional requirements for short period followed by necessary dietary adjustments to meet all needs. Fluid, soft or general diet, depending on severity.

Chronic—Compensated. Normal circulation maintained by heart enlargement and increased pulse rate. Normal diet with following adjustments:

Low calories if patient is overweight to keep weight normal or slightly below normal and to lessen burden on heart.

Carbohydrates furnish bulk of calories.

Five to six small meals rather than three regular meals.

Indigestible, bulky, or gas-forming foods prohibited to prevent pressure on heart.

Limited stimulants (tea and coffee). Avoid very hot or very cold beverages.

Good choice of foods to prevent constipation.

Possible salt restriction if edema is a possibility.

Vitamins and minerals may be ordered in concentrated form.

Diet gradually increased.

Chronic—decompensated. Heart unable to maintain normal circulation (to carry oxygen and nutrients to tissues and waste products from tissues). Edema may be present as sodium and water are held in tissues. Possibly liver and kidney involvement.

More rigid diet to relieve strain and prevent further damage.

Calories to cause loss of overweight or maintain weight at normal or slightly below normal.

Carbohydrates used as chief source of calories because they are digested and leave stomach quickly.

Protein normal—1 gram per kilogram of body weight.

No bulky or gas-forming vegetables; easily digested foods.

Vitamin and mineral supplements may be ordered.

Small meals to prevent stomach pressure on heart.

Salt and fluid restriction as edema is usually present—adjusted to individual needs of patient. Diuretics may be part of the treatment.

Hypertension. (symptom accompanying cardiovascular and renal disease).

Low calorie diet or diet to maintain normal weight (obesity is a predisposing factor in hypertension).

Sodium restricted diet if hypertension accompanies cardiac disease.

Further adjustments in protein, salt, and fluids if there is kidney involvement.

WHAT ARE THE PURPOSES AND INDICATIONS FOR SODIUM-RESTRICTED DIETS?

Purposes	*Indications*
To aid the body in eliminating sodium and fluids (prevent edema) in disorders where there is abnormal retention.	Hypertension
	Congestive heart failure
	Renal disorders with edema
	Edema from any cause
To control sodium intake.	Toxemias of pregnancy
To relieve severely elevated blood pressure.	ACTH and cortisone therapy
	Cirrhosis of liver
	Meniere's disease

WHAT IS A SODIUM-RESTRICTED DIET?

A sodium-restricted is a normal adequate diet modified in sodium content, from a very low amount of 250 milligrams to 2000 milligrams or more.

An average diet prepared in the kichen with some commercially prepared foods, foods salted during cooking, and some salt added at the table, provides about 3000 to 7000 milligrams of sodium daily. For therapeutic purposes, sodium may vary from 250 milligrams daily to 2000 milligrams or more. Diets in which sodium is limited were formerly called "low-salt" diets when salt was omitted only in the preparation of food, and "salt-free" when it was allowed neither in cooking nor at the table. Such diets are now named in terms of the level of salt restriction, the most usual being the 500 milligram sodium diet (strict), the 1000 milligram sodium diet (moderate), and the 2400–4500 milligram sodium diet (mild restriction).

WHAT ARE SODIUM AND SALT AND WHERE ARE THEY FOUND?

Sodium (Na), an essential mineral nutrient required daily in a small but nutritionally significant amount, is found in nearly all plants and animals used as food. Salt or sodium chloride (NaCl) is nearly half sodium. An average healthy person receives more sodium through food and water than he requires, but the excess is excreted through the kidneys. In certain disorders water is retained in the body and some sodium along with it. A reduction of the sodium in the diet under these conditions helps the body to reduce its salt content to approximately the amount it needs daily. Sodium in food is naturally present or is added during processing, cooking, or both, usually as table salt or monosodium glutamate (MSG), both of which are high in Na. Foods labeled "low sodium" may still be high in Na for very restricted diets. The list below shows sources of sodium in the diet.[9]

Natural Sources of Na[10]

Small amounts: fruits.

Large amounts: meat, fish, poultry, milk, milk products, eggs. Canned, smoked, salted, seasoned meats.

Small to large amounts: vegetables.

Read labels for sodium in cereals (some have no added sodium).

High amounts: Average drinking waters, "Softened" waters.

Low amounts: Distilled water.

Sodium Compounds Added to Foods in Processing and Preparation[10]

Salt (sodium chloride)

Baking soda (sodium bicarbonate)

Brine (table salt and water)

Monosodium glutamate   Sodium alginate

Disodium phosphate   Sodium benzoate

Sodium hydroxide   Sodium sulfite

Sodium propionate   Baking powder

(read labels on processed foods)   Sodium saccharin

1 level tsp. salt (NaCl) contains about 2300 mg. Na.

1 level tsp. baking soda contains about 1000 mg. Na.

1 level tsp. regular baking powder contains about 370 mg. Na.

1 level tsp. monosodium glutamate contains 750 mg. Na.

Medicines and Dentifrices[10]

"Alkalizers"

Antibiotics

Cough medicines

Laxatives

Pain relievers

Sedatives

Tooth pastes and powders

Mouth washes (read label)

HOW DO SODIUM-RESTRICTED DIETS DIFFER AT THE VARIOUS SODIUM LEVELS?[11]

2400–4500 mg. Na Diet (Mild restriction)

No salt at table.

Only light salting of food during cooking. About half as much salt as most people are ac-

1000 mg. Na Diet (Moderate restriction)

Small amount of salt each day, either in cooking or at the table; alternatives: either add 1/4 *level* teaspoon *only*

500 mg. Na Diet (Strict restriction)

Limited quantities of foods with natural sodium.

See following menus

The use of low-sodium

---

[9] Your 500 Milligram Sodium Diet, New York, The American Heart Association, 1970, p. 8, adapted.

[10] Ibid., p. 8–9, 10, adapted, and booklet.

[11] Three Sodium-Restricted Diet Books, American Heart Association.

customed to is about right.

Canned and processed foods are already lightly salted.

No foods that are very salty, that are preserved in salt or brine.

No monosodium glutamate or soy sauce to be added to foods.

Check with doctor about any unprescribed medicines.

to the 500 mg. Na Diet to make it a 1000 mg. Na Diet or use regular bakery bread and some salted butter.

Drinking water if it contains no more than 5 mg. Na to each 8 oz. (otherwise, use distilled).

No "softened water" as it contains too much Na.

milk instead of regular milk will reduce amount of sodium to 250 mg.

Sodium restricted diets require careful planning to include just the right amounts of the foods permitted. The booklets available from local Heart Associations or the American Heart Association show the correct amounts of foods and sample menus for 500 milligram, 1000 milligram, and mild sodium restricted diets. A diet plan with foods to use and not to use for the 1800 calorie, 500 milligram sodium diet follows. On page 244 are shown two sets of menus for this diet plan. See page 245 for note about the American Dietetic Association's Na-restricted Diabetic Diet based on the Food Exchange Lists.

WHAT IS A DAILY DIET PLAN FOR A 500 MG. SODIUM-RESTRICTED, 1800 CALORIE DIET?[12]

FOLLOW THIS DIET EVERY DAY

Foods and Amounts	*Use*	*Do Not Use*
Milk 2 glasses Each glass contains about 170 calories, 120 mg. sodium. 1 glass milk = 8 oz. 1/2 cup evaporated milk = 1 glass milk.	Regular (whole) milk; evaporated milk; skim milk; powdered milk. If skim milk used, add 2 servings fat to diet for each glass milk. Substitute for not more than one glass milk a day: 2 oz. meat, poultry, or fish or 6 oz. yogurt 3/4 container). Count milk used in cooking from day's allowance. Check dairies for use of milk in buttermilk.	Ice cream; sherbet; malted milk; milk shake; instant cocoa mixes; chocolate milk; condensed milk; all other kinds of milk and fountain drinks. These foods are high in calories and the sodium content is unknown.
Meat, Poultry, Fish	Fresh, frozen, or dietetic	Brains or kidneys; canned,

---

[12] Sodium Restricted Diet—500 milligrams, Leaflet, New York, American Heart Association, 1969 centerfold, adapted.

Foods and Amounts	*Use*	*Do not Use*
5 oz. cooked Each oz. contains average of 75 calories, 25 mg. Na.	canned meat or poultry; beef; lamb; pork; veal; fresh tongue; liver; chicken; duck; turkey; rabbit. Fresh or dietetic (not frozen) fish: any kind except those listed at right. Substitutes for 1 oz. meat, poultry, fish: an egg (limit is 1 egg a day); 1/4 cup unsalted cottage cheese; 1 oz. low-sodium dietetic cheese; 2 tbsp. low-sodium dietetic peanut butter. Use beef liver not more than once in two weeks.	salted, or smoked meat (bacon, bologna, chipped or corned beef, frankfurters, ham, meats koshered by salting, luncheon meats, salt pork, sausage, smoked tongue). Frozen fish fillets: canned, salted, or smoked fish (anchovies, caviar, salted cod, herring, sardines); canned tuna or salmon unless low-sodium dietetic; shellfish (clams, crabs, lobsters, oysters, scallops, shrimp). Regular cheeses, peanut butter and salted cottage cheese.
Vegetables At least 3 servings Each starchy vegetable contains about 70 calories, 5 mg. sodium. Other vegetables contain from 5 to 35 calories, about 9 mg. sodium. Count as serving: about 1/2 cup vegetable.	Any fresh, frozen, or dietetic canned vegetables or vegetable juices, except those listed at right. Check label on frozen peas and lima beans—may have had salt or other sodium compound added during processing. Avoid ordering vegetables when eating out, because of salt and MSG additions.	Canned vegetables or vegetable juices unless low-sodium dietetic; frozen vegetables if processed with salt; the following vegetables in any form: artichokes, beet greens, beets, carrots, celery, chard, dandelion greens, whole hominy, kale, mustard greens, sauerkraut, spinach, white turnips.
Fruit At least 3 servings Each serving contains about 40 calories, 2 mg. sodium. Size of fruit serving varies, depending on the fruit and the calories.	Any kind of fruit or fruit juice—fresh, frozen, canned or dried—if sugar has not already been added. Substitute for fruit juice: low-sodium dietetic tomato juice. If you do want sweetened fruit or juice, add an allowed sugar substitute or the amount of sugar, honey, etc., allowed on list headed "And . . . take your choice."	Fruits canned or frozen in sugar syrup because of extra calories they contain.

Foods and Amounts	*Use*	*Do not Use*
Low-Sodium Breads, Cereals and Cereal Products 7 servings Each serving contains about 70 calories, 5 mg. sodium. 1 serving: 1 slice bread; 1 roll or muffin; 4 crackers or pieces melba toast; 1/2 cup cooked cereal, noodles, rice; 1 1/2 cups popcorn; 2 1/2 tablespoons flour.	Low-sodium bread, rolls, crackers; unsalted cooked cereals (farina, hominy grits, oatmeal, rolled wheat, wheat meal); dry cereals (puffed rice, puffed wheat, shredded wheat); plain unsalted matzo; unsalted melba toast; macaroni; noodles; spaghetti; rice; barley; unsalted popcorn; flour. Substitute for a serving of bread or cereal; a starchy vegetable.	Regular breads, crackers; commercial mixes; cooked cereals containing a sodium compound (read label); dry cereals other than those listed or those that have more than 6 mg. sodium in 100 gm. cereal (read label); self-rising corn meal or flour; potato chips; pretzels; salted popcorn.
Unsalted Fat 4 servings Each serving contains about 45 calories, practically no sodium. 1 serving: 1 teaspoon butter, margarine, fat, oil, mayonnaise; 1 tbsp heavy cream (sweet or sour); 2 tbsp light cream; 1 tbsp. French dressing; 6 small nuts; 1/3 of a 4 inch avocado.	Unsalted butter or margarine; unsalted cooking fat or oil; unsalted French dressing; unsalted mayonnaise; heavy or light cream; unsalted nuts; avocado. Limit cream to 2 tablespoons a day.	Regular butter or margarine; commercial salad dressings or mayonnaise unless low-sodium dietetic; bacon and bacon fat; salt pork; olives; salted nuts; party spreads and dips.
And...Take Your Choice Choose 2—each choice contains about 75 calories, practically no sodium.	Each of these is one choice: 2 servings fruit; 1 serving bread, cereal, or starchy vegetable; 2 servings fat; 4 tsp. sugar, honey, syrup, jelly, jam, marmalade; candy made without salt or other Na compounds— 75 calories worth.	These choices are part of the diet. They are intended to give more freedom in planning the day's meals, but they must be included every day. Choices may be split, if desired. For example, 1 serving fruit and 2 tsp. sugar make 1 choice.
Miscellaneous	Use as desired: regular and instant coffee, tea, coffee substitutes; lemons; limes; plain unflavored gelatin; vinegar; cream of tartar, potassium bicarbonate; sodium-free baking powder; yeast.	Instant coffee treated with a sodium compound as sodium hydroxide. Instant cocoa mixes; other beverage mixes, including fruit-flavored powders; fountain beverages. Malted milk; soft drinks, reg-

Foods and Amounts	Use	Do Not Use
	Almost every seasoning may be used except celery, garlic, onion salt, catsup, chili sauce, prepared mustard, horseradish sauce with salt, barbecue sauces, meat sauce, meat tenderizers, soy sauce, Worcestershire sauce. Do not use celery leaves and flakes, celery seed, olives, pickles, relishes, cooking wine.	ular or low-calorie; any kind of commercial bouillon (cubes, powders, liquids); sodium saccharin; commercial candies; commercial gelatin desserts; regular baking powder; baking soda (sodium bicarbonate); rennet tablets; molasses; pudding mixes; seasonings noted below. See Na compounds on page 240.

Do not use salt, MSG, etc. in cooking or at table.

Become a label reader to spot products that contain sodium. Canned vegetables contain sodium usually but label may not say so.

If doctor prescribes 250 mg. sodium instead of 500, use low-sodium milk (whole or powdered) instead of regular milk.

For low-sodium baking commercially prepared low-sodium baking powder is available in some stores; also available in same stores may be potassium bicarbonate to use in place of baking soda (sodium bicarbonate).

Consult The American Heart Association's Sodium-Restricted Booklets for ways of adding flavor to Sodium-Restricted Diets.

1800-CALORIE DIET MENUS (500 MG. SODIUM)[13]

Sample menus for two days.

Breakfast	Lunch	Dinner
2 medium prunes with 2 tbsp. juice	2 oz. broiled liver	Baked casserole of beef with whipped potato topping made with:
3/4 cup puffed wheat	Baked acorn squash with 1 small pat unsalted butter	3 oz. cooked beef
1 cup milk		1/2 cup broth from beef
1 slice low-sodium toast	Cabbage slaw with caraway seeds, green pepper, and vinegar	1/2 cup potato
1 small pat unsalted butter		Green beans
Coffee or tea, if desired	2 medium low-sodium muffins, 1 small pat unsalted butter	Tomato and cucumber salad on lettuce leaf with 1 tbsp. low-sodium French dressing
Mid-morning snack: 1/2 cup milk	Apricot bread pudding made with:	2 medium low-sodium rolls
Mid-afternoon snack: 1 small orange	1 slice low-sodium bread 4 dried apricot halves 1/4 cup milk	1 small pat unsalted butter
Evening snack: 1 small sliced banana with 1/4 cup milk	1 small pat unsalted butter	Fruit gelatin made with: unflavored gelatin lemon juice
	Coffee or tea, if desired	1/2 cup mixed fruit artificial sweetener
		Coffee or tea, if desired

---

[13] Ibid., 500 Milligram Sodium Diet, pp. 24–25.

Breakfast	Lunch	Dinner
1/2 cup grapefruit juice	2 oz. sliced roast chicken	Home-made bean soup
1 medium egg, scrambled	1/3 cup low-sodium bread	made with 1/2 cup
1/2 cup applesauce	dressing	cooked dried beans
2 slices low-sodium toast	1 tbsp. cranberry sauce	2 oz. broiled halibut with
1 small pat unsalted but-	1/2 cup cauliflower	lemon
ter	Lettuce salad	1/2 cup green peas
Coffee or tea, if desired	1 medium low-sodium roll	1 small broiled tomato
Mid-morning snack:	1 small pat unsalted but-	1/2 baked sweet potato
1/2 cup milk	ter	1 small low-sodium corn-
5 low-sodium crackers	1 cup milk	meal muffin
(2″)	Coffee or tea, if desired	2 small pats unsalted
Mid-afternoon snack:	Evening snack:	butter
1 small pear	12 grapes, coffee or	Rice-raisin pudding made
Coffee or tea, if desired	tea, if desired	with:
		1/2 cup cooked rice
		2 tbsp. raisins
		1/2 cup milk
		Coffee or tea, if desired

Do not use salt or other seasonings not allowed at the table or in preparing these foods.

You may eat the between-meal snacks at mealtime if you like.

1 small pat of butter=1 tsp. butter (1 unit).

ACTIVITIES

If possible, observe patients on sodium restricted diets at various sodium levels. Follow observations with class discussion on progress of patients.

SUPPLEMENTARY READING

Howe: Chapter 22. Mowry: Chapter 20. Peyton: Chapter 25. Robinson: Chapter 25.

Your 500 Milligram Sodium Diet. New York, American Heart Association, 1968.

Your 1000 Milligram Sodium Diet. New York, American Heart Association, 1969.

Your Mild Sodium Restricted Diet. New York, American Heart Association, 1969.

A. S. Payne and D. Callahan, *Low Sodium Cook Book.* Boston, Little, Brown and Co., 1953.

R. A. Hasker, *The Cook Book for the Low Sodium Diet.* New York, American Heart Association, 1955.

American Dietetic Association Sodium-Restricted Diabetic Diet, Chicago, American Dietetic Association and American Diabetes Association.

Hypertension, National Institutes of Health Bulletin No. 1714, Washington, D. C., U. S. Department of Health, Education and Welfare, 1969.

PART 3.   DIET IN KIDNEY DISORDERS

(Diet Modifications: *Protein-Modified Diet; Mineral-Modified* [Na, K, Ca, P] *Diet*)

WHAT ARE THE FUNCTIONS OF THE KIDNEY? AND TYPES OF KIDNEY DISORDERS

Kidney functions. Kidneys act as a selective filter, removing waste materials of metabolism from the blood and other substances (to form urine collected in the bladder and eventually discharged from the body), and retaining other useful materials to be reabsorbed and returned to the circulation.

Filtering unit is the nephron, which contains a tuft of capillaries called the glomerulus surrounded by a membrane or funnel-like capsule which leads to a long winding tubule.

Maintains acid-base balance and water balance in body.

Helps to maintain normal composition and volume of blood.

Maintains water balance and acid-base balance (body neutrality).

WHAT ARE THE CAUSES AND TYPES OF KIDNEY DISORDERS?

Causes.   Anything which alters normal kidney functioning, particularly that of the filtering unit: cysts, infections and inflammation; cardiovascular disorders; degenerative changes; renal calculi (kidney stones). The condition may be acute, recurrent or chronic.

Nephritis or Bright's disease: general term to cover kidney disorders of the inflammatory type. Glomerulonephritis (acute or chronic): more specific term as glomeruli are primarily affected following infections.

Nephrosis (degenerative Bright's disease).

Nephrosclerosis (arteriosclerotic Bright's disease): due to vascular disease and hardening of renal arteries occurring in older age groups, with albuminuria and edema.

Renal calculi (nephrolithiasis of kidney stones): calcium, oxalate, uric acid or cystine-containing stones.

Renal failure: kidney unable to excrete waste products of metabolism with resulting uremia.

WHAT ARE THE PRINCIPLES OF DIETARY TREATMENT FOR KIDNEY DISORDERS?

Calories.   Adequate, particularly when the diet is restricted in protein so body protein will not be used to meet energy need. Restricted in overweight and obesity.

Protein.   Adequate amount as long as kidney functions remain unimpaired. Range from very low (20 gm.) to low (40–50 gm.) to high (100–125 gm.) depending on disorder. Increased to meet unusual nutritional needs to make up for albumen loss in urine; restricted to various levels with lessened kidney function and retention of end products of protein metabolism in blood.

Minerals.   To combat edema in hypertension, *sodium* is restricted to 500 mg. A low protein diet will be a restricted sodium diet also because protein foods are high in sodium.

Potassium is restricted because its excretion lessens with progressive kidney damage and it is retained in blood with renal failure—usually to the 1.5 gm. level. (A normal diet may contain as much as 3 to 8 gm. because potassium is widely distributed in foods (meats, fruits, whole grain breads and cereals, and dark green leafy vegetables). Cooking water and canned fruit and vegetable juices must be discarded because potassium is water soluble. A usual diet order might read: protein, 40 gm., Na, 500 mg., and potassium, 1.5 gm. Diet plans have been formulated for such controlled diets as this, using Food Exchange Lists similar to those used for calculating diabetic diets.

Fluids.   Fluids are restricted in kidney failure; a balance must be made between intake and output.

Special Modifications to Prevent Kidney Stone Formation.   Restricted calcium and phosphorus to prevent calcium stones; acid-ash to prevent calcium and magnesium stones; alkaline-ash to prevent oxalate and uric acid stones; oxalates or oxalic acid in foods to prevent oxalate stones; purines to prevent uric acid stones; and sulfur-containing protein to prevent cystine stones.

WHAT ARE FOOD ALLOWANCES FOR DIETS AT LOW, MODERATE, AND HIGH-PROTEIN LEVELS?[14]

Foods	*Daily Protein*			
	20 gm.	40 gm.	60 gm.	125 gm.
Milk, cups	0	1/4	2	4
Cream, light, cups	1/2	1/2	0	0
Lean meat, poultry, fish, or cheese, ounces	0	1	$2\frac{1}{2}$	7–9
Eggs	0	1	1	1–3
Vegetables, one raw				
Potato or substitute, servings	2	2	2	1–2
Green leafy or deep-yellow, servings	1	1	1	1
Other, servings	1–2	1–2	1–2	1–2
Fruits				
Citrus, servings	1	1	1	1
Other, fresh, canned, frozen, servings	2	2	2	1–2
Juice, cups	2	1	0	0
Cereals and breads, enriched or whole-grain, servings	4	5	5	6–7
Butter, margarine, salad dressings, tablespoons	3	3	3	6
Sugar, jelly, jam, tablespoons	7	4	4	4 or more
Daily calories	1990	2025	2020	2500

[14] C. H. Robinson, *Basic Nutrition and Diet Therapy,* 2nd edition, New York, The Macmillan Company, 1970, p. 241.

WHAT ARE TYPICAL MENUS FOR VERY-LOW-PROTEIN AND VERY-HIGH-PROTEIN DIETS?[15]

Very-Low Protein Diet (20 gm.)
Breakfast
Stewed prunes
Cooked rice with cream, 1/2 cup
Brown sugar
Toast, enriched, 1 slice
Butter
Jelly
Coffee with cream, sugar
Midmorning
Grape juice with ginger ale, 1 cup
Luncheon
Baked potato with butter
Zucchini squash
Lettuce with sliced tomato
Mayonnaise
Roll
Butter, jelly
Fresh peaches
Tea with sugar
Midafternoon
Orangeade, 1 cup
Dinner
Parsley-buttered noodles
French green beans
Grapefruit avocado salad on water
cress
French dressing
Dinner roll with butter, jelly
Raspberry ice
Tea or coffee with sugar
Bedtime
Grapefruit juice with glucose, 1 cup

Very-High Protein Diet (125 gm.)
Breakfast
Stewed prunes
Scrambled eggs, 2
Wheat flakes with milk, 1 cup
Sugar
Toast, enriched, 1 slice
Butter
Jelly
Coffee with cream, sugar
Luncheon
Cold sliced ham, bologna, cheese,
3 oz.
Potato salad
Lettuce, sliced tomato
Mayonnaise
Roll
Butter
Fresh peach ice cream
Cookie
Milk, 1 cup
Tea, if desired
Dinner
Swiss steak, 4 oz.
Parsley-buttered noodles
French green beans with slivered
almonds
Grapefruit avocado salad on water
cress
French dressing
Dinner roll with butter
Floating Island
Milk, 1 cup
Tea or coffee, if desired
Bedtime
Egg salad sandwich
Milk, 1 cup

SUPPLEMENTARY READING

Howe: Chapter 24   Mowry: Chapter 18   Robinson: Pages 238–243; Chapter 25

---

[15] C. H. Robinson, *Basic Nutrition and Diet Therapy,* 2nd edition, New York, The Macmillan Company, 1970, p. 242.

Unit Five

DIET IN DISEASES OF THE GASTROINTESTINAL TRACT

PART 1. **DIET IN DISEASES OF THE STOMACH**

PART 2. **DIET IN DISEASES OF THE INTESTINE**

PART 3. **DIET IN DISEASES OF THE LIVER AND GALLBLADDER**

Object

To understand the relation of diet to the treatment of diseases of the stomach, intestines, liver and gallbladder and how the basic normal diet is modified in each case for therapeutic purposes.

PART 1. DIET IN DISEASES OF THE STOMACH

(Diet Modification: *Bland, Fiber-Restricted Diet*)

WHAT ARE IMPORTANT FUNCTIONS OF THE STOMACH?

The stomach is the first important organ of digestion, carrying on its work through its secretory (chemical) and motor (physical) functions:

Chemical Functions. Stomach secretes gastric juice which contains:

Hydrochloric acid (HCl)

Protein-splitting enzyme

Small amount of a fat-splitting enzyme

"Intrinsic factor" to aid in the absorption of vitamin B_{12}.

Digestion of protein is started.

Emulsified fats are digested.

Physical Functions. Contraction and relaxation of the muscular wall of stomach.

Peristaltic action: Deep waves assist in mixing food mass with digestive juice and passing it into intestine for further digestive action and absorption.

The following factors modify acid secretion and gastrointestinal motility and tone:[1]

---

[1] F. T. Proudfit, and C. H. Robinson, *Normal and Therapeutic Nutrition,* 13th edition. New York, The Macmillan Company, 1967, p. 521.

*Increased Flow of Acid
and Enzyme Production*

Chemical stimulation—meat extractives, seasonings, spices, alcohol, acid foods

Attractive, appetizing, well-liked foods

State of happiness and contentment

Pleasant surroundings for meals

*Decreased Flow of Acid
and Enzyme Production*

Large amounts of fats, especially in fried foods, pastries, nuts, etc.

Large meals

Poor mastication of food

Foods of poor appearance, flavor, or texture

Foods acutely disliked

Worry, anger, fear, pain (These may stimulate flow of gastric juice in certain individuals)

Increased Tone and Motility

Warm foods

Liquid and soft foods

Fibrous foods, such as certain fruits and vegetables

High-carbohydrate, low-fat intake

Seasonings; concentrated sweets

Fear, anger, worry, nervous tension

Decreased Tone and Motility

Cold foods

Dry, solid foods

Low-fiber foods

High-fat intake, especially in fried foods, pastries, etc.

Vitamin B complex deficiency, especially thiamine

Sedentary habits

Fatigue

Worry, anger, fear, pain

WHAT ARE COMMON GASTRIC DISORDERS?

Functional or Reflex
(Secretory and motor activity may be affected in either)

Usually caused by errors in diet or by neuroses—no lesions present

Indigestion or "dyspepsia"

Acute and chronic gastritis

Hyperchlorhydria

Hypochlorhydria

Organic

Pathologic lesions present

Peptic ulcer
(gastric or duodenal)

Carcinoma

WHAT ARE THE MEANING, CAUSE, AND SYMPTOMS OF PEPTIC ULCER?

Meaning. Peptic ulcer is an eroded lesion in mucosa of stomach (gastric ulcer) or duodenum (duodenal ulcer). The stomach has low resistance to the action of the gastric (digestive) juice.

Causes. (theories.)

Poor dietary habits.

Excessive alcohol.

Excessive smoking.

Irregular and hurried eating.

Emotional and nervous factors.

Symptoms. Burning or gnawing pain in the pit of the stomach, occurring, after the same interval, every time food is eaten.

Hypersecretion of hydrochloric acid.
Hyperacidity of stomach contents.
Weakness and sometimes loss of weight.
Hunger contractions when stomach is empty; increased tonus.
Possible hemorrahge.
Methods of Diagnosis.   Gastric analysis; x-ray or fluoroscopic examination; gastroscopy.

WHAT PRINCIPLES UNDERLIE THE DIETARY TREATMENT OF PEPTIC ULCER?

General: physical and mental rest.
Medication: to reduce excessive acidity.
            to reduce secretion of gastric juice.
            to reduce motor activity.
Diet: extremely important.

Dietary Principles

1. Feedings: small to prevent pressure in stomach and frequent to keep some food in stomach constantly.
2. High protein to combine with (buffering) stomach acid, thereby preventing irritation of the ulcerated area.
3. High fat to inhibit gastric secretion and delay stomach emptying.

Bland Diet

4. No *mechanically* irritating foods—meat residue, whole cereals, unstrained fruits or vegetables.
5. No *chemically* irritating foods—meat extractives, tea, coffee, spices, alcohol, or acids.
6. No *thermally* irritating food—very hot or very cold foods.
7. Gradual progression to a more nutritionally adequate soft diet and intermediate diets to regular full but bland diet.

These principles represent the bases for the traditional "Sippy" progressive peptic ulcer regimen and its various modifications. The steps include alternate hourly feedings of milk and cream (in later years homogenized milk and skim milk are variations), and antacids during the acute stage, then six meals a day of selected foods and a gradual return to a regular diet with a few restrictions.

Today, the trend is toward more liberal diets with regular meals, more suited to patients' tastes. They have proved effective in treatment and meet some of the criticisms leveled at the Sippy regimen — monotonous, flavorless, unattractive, unappetizing, and too high in fat.

Stages in Treatment

Usually referred to as the Four-Stage Bland, Fiber-Restricted Diet with gradual increases in the kinds and amounts of foods.

1. Frequent small feedings (3 ounces) of milk or milk and cream, or a high protein mixture alternated with alkaline medication (for a few days only).

2. Other foods added, one at a time, as three small meals with limited size feedings (6 ounces): soft egg, refined or strained cereal, strained cream soup, junket, etc.

3. Three small meals at usual times with same foods as in stage two plus cream or cottage cheese, or strained cooked fruit and fruit juice.

4. Six meals a day with feedings between of above foods and added ground meat, strained vegetables, puddings, etc. Then a gradual return to regular diet with between-meal feedings without high residue or stimulating foods. See the diet progression below.

WHAT FOODS ARE GIVEN ON THE PROGRESSIVE REGIMEN OF THE BLAND DIET?[2]

BLAND I		BLAND II		BLAND III	
90 cc. of half milk and half light cream	EARLY MORNING, WHEN AWAKE - EVERY HOUR -	*Milk and cream	90 cc.	*Milk and cream	90 cc.
	BREAKFAST	Cereal, refined or strained Sugar Milk	1/2 cup 1 teaspoon 1/4 cup	Cereal, refined or strained Sugar Milk Egg	1/3 cup 1 teaspoon 1/3 cup 1
every hour	BETWEEN BREAKFAST & LUNCH--EVERY HOUR-	*Milk and cream	90 cc.	*Milk and cream	90 cc.
from 6-7 A.M. to 9-10 P.M.	LUNCHEON	Cream soup White crackers Butter Dessert	1/2 cup 2 1 teaspoon 1/4 cup	Cottage cheese Toast, white Butter Strained fruit	2 ounces 1 slice 1 teaspoon 1/3 cup
and during the night if necessary	BETWEEN LUNCHEON & DINNER - EVERY HOUR-	*Milk and cream	90 cc.	*Milk and cream	90 cc.
	DINNER	Egg, soft cooked Toast, white Butter Dessert	1 1 slice 1 teaspoon 1/2 cup	White potato Butter Dessert Fruit juice	1/3 cup 1 teaspoon 1/4 cup 1/4 cup
	AT NIGHT, WHEN AWAKE - EVERY HOUR-	*Milk and cream	90 cc.	*Milk and cream	90 cc.

*This mixture is half milk and half light cream. (Commercial "Half and Half" may be used.)

Bland IV

Purpose.

1. To provide essentials for good nutrition using bland, easily digested foods, moderately low in residue.
2. To provide a diet which avoids mechanical irritation and stimulation of gastric activity and provides dilution and neutralization of stomach contents by giving frequent feedings.

General Rules. Include the following foods daily:

Milk: 4–6 Cups

Egg: 1

Meat, poultry, or fish, ground unless tender

---

[2] *Diet Manual.* New York, Nutrition Department, Presbyterian Hospital, Columbia-Presbyterian Medical Center, 1963, pp. 32, 33, 35.

Mild soft cheese, egg, meat, poultry, or fish
Potato, without skin, or rice, noodles, macaroni, or spaghetti
Suggested Meal Plan
Breakfast
Fruit juice, strained fruit, or ripe banana
Cereal, strained whole grain or enriched refined
Egg
Toast, enriched white
Butter or fortified margarine
Bland coffee or tea, cocoa, or milk
Midmorning
Milk
White crackers
Luncheon or Supper
Strained cream soup, no stock
Mild soft cheese, egg, meat, poultry, or fish (grind meat and poultry unless tender)
White potato, without skin, or substitute
Bread, enriched white
Butter or fortified margarine
Strained vegetable: 1 serving *no more*
Strained fruit: 1 serving *no more*
Orange, grapefruit, or tomato juice: 1 cup
Bread, enriched white
Cereals, enriched, refined, or strained whole grain

Butter or fortified margarine
Other foods as allowed to provide adequate calories
Include between-meal nourishment of milk and white crackers.

Note: 1/2 cup tea or coffee with 1/2 cup hot milk is allowed only once a day. More is given only upon order of a physician.
Milk may be given at any time the patient requests.
Whole fruits and vegetables given only upon request of a physician.
Strained fruit
Milk
Midafternoon
Milk
White crackers
Dinner
Orange, grapefruit, or tomato juice
Tender meat, poultry, or fish (ground unless tender)
White potato, without skin, or substitute
Strained vegetables
Bread, enriched white
Butter or fortified margarine
Dessert (not fruit)
Milk
Bedtime
Milk
White crackers

FOODS TO AVOID[3]

Meat with gristle, tough fibers, and excessive fat
Smoked and salted meats and fish
Fish with small bones
Fried meat and fish
Strongly flavored cheese
Fried potatoes
Raw vegetables

Coarse and strongly flavored vegetables: broccoli, Brussels sprouts, cabbage, cauliflower, chives, corn, onions, green peppers, turnips
All raw fruit except banana, avocado, strained fruit juices
Fresh or hot breads
Coarse whole grain breads

[3] *Diet Manual.* Nutrition Department, Presbyterian Hospital, Columbia-Presbyterian Medical Center, 1963, pp. 33–37, adapted.

Whole grain crackers such as graham

All dry cereals except: Corn Flakes, Puffed Rice, Rice Krispies, Rice Flakes

Whole grain cereal unless strained

All fats except butter, cream, fortified margarine, vegetable oil, cooking fats, smooth peanut butter, mild mayonnaise

Fried foods

Desserts containing nuts, raisins, coconut, or whole fruit

Rich pastries

All soups (except cream soups made with vegetables other than those listed at left and without stock or broth)

Coffee, tea, except in amounts of diet

Decaffeinated coffee

Cereal beverages such as Postum

Carbonated and cola drinks

Fried food

Meat gravies and sauces

Olives and pickles

Vinegar

Seasonings, spices and condiments such as catsup, chili sauce, garlic, horseradish, mustard, Worcestershire sauce

SUPPLEMENTARY READING

Howe: Chapter 19; Pages 431–433
        Chapter 16

Mowry:

Peyton: Chapter 22: pp. 191–196.
Robinson: Pages 206–210
Review: Section One, Unit Two, Part 7, Page 93

PART 2. DIET IN DISEASES OF THE INTESTINE

(Diet Modifications: *Residue-Modified Diet; Gluten-Free Diet*)

WHAT ARE THE FUNCTIONS OF THE INTESTINES AND TYPES OF INTESTINAL DISEASES?

Intestinal Functions

Small Intestine:

Receives food from stomach for completion of digestion.

Digestion of food is completed with aid of enzymes from the pancreatic and intestinal juices (bile aids fat digestion).

Propels food mass along intestinal tract by peristaltic action.

End products of digestion absorbed in lower portion.

Large intestine:

Water and salt absorbed.

Feces formed.

Peristaltic action propels waste products to colon for excretion as feces.

Intestinal Diseases

Diarrhea: frequent bowel movements interfering with digestion and absorption of food. May be a disease symptom.

Ileitis (enteritis): inflammation of ileum.

Ulcerative colitis (organic): chronic condition of inflammation; frequent stools with blood, possible anemia and underweight; distention and cramps.

Diverticulitis: inflammation usually in colon.

Atonic constipation: sluggish intestine; decreased muscle tone.

Spastic constipation: overactive and irritable colon; increased muscle tone with narrowing of colon.

Sprue: similar to celiac disease in children—diarrhea, distention, fatty stools.

WHAT ARE PRINCIPLES OF DIETARY TREATMENT FOR INTESTINAL DISEASES?

Disease	*Diet*
Diarrhea (long duration)	Low residue diet with liberal protein and calories.
Ileitis	Low residue diet high in protein and calories.
Ulcerative colitis	Very low residue diet or moderately low residue diet followed by a *bland high-protein diet.*
Atonic constipation	High residue diet
Spastic constipation	Soft residue diet.
Sprue (non-tropical) (adult "celiac")	Low gluten diet (wheat, rye, oat, and barley free diet)

Disease	*Diet*
Diverticulitis	Very low residue diet— followed by moderate restriction.

WHAT ARE THE MEANING, PURPOSE, AND USE OF A LOW RESIDUE DIET?

Meaning

Diet with a minimum of residue "Residue" and "fiber" sometimes used interchangeably; *fiber* refers to indigestible products such as skins and seeds of fruits, bran layers on cereal grains, and stringy parts (structural) of vegetables. *Residue* refers to any of the above substances, incompletely digested foods, meat fibers (connective tissues) left in intestinal tract.

Purpose

To prevent stimulation of peristalsis and avoid distention of intestine by restricting residue to a minimum

Use

Spastic constipation
Colitis
Diverticulitis
Dysentery and diarrhea
Surgery on large intestine
Partial intestinal obstruction
To prevent peristalsis
To prevent distention.

WHAT FOODS ARE ALLOWED AND OMITTED ON LOW RESIDUE DIETS?

	Allowed	*Omitted*
Beverages	Tea, coffee, Postum in limited amounts	Milk and milk beverages may be limited or omitted in certain instances
Breads	White enriched (bread or toast) Plain crackers (white), zwieback, Melba toast	Whole grain bread, crackers, graham crackers, hot breads
Cereals	Enriched refined, rice, cornmeal, farina, strained oatmeal, Cream of Wheat, Corn Flakes, Rice Krispies, Puffed Rice, Rice Flakes	Whole grain cereals unless strained Any dry cereals not listed
Vegetables	Strained cooked vegetables: green beans, asparagus, beets, peas, limas, carrots, squash	Raw vegetables Salads Strong flavored vegetables: broccoli, brussels sprouts, cabbage, cauliflower, onions, turnips, green peppers
Fruits	Strained fruits and to-	Coarse vegetables: corn

	Allowed	Omitted
	mato juices	Raw fruit—ripe banana, avocado may be used
	Ripe banana, avocado	
	Strained cooked (or canned) apricots, apples, peaches, prunes, plums	Fruits with skins or seeds
Potato or substitute	Mashed, baked (without skin) macaroni, noodles, rice	Fried potatoes
Meat, eggs, cheese	Beef, lamb, chicken— tender or ground— also liver	Smoked meat, tough meat, strong flavored cheese
	Fish without bones	
	Cottage, cream, mild American cheese	
	Eggs	
Desserts	Plain cake: pound, angel, sponge	Rich cake, pies, doughnuts, rich puddings
	Plain cookies, plain ice cream	Desserts with nuts, raisins, coconut, fruit
	Custards, gelatin desserts, sherbets and ice cream without nuts or fruits	
	Junket, tapioca, cornstarch, rice pudding	
Fats	Butter, fortified margarine, oils, cream	Fried foods
Soup	Strained cream soup made with vegetables allowed above	
	Broth	
Miscellaneous	Moderate sweets, jelly, syrups	Condiments: spices, pepper, pickles, nuts, olives, popcorn, rich gravies and sauces, coconut, seeds
		Jams, marmalades

Note: All fruit and fruit juices, vegetables and vegetables juices, are omitted on a very low residue diet; sweets and fats are permitted in limited amounts and milk may be boiled.

WHAT IS A SAMPLE MEAL PLAN FOR A LOW RESIDUE DIET?

Breakfast   Strained orange juice or ripe banana
Cream of Wheat with cream and sugar
Soft cooked egg
Enriched toast and butter
Tea or coffee with cream and sugar

Luncheon   Cream soup
    or   Ground or tender meat, poultry, fish or cottage cheese or egg
Supper   Enriched white bread or roll and butter
             Strained fruit
             Milk
             Beverage
Dinner   Ground or tender meat
             White potato without skin
             Strained vegetables.
             Enriched white bread or roll and butter
             Simple dessert
             Milk
             Beverage

WHAT ARE THE MEANING, PURPOSE OF, AND FOODS USED ON A HIGH RESIDUE (FIBER) DIET?

Meaning

A normal diet in which fiber content is increased from 5 to 6 grams to 10 to 11 grams

Purpose

To stimulate muscle tone of intestine and encourage evacuation in atonic constipation

Thiamine may be given as supplement to stimulate intestinal wall

Note: Good health habits also important:
    Rest and relaxation

Exercise
Regularity of meals
Regular time for elimination

Foods

Foods high in indigestible cellulose: vegetables with fibers and skins, fruits with tender skins, whole grain cereals and breads, connective tissues of tougher meats

Bran in moderation
Plenty of fluids
High fat if no overweight
Salads at noon and night meals with raw fruits and vegetables

WHAT IS A BLAND HIGH PROTEIN DIET?

Refer to Bland Diet IV on page 251 and to Ways of Increasing Food Value—Protein on page 203.

WHAT FOODS ARE ALLOWED AND OMITTED ON A LOW GLUTEN DIET?[4]

(Diet Free of Wheat, Rye, Oats, and Barley Protein)

	Foods Allowed	*Foods Omitted*
Beverages	Coffee, tea, decaffeinated coffee (read label to be sure that no wheat flour has been added), carbonated beverages	Cereal beverages such as Postum, Ovaltine; beer, ale

---

[4] From Arthur B. French, Instructions and Tested Recipes for Low-Gluten Cooking. *Modern Treatment* 2:408, March, 1965. Courtesy of Hoeber Medical Division, Harper and Row, Publishers.

	Foods Allowed	*Foods Omitted*
Bread	Only those made from arrowroot, buckwheat, corn, potato, rice, soybean and low gluten wheat starch flours, breaded foods made with crushed ready to eat corn or rice creals	All bread, rolls, crackers etc. made from wheat, rye, oats, and barley; commercial gluten bread; commercially prepared mixes for biscuits, cornbread, muffins, pancakes, buckwheat pancakes, waffles, etc.; rusks, zwieback, pretzels, bread and cracker crumbs, breaded foods
Cereals	Cornmeal, hominy, rice, cream of rice, ready to eat corn and rice cereals (these cereals may contain a small amount of malt as flavoring, however in most instances they have been well tolerated)	All wheat and rye cereals, wheat germ, barley, oatmeal, kasha
Desserts	Custard, junket; homemade cornstarch and rice, puddings; gelatin desserts, ices, ice cream and sherbet if they do not contain gluten stabilizers; cakes, cookies, pastries, etc. prepared with permitted low gluten flours, or instant potato granules	Cakes, cookies, doughnuts, pastries, etc. prepared with wheat, rye, oats, or barley flours; commercial ice creams unless they do not contain gluten stabilizer (check with supplier); ice cream *cones;* all commercially prepared mixes for cakes, cookies, puddings, etc.; bread puddings thickened with flour
Egg	As desired	
Fat	Butter and other fats as desired, pure mayonnaise and other commercial salad dressings if they do not contain a gluten stabilizer (*read labels*)	Commercial salad dressings, except pure mayonnaise, which contains gluten stabilizers
Fruits	As desired: at least three servings a day, including one citrus fruit	Fruits in combination with wheat, rye, oats, or barley flours or cereals

	Foods Allowed	*Foods Omitted*
Meat, Fish, cheese	Meat, fish, and poultry prepared without the addition of wheat, rye, oats, or barley; at least two servings daily; gravy only when thickened with cream, cornstarch, potato or low gluten wheat starch flour. Meats, fish, and poultry may be combined or breaded with cornmeal or crumbs from crushed ready to eat corn and rice cereals. Stuffings may be made with cornmeal or rice. Bacteria ripened cheeses, cottage cheese, cream cheese, processed cheese products if they do not contain a gluten stabilizer (*read labels*)	Meat, fish or poultry patties or loaves made with bread or bread crumbs; croquettes; breaded meat, fish, poultry; chili con carne; canned meat dishes; all prepared meats such as cold cuts, sausages and frankfurters unless guaranteed pure meat; bread dressings; gravy and cream sauce thickened with wheat flour; stews with noodles, dumplings or sauce prepared with wheat flour. Processed cheese, cheese foods and cheese spreads which may contain a gluten stabilizer
Milk	At least 1 pint a day; more if desired	Malted milk, commercial chocolate milk which may have a cereal additive
Potato or Substitute	Potato as desired except when prepared with a wheat flour white sauce such as creamed or scalloped; rice; home made noodles prepared with allowed low gluten flours or starches; rice sticks (usually obtainable at oriental specialty stores)	Macaroni, spaghetti, noodles
Soup	Clear meat soups and vegetable soups (some canned and frozen soups are allowed) (*read labels*); cream soups thickened with cream or allowed low gluten flours or starches	All soups containing wheat, rye, oats, or barley in any form

	Foods Allowed	*Foods Omitted*
Vegetables	As desired except when prepared with wheat flour or products such as cracker crumbs	Vegetables prepared with wheat, rye, oats, or barley flours or products
Sweets	Sugar, honey, corn syrup, molasses, jelly, jam, homemade and certain commercial candies free of wheat, rye, oats, and barley	Commercial candies containing wheat, rye, oats, or barley (*read labels*)
Miscellaneous	Salt, pepper, spices, monosodium glutamate, vinegar, olives, nuts, peanut butter, coconut, tapioca, chocolate, pure cocoa, marshmallows	Any foods containing wheat, rye, oats, or barley as fillers or stabilizers such as commercial meat sauces and seasonings.

Special Hints.

1. Arrowroot, corn, potato, rice, soybean and low gluten wheat starch flours may be used in place of wheat flour in many recipes.

2. Recipes are readily available for products using cornstarch, gelatin, tapioca, and corn and rice cereals which can be used to add variety to the low gluten diet. These recipes can be found in standard cookbooks and can be obtained from certain food companies.

3. A list of some packaged and prepared foods, known to be acceptable for the low gluten diet, can be obtained from the Clinical Research Unit, University of Michigan Hospital, Ann Arbor, Michigan.

4. Unlike wheat gluten most of the flours permitted in the Low-Gluten Diet contain mainly starches and non-sticky proteins. Suggestions for use and handling of these flours are included in the reference at the bottom of this page.

SUPPLEMENTARY READING:

Howe: Chapter 19   Mowry: Chapter 16   Peyton: Chapter 22: pp. 196–202
                                                   Robinson: Pages 205–210
Low Gluten Diet with Tested Recipes, Ann Arbor, Michigan, The University of Michigan, 1969.

PART 3. DIET IN DISEASES OF THE LIVER AND GALLBLADDER

(Diet Modifications: *High Protein, High Carbohydrate, Moderate Fat—Liver Diseases; Fat-Restricted—Gallbladder Disease*)

WHAT ARE THE FUNCTIONS OF THE LIVER AND TYPES OF LIVER DISEASES?

Liver Functions. Liver is the largest glandular organ and performs more functions than any other organ.

Produces bile which aids the digestion and absorption of fat.

Aids in metabolism of carbohydrates, fats and proteins.

Stores some minerals and vitamins.

Aids in storage and metabolism of iron and copper.

Storehouse for glycogen.

Detoxifies harmful substances.

Performs numerous other functions.

When liver is diseased, carbohydrate storage, fat metabolism, serum protein, and prothrombin production are abnormal .

Liver Diseases (requiring dietary adjustment).

Jaundice: a symptom of liver and biliary tract diseases.

Hepatitis: inflammation and injury to liver cells caused by infections, drugs, and toxins. Infectious: viral hepatitis.

Cirrhosis: chronic condition with scar tissue replacing liver cells. Caused by infectious hepatitis, alcoholism, certain agents. Fat metabolism impaired.

WHAT ARE PRINCIPLES OF DIETARY TREATMENT FOR LIVER DISEASES?

Hapatitis. Object of diet:

To reduce liver strain and injury.

To build up liver tissue.

To permit liver to function as easily and efficiently as possible.

Acute stage: liquid to soft diet.

Convalescence: Liberal diet.

High-protein: 100 to 125 gm. to build liver tissue.

High carbohydrate: to furnish calories, build up glycogen store, and spare protein.

Moderate fat: to help with calories and make diet more palatable.

Cirrhosis. Liberal diet:

High protein to rebuild liver tissue, move fat from liver cells, increase serum albumin.

High carbohydrate to spare protein.

Moderate fat to increase calories and make diet palatable.

Liberal vitamins in foods and possibly as supplements.

Restricted salt if ascites and edema.
Soft or semiliquid diet.

WHAT MEAL PLAN WITH SAMPLE MENU MAY BE USED FOR A HIGH PROTEIN (100 GM.), HIGH CARBOHYDRATE (400 GM.), MODERATE FAT (100 GM.) DIET?[5] TOTAL CALORIES 2900

MEAL PLAN	SAMPLE MENU	SERVINGS Weight Grams	Household Measure
	BREAKFAST		
Fruit	Orange juice	124	1/2 glass (4 oz.)
Cereal	Cooked oatmeal	177	3/4 cup
Eggs	Poached eggs	100	2
Bread	Toasted whole wheat bread	46	2 slices
Butter or margarine	Butter or margarine	7	1 pat
Jelly	Jelly	20	1 tablespoon
Coffee	Coffee	200	1 pot
Cream, 20%	Cream, 20%	60	2 ounces
Sugar	Sugar	12	1 tablespoon
	MID-MORNING		
Fruit juice	Lemon and pineapple juice	248	1 glass (8 oz.)
with lactose	with lactose	16	2 tablespoons
	LUNCHEON		
Soup	Broth	120	1/2 cup (4 oz.)
Meat	Cold sliced turkey	85	3 ounces
Vegetable	Cooked green snap beans	63	1/2 cup
Salad	Sliced tomato salad	150	1 medium
Bread	Whole wheat bread	46	2 slices
Butter or margarine	Butter or margarine	7	1 pat
Jelly	Jelly	20	1 tablespoon
Dessert	Mixed fruit cup	128	1/2 cup
Beverage	Milk	244	1 glass (8 oz.)
	MID-AFTERNOON		
Fruit juice	Grapefruit juice	248	1 glass (8 oz.)
with lactose	with lactose	16	2 tablespoons
	DINNER		
Meat	Roast lamb	85	3 ounces
Potato or alternate	Boiled potato with parsley butter	122	1 medium
Vegetable	Baked winter squash	103	1/2 cup
Bread	Whole wheat bread	46	2 slices
Butter or margarine	Butter or mrgarine	7	1 pat
Jelly	Jelly	20	1 tablespoon
Dessert	Bananas and strawberry gelatin	194	1 sauce dish
Beverage	Milk	244	1 glass (8 oz.)
	BEDTIME		
Fruit juice	Orange juice and lemon juice	247	1 glass (8 oz.)
with lactose	with lactose	16	2 tablespoons

[5] From M. V. Krause, *Food, Nutrition and Diet Therapy,* 4th edition. Philadelphia, W. B. Saunders Co., 1966, p. 263.

WHAT ARE FUNCTIONS OF THE GALLBLADDER AND COMMON GALLBLADDER DISEASES?

Gallbladder Functions.
Concentrates and stores bile until needed in intestine to aid fat digestion.

Fat in the intestine stimulates a hormone (in duodenal cells) which goes by way of the blood to gallbladder and causes it to contract and release bile.

Bile is required for the absorption of fat and fat-soluble vitamins in the intestine.

Gallbladder Diseases.
Cholecystitis: inflammation of the gallbladder. Fatty meal brings on pain when gallbladder is inflamed.

Cholelithiasis: gallstones (block bile duct and interfere with the flow of bile).

WHAT ARE PRINCIPLES OF DIETARY TREATMENT FOR GALLBLADDER DISEASES?

Diet modification: Low Fat Diet. Moderately Low Fat: 60–65 gm. fat. Strict Low Fat: about 30 gm. fat.

Low calories if patient is overweight.

Bland flavor, non-stimulating, easily digested, nonirritating foods.

Limited coarse fiber, Non-distending foods.

Heated fats less well tolerated than non-heated fats.

Additional fruit and non-distending vegetables if patient constipated.

Low fat diet may be further modified for high residue, low residue, or bland low fat.

Easily digested fats: butter, margarine, egg yolk, whole milk.

On *strict* low fat diet: skim milk in place of whole milk; butter, margarine, and egg yolk omitted; only very lean meats allowed and also uncreamed cottage cheese.

WHAT FOODS ARE ALLOWED AND AVOIDED ON A LOW FAT DIET?

	Foods Allowed	*Foods Avoided*
Milk	Skim milk and buttermilk as desired; whole milk may be limited to 1/2 to 1 pint	Beverages with cream, milk, ice cream
Egg	One, if tolerated and ordered by physician; egg white preferable	
Meat, fish, poultry	Lean meat and low fat fish: 3 to 4 ounces without added fat	Fat meat and fish: bacon, pork, sausage, duck, mackerel; fish canned in oil
Cheese	Uncreamed cottage	All except cottage

	Foods Allowed	*Foods Avoided*
Fruits	All except avocado, if tolerated	Avocado; raw apples, melons, pineapple if not tolerated
Vegetables	All without added fat or sauces as tolerated	Cauliflower, cabbage, broccoli, onion, turnips, brussels sprouts, cucumbers, radishes, dried beans, peppers, pickles
Soups	Fat free broth, bouillon Skim milk soups without fat	Cream soups with whole milk and fat
Cereals	Whole grain and enriched rice, macaroni, spaghetti, noodles	Coarse or excessive bran. Avoid all bran unless tolerated
Bread	Whole grain and enriched breads, crackers without shortening	Muffins, biscuits, pastries, hot breads
Fats	One teaspoon at each meal, butter or fortified margarine	Sweet and sour cream, mayonnaise, peanut butter, other fats and oils, salad dressings
Desserts	Fruit, jello and gelatin desserts, puddings made with skim milk, angel food cake, sherbet, ices, fruit whips (egg whites), skim milk junket	Cake, pies, doughnuts, ice cream, rich cookies, rich desserts
Beverages	Tea, coffee, cocoa with skim milk, carbonated beverages, if tolerated	Chocolate, malted milk drinks, milk shakes, sodas
Miscellaneous	Jelly, jam, molasses, plain candies	Nuts, peanut butter, olives, gravies, sauces, excess condiments and spices, chocolate candies, candies with nuts

WHAT MEAL PLAN AND SAMPLE MENUS MAY BE USED FOR A LOW FAT DIET?

Meal Plan	*Sample Menus*
	Breakfast
Fruit	Grapefruit
Whole grain or enriched cereal (1/2 cup)	Ralston cereal
	Skim milk or 1/2 cup whole milk
Egg (1)	Soft cooked egg
Whole grain or	Whole wheat toast

Meal Plan	*Sample Menus*
enriched bread or toast (2 slices)	Butter or fortified margarine
Butter (1 teaspoon)	Jelly
Jelly (1 tablespoon)	Coffee
Milk (1/2 cup) or skim milk	Sugar
Coffee	
Sugar	

Luncheon or Supper

Lean meat, fish, poultry, or uncreamed cottage cheese	Tomato bouillon
Potato or substitute	Baked potato
Vegetable	Asparagus tips
Salad	Whole wheat bread
Whole grain on enriched bread	Cottage cheese and peach salad
Butter (1 teaspoon)	Butter or fortified magarine
Jelly (1 tablespoon)	Fruit jello
Fruit	Jelly
Skim milk or 1/2 cup whole milk	Skim milk or 1/2 cup whole
Tea or coffee	
Sugar	

Dinner

Lean meat, poultry, fish	Roast lamb
Potato or substitute	Steamed rice
Vegetable	Cooked carrot strips
Salad	White enriched roll
Enriched bread	Butter
Butter	Lettuce wedge with lemon juice
Jelly	Jelly
Fruit or sherbet	Canned cherries
Beverage	Angel food cake
Sugar	Tea
	Sugar

SUPPLEMENTARY READING

Howe: Chapter 20   Mowry: Chapter 17   Peyton: Chapter 23
Robinson: Pages 248–251

Unit Six

DIET IN MISCELLANEOUS DISEASES AND CONDITIONS

Object

To bring to the attention of the practical nurse the importance of certain modifications of the normal basic diet in the therapeutic treatment of various additional diseases; also in surgery and burns.

DIET IN MISCELLANEOUS DISEASES AND CONDITIONS

Allergies and Skin Disorders. Hypersensitivity to one or more food substances (allergens usually proteins). Evidenced in skin lesions, gastrointestinal disturbances, headaches, asthma, etc. Usual allergens: milk, eggs, wheat, oranges, tomatoes, grapefruit, chocolate, spinach, oatmeal, corn.

Different test diets—Four Rowe Elimination Diets—containing a few carefully chosen foods, with common allergens omitted from one or more of the diets, are used to determine the causative food allergen. Diets 1 to 3 contain a cereal or starch, 1 or 2 meats, a selected small group of fruits and vegetables, seasonings, and condiments; diet 4 contains only milk, tapioca, and cane sugar. A nutritionally adequate diet is then planned to exclude the specific foods to which the individual is allergic. Below are listed common foods to be omitted on a wheat-free diet, an egg-free diet, and a milk-free diet, and the recipes that are available.[1] Additional commercial products for allergy diets are now available. Careful reading of labels on such products is necessary to detect any specific allergen to be omitted in the diet.

Common Foods Containing Wheat.[2] Omit these foods on a wheat-free diet.

Beverages: Malted Milk, Postum, Hemo, Nestle's Food.

Bread: All breads including rye, oatmeal, nut breads, hot breads, muffins, cornbread, baking powder biscuits, zwieback, rusks, pretzels, matzoh, rolls, gluten bread, bagels.

Cereals:

All-Bran	Cream of Wheat	Kellogg's K
Beemax	Farina	Kix
Bran Flakes	Grapenuts	Krumbles
Cheerios	Grapenuts Flakes	Maltex
Cocoa Puffs	Infant-type mixed	Maypo
Crackles	Jets	Mello-wheat

---

[1] *Allergy Recipes*, Chicago, American Dietetic Association, 1957.

Baking for People with Food Allergies, Home and Garden Bulletin No. 147, U. S. Department of Agriculture, Washington, D. C., 1968.

C. G. Emerling and E. O. Jonckers, *The Allergy Cookbook*, New York, Doubleday Company, 1968.

[2] *Diet Manual.* New York, Nutrition Department, Presbyterian Hospital, Columbia-Presbyterian Medical Center, 1963, p. 57.

Muffets	Trix
Pop	Wheat Chex
Pettijohn	Wheat Flakes
Protein Plus	Wheat Honeys
Puffed Wheat	Wheat germ
Ralston; regular,	Wheat Puffs
instant, shredded	Wheaties
Shredded Wheat	Wheatsworth
Sugar Crisp	Wheatena
Sugar Smacks	Whole Bran

Flours: Wheat flour in any form including graham, white or whole wheat.

Desserts: Cakes, cookies, doughnuts, pies, ice cream cones, puddings and prepared mixes except those especially made without wheat.

Miscellaneous: Macaroni, spaghetti, noodles, vermicelli, pastina and other pasta.

Dumplings, griddle cakes, waffles, pancakes, pizza.

Commercial candies that contain wheat.

Gravies and sauces thickened with flour, commercial spaghetti and other sauces made with wheat.

Soups containing wheat or wheat products, including canned broth or consomme.

Fish or meats prepared with flour, bread or cracker crumbs such as: croquettes, meat loaf, and stew thickened with flour.

Commercially prepared meat such as frankfurters, sausages, and cold cuts where wheat may be used as a filler.

Salad dressings—cooked or boiled—where flour is used for thickening.

Note 1:   Bread and other baked products can be made with soy, rice, corn or potato flour or cornmeal.

Note 2:   100% rye bread, crackers and wafers are available in some stores.

Common Foods Containing Egg.[3]   Omit these foods on an egg-free diet:

Breads prepared with egg	Marshmallow Fluff
Cake	Mayonnaise
Cookies	Meringue
Custard	Milk puddings containing egg
Doughnuts	Muffins
Eggs (any form)	Noodles
Eggnog or other egg drinks	Pretzels
Fritters	Ravioli
Frosting prepared with egg	Rolls, soft prepared with egg
Griddle cakes	Waffles
Hollandaise sauce	Zwieback
Ice cream	

Cream type pies such as lemon, custard, pumpkin, coconut, etc.

Soft candy such as chocolate cream, nougat, fondant.

Fish or meat prepared with egg: meat loaf, croquettes, breaded meat.

Foods containing albumin.

---

[3] *Diet Manual.* New York, Nutrition Department, Presbyterian Hospital, Columbia-Presbyterian Medical Center, 1963, p. 57.

Common Foods Containing Milk.[3] Omit these foods on a milk-free diet.

Bread made with milk
Butter
Buttermilk
Cake and cookies made with milk
Candies made with milk or milk products
Caramels
Cheese
Chocolate candy
Cocomalt
Crackers made with milk
Cream
Cream or soft pies
Cream sauces
Cream soup
Custard
Doughnuts
Frosting prepared with milk
Ice cream

Malted milk
Margarine
Milk
Milk, condensed
Milk, evaporated
Milk, skimmed
Milk puddings
Nestle's Sweet Milk Cocoa
Ovaltine
Pie crust made with butter or margarine
Potato mashed with milk or butter
Pream
Rarebit
Rusks
Yogurt
Zwieback

Vegetables with butter, margarine, milk or cream.
Gravies with butter, margarine, milk, or cream.
Creamed or scalloped foods.
Any foods or commercial mixes containing milk, dried milk solids, casein, lactalbumin, or curds and whey.

Skin Diseases.[4] There is evidence that dietary changes may affect the skin in health and disease. In the chronic skin infection psoriasis, where there is a rapid turnover of epidermis, attempts have been made to control the process by dietary modification. Moderate restriction of protein intake, as well as restriction of the intake of the amino acid taurine, has been advocated by Dr. Daphne A. Roe.

As foods of animal origin all contain taurine in varying amounts (it is partially removed by boiling), gravies, juices, and soups from meat and fish are completely restricted, commercially prepared cold cuts are also excluded, and eggs and egg-containing foods are limited. Recommended as protein sources are milk and cheese (lower in taurine than meats) and vegetable protein foods—legumes, nuts and nut products to supplement but not replace animal protein foods. The diet needs to be administered under the direction of a physician.

Gout. (Purine-Restricted Diet) A disturbance in the metabolism and excretion of purines (end products of nucleo-proteins). Sodium urate crystals are deposited in and around joints. There is increased uric acid in the blood.

Normal diet with purines restricted to 100–150 mg. (average diet contains 600–1000 mg.). Low calorie diet if patient is overweight.

---

[4] Personal communication from Dr. Daphne A. Roe, Cornell University Graduate School of Nutrition.

FOODS GROUPED ACCORDING TO PURINE CONTENT[5]

GROUP 1:   HIGH PURINE CONTENT
(100 TO 1,000 MG. OF PURINE NITROGEN PER 100 GM. OF FOOD)

Anchovies

Bouillon

Broth

Consomme

Goose

Gravy

Heart

Herring

Kidney

Liver

Mackerel

Meat extracts

Mincemeat

Mussels

Partridge

Roe

Sardines

Scallops

Sweetbreads

Yeast, baker's
    and brewer's

Foods in this preceding list should be omitted from the diet of patients who have gout (acute and remission stages).

GROUP 2:   MODERATE PURINE CONTENT
(9 TO 100 MG. OF PURINE NITROGEN PER 100 GM. OF FOOD)

Meat and fish
(except those on Group 1):

Brains

Fish

Fowl

Meat

Shellfish

Vegetables:

Asparagus

Beans, shell

Lentils

Mushrooms

Peas

Spinach

One serving (2 to 3 ounces) of meat, fish or fowl or 1 serving ($\frac{1}{2}$ cup) vegetable from this group is allowed each day or five days a week (depending upon condition) during remissions.

GROUP 3:   NEGLIGIBLE PURINE CONTENT

Bread,
    enriched white
    and crackers

Butter or fortified
    margarine
    (in moderation)

Cake and cookies

Carbonated
    beverage

Cereal beverage

Cereals and
    cereal products
    (refined and
    enriched)

Cheese

Chocolate

Coffee

Fruit

Gelatin desserts

Herbs

Ice cream

Milk

Nuts

Olives

Pickles

Popcorn

Puddings

Relishes

Rennet desserts

Rich desserts
    (in moderation)

Salt

Spices

Sugar and sweets

[5] M. V. Krause, *Food, Nutrition and Diet Therapy,* 4th edition, Philadelphia, W. B. Saunders Company, 1966, p. 319.

Condiments
Cornbread
Cream
   (in moderation)
Custard
Eggs
Fats
   (in moderation)

Tea
Vegetables
   (except those in
    Group 2)
Vinegar
White sauce

Foods included in this group may be used daily.

Anemia (Iron-deficiency anemia).   Decrease in quantity of hemoglobin or in number of red blood cells and decrease in number of smaller sized red blood corpuscles (hypochromic: low color; microcytic: small sized cells). Causes: loss of blood (hemorrhage) or inadequate intake or absorption of iron and protein, nutrients essential for hemoglobin formation.

High-Protein, High-Iron diet, nutritionally adequate otherwise. Absorption of iron from the intestinal tract is aided by liberal amounts of ascorbic acid. Iron-rich foods are stressed, possibly supplemented by iron salts therapy.

Liver, lean meat, eggs, kidney, heart   Whole grains and enriched breads
                                          and cereals

Green leafy vegetables   Potatoes
Dried fruits, legumes   Molasses
Liberal citrus fruits for ascorbic acid

Other anemias. (Macrocytic: large cell). Diet to meet or exceed recommended allowances, supplemented by folic acid therapy in Folic Acid Deficiency Anemia, and with vitamin B_{12} by injection in Pernicious Anemia (absence of an "intrinsic factor" needed for absorption of diet B_{12}).

Diseases Due To Malabsorption

Thought to be due to lack of one or more enzymes.

Celiac Disease.   Inability to absorb carbohydrates (simple or monosaccharides) or fat or both. Poor appetite. Hypersensitivity to gluten of grains.

High-Protein diet with restricted fat, restricted carbohydrate, or Low-Gluten diet (see page 258). High vitamins.[6]

Cystic Fibrosis.   Deficiency, absence, or failure of pancreatic enzymes to reach intestinal tract. Utilization of proteins, carbohydrates, and fats interfered with. Digestion very slow and much undigested food lost in feces.

High-Calorie, High-Protein, Moderate-Fat diet; vitamin supplements; salt in summer months to replace that lost in perspiration.

Other Diseases

Tropical sprue and the more recently discovered deficiency disease due to absence of enzymes to break down double sugars or disaccharides.

---

[6] *Celiac Disease Recipes,* Hospital for Sick Children 555 Shop, Toronto 2, Ontario.

Diseases Due To Inborn Errors Of Metabolism

Diseases Due To a Genetic Defect in Metabolism

Galactosemia. Inability to metabolize galactose (formed from lactose in milk). Galactose-free diet. Nonmilk formula products used in place of milk: casein hydrolysate, soybean mixture, or meat-base mixture.

Milk and all foods containing milk are excluded from diet. See "Foods containing milk," page 269.

Phenylketonuria. Absence of an enzyme necessary for the metabolism of the amino acid phenylalanine. Phenylalanine accumulates in the blood and causes mental retardation.

Very restricted diet since all proteins contain phenylalanine. Early treatment to prevent mental retardation. Diet low in natural protein supplemented by commercially prepared synthetic protein products with no phenylalanine. A commercial formula "Lofenalac" may serve as a protein main source because it contains very small amounts of phenylalanine.

Phenylalanine, a Diet Guide for Parents of Children with Phenylketonuria, California, State Department of Health, 1965

Parents' Guide for the Galactose Free Diet, California, State Department of Health.

Other Inborn Errors. Diabetes, gout and the more recently recognized histidinemia, maple sugar urine disease, and a certain type of hypoglycemia—all amino acid metabolic errors.

Nutritional Deficiencies

Any pathological condition brought about by a diet lacking in one or more nutrients due to inadequate intake, incomplete absorption, or incomplete utilization as diagnosed from medical history, physical examination, certain laboratory tests, and history of dietary practices. Treatment in each case: nutritionally adequate diet with special emphasis on the nutrient or nutrients lacking.

Vitamin Deficiencies	*Mineral Deficiencies*
Vitamin A: night blindness (nyctalopia) day blindness (hemeralopia) xerophthalmia	Ca and P: rickets, dental caries, osteomalacia, osteoporosis
Vitamin D: rickets osteomalacia (adult rickets) osteoporosis (other factors also) dental caries (?)	Fe: nutritional anemia (other factors also)
Thiamine: beriberi	Iodine: simple or endemic goiter
Riboflavin: ariboflavinosis	Fluorine: dental cavities
Niacin and tryptophan: pellagra	*Protein Deficiencies*
Ascorbic acid: scurvy	Hypoproteinemia
Vitamin K: hemorrhagic disease of newborn	Nutritional edema Protein Calorie Malnutrition Kwashiorkor Marasmus

DIET IN SURGERY

A good state of nutrition before and following surgery is a health asset to any surgical patient. It can determine the success of an operation as well as postoperative progress in withstanding stresses imposed by surgery and the period of convalescence. Fewer complications, quicker and better wound healing, and a shorter convalescence can be expected.

Preliminary dietary treatment may be required for a time, dependent upon the condition of the patient, and the type of operation—major or minor—with special attention given to high protein, high carbohydrate and minerals and possibly vitamin supplementation, particularly of ascorbic acid, and fluids. Obese patients, anemic patients, and diabetics may need special diet adjustments. Preoperative diet is equally important for the patient in good nutritive condition to meet the shock of surgery and the few days following when food is curtailed and nutritive balance impaired.

WHAT IS USUAL PREOPERATIVE AND POSTOPERATIVE DIET PROCEDURE?

Preoperative.   No food allowed immediatly before operation—time dependent on type of operation and anesthesia.

Minor sugery: no food day of operation unless scheduled for P.M.

GI tract surgery: fluid diet for several days preceding operation. No fluid or food after midnight of day previous to operation.

Postoperative.   Intravenous feedings to prevent dehydration and furnish very small amounts of nutrients—first physiologic saline and possibly glucose, protein hydrolysates, amino acids, water soluble vitamins, fat emulsions or glucose-fat emulsions, depending on individual patient and his surgeon.

Progression of sips of water or bits of ice in mouth, then clear liquid, full liquid, soft, and full diet, rapidity of increase determined by patient's progress and surgeon, and operation. For any but very special types of surgery, progression from liquid to full diet may be rather rapid.

Note to Instructor: It is desirable to provide each student with a copy of the preoperative and postoperative procedures followed in her own hospital to be attached to this page; also, any special routines individual surgeons request following certain types of surgery.

Dumping Syndrome

The "dumping syndrome" refers to certain symptoms experienced by some patients when they return to a full diet following gastric surgery involving a partial or total gastrectomy. The foods eaten are not held in the new pouch formed by the remaining stomach tissue and pass very quickly into the jejunum before any digestion takes place in the stomach—giving rise to pain and other symptoms. Dietary treatment is of extreme importance and includes high protein, high fat, and low carbohydrate foods in 6 to 8 small meals per day, eaten regularly, and no fluids at meals. Whole milk may not be tolerated.

Fractures[7]

Following fractures of the long bones there is an increase in protein breakdown in well-nourished individuals, aggravated still further by prolonged immobilization. Loss of protein (nitrogen) is accompanied by loss of potassium, phosphorus and

---

[7] M. V. Krause, *Food ,Nutrition and Diet Therapy,* 4th edition, Philadelphia, W. B. Saunders Company, 1966, p. 280

sulfur; osteoporosis will develop with loss of calcium due to immobilization; loss of fluids and imbalance among minerals (Na, K, Cl electrolytes) may also occur. The aim of dietary treatment is to replace losses by a diet high in protein—about 150 grams—plus 3000 non-protein calories (unless problems of obesity occur) in regular meals; high protein - high calorie beverages between meals if appetite limited at mealtime. Liberal protein in the diet favors deposition of calcium in the bones and formation of good callus.

WHAT ARE SPECIAL DIETARY NEEDS FOLLOWING BURNS?

To meet large losses of protein, salts, and fluids and wide tissue breakdown: high protein, high calorie, high vitamins (as supplements), ascorbic acid for wound healing and B complex vitamins because of increased metabolism, all supplemented with high calorie beverages.

Note: Refer to page 203 for information about fluid and tube feedings.

CLASS ACTIVITY

For purposes of review of Therapeutic Diets, each student may be supplied with a current copy of her hospital's menus for patients. This copy may be attached to this page for reference. On the back of this page may then be shown how the day's menu was adapted for therapeutic diets served on the particular day.

SUPPLEMENTARY READINGS

Howe: Surgery, Chapter 17; Allergy, Chapter 26, and pages 397–401; Children's Diseases, Chapter 27; Nutrient Deficiencies, Chapter 16; Mowry: Chapters 19, 24; Peyton: Chapter 27; Robinson: Consult Index for various diseases.

Section Three

FOOD PREPARATION AND SERVICE

Object

To help the practical nurse, through discussion, observation of demonstrations and/or some practice in simple food preparation, to acquire the appreciation and knowledge of the basic principles involved in the selection and cookery of foods that will be palatable and high in original nutritive value, and to develop simple food preparation skills.

NOTE TO INSTRUCTOR

Recipes for dishes suitable to be prepared or demonstrated in food preparation classes will be found in the following references:

Food preparation sections in references marked with asterisk on page 291.

Standard cookbooks.

The Basic Cookbook, by M. Heseltine and U. Dow, Boston, Houghton Mifflin Company, 1967.

Cookbook of the United Nations, United Nations Association of the United States, New York, John Wiley and Sons.

U. S. Department of Agriculture Yearbooks:

Food–1959, pages 519–554, *"What and How to Cook"*. Recipes arranged according to the Four Food Groups in the Daily Food Guide.

Food for Us All—1969. Recipes scattered throughout book.

Family Fare, Home and Garden Bulletin No. 1, Washington, D. C., U. S. D. A., 1970.

Money-Saving Dishes, Home and Garden Bulletin No. 43, Washington, D. C. U. S. D. A., 1970.

Bulletins: U.S. Department of Agriculture. See page 116. State Extension Offices.

The information listed below will be found in:

Standard cookbooks.

Handbook of Food Preparation, American Home Economics Association, Washington, D. C., 1971.

Foods, by G. E. Vail, R. M. Griswold, M. M. Justin, and L. O. Rust, Boston, Houghton Mifflin Company, 1967.

Information about recipe ingredients and how to substitute one for another

Terms used in preparing, combining and cooking foods

Cooking and baking guides and tips for all groups of foods

Meal planning tips and service

Number of servings in common units of food

LESSON 1. INTRODUCTION TO LABORATORY

Object: To become familiar with the food laboratory.

To discuss the fundamentals of food preparation.

To discuss table and tray service.

To discuss nutritive value and preparation of beverages and toast.

Become Familiar With The Food Laboratory

1.   Check your desk and note arrangement of equipment.

2.   Become familiar with general equipment in the laboratory: the location and arrangement of larger utensils, china, glassware, and silver; location and arrangement of supplies.

3.   Read carefully bulletin board items: general and individual housekeeping duties; directions for care of equipment; rules for working; methods of dishwashing; other items. Get in the habit of checking bulletin board for nutrition items, illustrations, etc.

4. Jot down in your notebook dates you are responsible for geneal and specific duties.

Fundamentals of Food Preparation

Reasons for Cooking Foods. To make foods not ordinarily eaten raw more appetizing as to appearance, texture, and flavor.

To make foods more digestible by softening fruit and vegetable cellulose; softening meat fibers; bursting cereal and starch granules.

To destroy certain undesirable microorganisms and parasites.

To make foods and meals more interesting by increasing the variety in preparation.

General Principles. Use accurate measurements.

Use tested recipes.

Use low heat for all protein foods as eggs, cheese, meat, fish, poultry.

Do not overcook foods.

Economy Hints. Use margarine in place of butter.

Foods prepared at home are less expensive than packaged mixes, partly cooked and ready-to-eat foods.

Foods in season are cheaper than when out of season.

Use the equally nutritious lower grade foods where appearance is less important.

Use all juices from cooking: meat juices, vegetable cooking water, liquid from canned foods.

Use fat and meat drippings for cooking other foods.

Use inexpensive forms of milk.

BASIC METHODS OF COOKING

Moist Heat	*Dry Heat*	*Frying*
Boiling	Broiling	(cooking in fat)
Simmering	Pan-broiling	Sauteing
Stewing	Baking	Pan-frying
Braising	Roasting	Deep-fat frying
Steaming		

COOKING TERMS[1]

Bake	To cook in an oven or oven-type appliance. Covered or uncovered containers may be used.
Barbecue	To roast slowly on a spit or rack over coals or under a gas broiler flame or electric broiler unit, usually basting with a highly seasoned sauce. Also, foods cooked in or served with barbecue sauce.

[1] From *Family Fare.* Home and Garden Bulletin No. 1. Washington, D. C., U. S. Department of Agriculture, 1970, pp. 86–87.

Baste	To pour melted fat, drippings, or other liquid over food to moisten it during cooking
Boil	To cook in water, or other liquid, at boiling temperature (212° F. at sea level). Bubbles rise continually and break on the surface.
Braise	To cook meat or poultry slowly in steam from meat juices or added liquid trapped and held in a covered pan. Meat may be browned in a small amount of fat before braising.
Broil	To cook uncovered on a rack placed directly under heat or over an open fire. *Pan-broil.* To cook in uncovered pan over direct heat, pouring fat off as it accumulates.
Caramelize	To heat sugar or food containing sugar until a brown color and characteristic flavor develop.
Fold	To combine two mixtures (or two ingredients such as beaten egg white and sugar) by cutting down gently through mixture, turning it over, and repeating until well mixed.

Fry	To cook in fat without water or cover.
	    Pan-fry or *saute.*—To cook in a small amount of fat (a few tablespoons, up to $\frac{1}{2}$ inch) in fry pan.
	    Deep-fry or french-fry.—To cook in a deep kettle, in enough fat to cover or float food.

Grill	Same as broil.
Knead	To press, stretch, and fold dough or other mixture to make it elastic or smooth. Bread dough becomes elastic, fondant becomes smooth and satiny.
Marinate	To let foods stand in a liquid (usually mixture of oil with vinegar or lemon juice) to add flavor or make more tender.
Parboil	To boil until partly cooked.
Poach	To simmer gently in liquid so food retains its shape.
Pot-roast	To cook large pieces of meat by braising.
Reconstitute	To restore concentrated food such as frozen orange juice or dry milk to its original state; usually by adding water.
Rehydrate	To soak or cook dried foods to restore water lost in drying.
Roast	To cook in heated air (usually oven) without water or cover.
Simmer	To cook in liquid just below the boiling point, at temperatures of 185° to 210° F. Bubbles form slowly and break below the surface.
Steam	To cook food in steam, with or without pressure. Food is steamed in a covered container, on a rack or in a perforated pan over boiling water.
Stew	To cook in liquid, just below the boiling point.

Measures and Temperatures

Measuring foods
Part of cup.—Use tablespoons or the smaller measuring cups—$\frac{1}{2}$, $\frac{1}{3}$, $\frac{1}{4}$

—for greater accuracy.
    Brown sugar.—Pack firmly into cup or spoon.

Solid fats.—When fat comes in 1-pound rectangular form, 1 cup or fraction can be cut from pound, which measures about 2 cups.

Or measure cupful by packing fat firmly into cup and leveling off top with spatual or straight knife.

Water method may be used for part of cup. To measure 1/2 cup fat, for instance, put 1/2 cup cold water in 1-cup measure. Add fat, pushing it under the water until water level stands at 1-cup mark. Pour out water and remove fat.

White flour.—Sift once. Lift lightly into cup. Level off top with spatula or straight knife.

Other flours, fine meals, fine crumbs, dried eggs. dry milks.—Stir instead of sifting. Measure like flour.

Baking powder, cornstarch, cream of tartar, spices.—Stir to loosen. Fill spoon to overflowing, level with spatula or straight knife.

Common food measures

3 teaspoons . . . . 1 tablespoon
2 tablespoons . . . . 1 fluid ounce
4 tablespoons . . . . 1/4 cup
5 1/2 tablespoons . . . . 1/3 cup
8 tablespoons . . . . 1/2 cup
16 tablespoons . . . . 1 cup
1 cup . . . . 8 fluid ounces
2 cups . . . . 1 pint
2 pints . . . . 1 quart

Oven temperatures

Very slow . . . . 250° and 275° F.
Slow . . . . 300° and 325° F.
Moderate . . . . 350° and 375° F.
Hot . . . . 400° and 425° F.
Very hot . . . . 450° and 475° F.
Extremely hot . . . . 500° and 525° F.

From *Family Fare.* Home and Garden Bulletin No. 1. Washington, D. C., U. S. Department of Agriculture, 1970, pp. 26–27.

GOOD WORKING HABITS

Read recipe directions carefully
Plan work in correct sequence
Wash hands before preparing food
Preheat oven if baking a product
Assemble ingredients to be used
Assemble utensils to be used—use as few as possible
Use accepted measuring equipment and methods

Rinse cooking utensils as soon as used; cold water for protein foods, hot water for greasy and starchy foods
Follow approved methods of dishwashing
Work quietly.

Learn to observe your own and class products critically for appearance, texture, flavor, and temperature (hot foods hot and cold foods cold)

Complete assigned housekeeping duties

Demonstration. Methods of measuring in food preparation (dry ingredients, liquids, fats)

Special cooking procedures
Placement of utensils in oven for baking
Storage of food in the refrigerator

Food Service

Review page 187.

Setting a table. Rules for setting a table to make it inviting and to make the serving of the meal easy.

Glassware, dishes, and silverware for each person at the table are called a "cover."

Use a clean tablecloth or mat of a color that looks well with the dishes.

Place silver, napkin, and dishes about an inch from the edge of the table.

Place tines of the fork and bowls of the spoons with hollow part up; the sharp edge of the knife toward the plate; the hemmed edges of the napkin toward the plate and edge of the tables.

If both a salad plate and a bread and butter plate are used, place the salad plate just above the napkin. If a bread and butter plate is not used, put salad plate just above the fork.

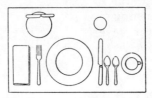

Exhibit. Place service properly arranged for one or three meals on dining table. Tray properly set up for breakfast, dinner, or supper service, or all three meals.

Bases for Judging Meals

SCORE SHEET FOR MEALS[2]

I. Selection of Food   Possible Score—138
   1. Balance: Different foodstuffs represented   _____   Use key (put in
   2. Texture: contrasting   _____   number which
   3. Flavor: contrasting   _____   corresponds to
           palatable   _____   quality)
   4. Color: colorful   _____   1. Very poor
           harmonizing   _____   2. Poor
   5. Adaptation: foods in season   _____   3. Fair
           foods suitable for the meal   _____   4. Satisfactory
II. Preparation of Food   5. Good
   1. Cooking: suitable method   _____   6. Superior
           neither overcooked nor underdone   _____
   2. Seasoning: pleasing   _____
   3. Organization: work well planned   _____
           (scored by instructor)
   4. Economy: no waste of time (scored by
           instructor)
           no waste of food   _____
III. Service of Food
   1. Punctual: ready at time set   _____
   2. Appearance: table or tray neat, attractive
           and correctly set   _____
           food inviting   _____

---

[2] G. E. Vail, R. M. Griswold, M. M. Justin, and L. O. Rust: *Foods*. 5th edition, Boston, Houghton Mifflin Company, 1967, p. 524-525.

3. Quietness: no rattling of silver or dishes   _____
4. Correctness: according to standards set   _____
5. Skill: quickly and easily done   _____
       silver handled correctly in
       serving and eating   _____
6. Atmosphere: at ease and pleasant   _____
7. Conversation: pleasant   _____

Beverages

Value. Relieve thirst
Stimulate appetite
Furnish body with fluids
Minerals and vitamins in fruit juices
   without too many extra calories
High nutrient value in milk beverages
Egg white, dried milk, cream, lactose
   increase nutritive value
Wines add extra caloric value
Refreshing. Water
Carbonated beverages
Fruit juices
Vegetable juices
Fruit ades
Iced tea
Ginger ale

Stimulating. Tea
Coffee
Eggnogs with rum, brandy, whiskey,
   coffee
Alcoholic beverages
Soothing. Warm milk
Hot tea
Nourishing. Milk—all forms
Eggnogs and other egg beverages
Fruit juices with lactose or glucose
Albuminized fruit juices
Fruit juice with whole eggs
Tube feedings

BEVERAGE SERVICE

Serve as soon as possible after preparation

Serve fruit juices on tart rather than sweet side

Serve hot beverages hot; cold ones cold

Standard sugar syrup may be used to sweeten beverages to save time

Garnishes add to attactiveness of beverage service: mint, fruit slices, cherries for fruit ades, etc.

Demonstration or student preparation: Coffee making: "boiled," percolator, drip, vacuum, automatic methods.

Cocoa: using cooked homemade or commercial syrup; using instant forms (more expensive).

Toast

Value. More readily digested than untoasted bread as starch is changed to dextrin by heat.

Dryness and hardness of toast require mastication.

Should be enriched or whole grain for maximum nutrients.

Preparation.   Follow manufacurer's directions with electric toaster.

May be broiler toasted with bread on rack under direct heat.

May be oven toasted but product dryer and crisper.

Use day old bread cut $\frac{1}{4}$ inch thick.

Should be golden brown and crisp.

Service.   Dry or buttered for breakfast.

Serve warm (cover with special cover or wrap in napkin).

Toast points, croutons, zweiback under creamed foods.

Cinnamon toast. Milk toast.

Toasted crackers and rolls.

Demonstration or student preparation: White and whole wheat toast: electric toaster; broiler; oven.

Service of Beverage and Toast

Exhibit.   Tray service for toast and beverage.[3]

LESSON 2. CEREALS AND FRUITS

Object: To study the nutritive value, preparation, and serving of cereals and fruits.

To study the importance of breakfast for good nutrition.

To study breakfast service.

Discussion

A. **Cereals.**   Review pages 112–114.

B. **Fruits.**   Review pages 109–110

C. **Breakfast.**   Plan and ideas on page 130.

Preparation of Fruits and Cereals for Breakfast Menus[4]

Breakfasts	I	II	III	IV
Fruit	Orange sections	Stewed prunes	Baked apple	Broiled grapefruit
Cereal (with milk and sugar) and/or	Oatmeal	Cream of wheat	Boiled white or brown rice	Maltex
Toast (with butter and marmalade, if desired)	Enriched	Whole wheat	Rye	Enriched
Milk to drink				
Beverage				

[3, 4] Where time or facilities do not permit preparation of complete meals, place proper dishes for foods not prepared on trays. Where no actual food preparation is possible, use food models.

Class Discussion of Breakfast Trays

Demonstration.   Sectioning grapefruit   Broiled grapefruit
Sliced oranges   Baked apples

LESSON 3. CREAM SAUCES AND SOUPS
FRUIT DESSERTS

Object: To study the properties and preparation of cream sauce as a basis for cream soups and other dishes.
To prepare simple fruit desserts.
To serve simple luncheon and supper trays.

Discussion

A. Fats.   Review pages 41 and 115.
B. Cream (white) sauces.   Review page 115.
Demonstration   or student preparation: Cream sauce (thin to medium).
Cheese souffle (use of thick white sauce)
C. Fruit desserts.   Types: Whips—sweetened fruit pulp and beaten egg white.
Souffles—whips baked at low temperatures.
Baked fruit puddings: Fruit Betty—fruit combined with bread.
Fruit crisp—fruit topped with crumb mixture.
Fruit cobbler—fruit topped with biscuit or pastry.
Fruit pudding—fruit combined with uncooked batter before baking.
Gelatin desserts—unflavored gelatin plus fruit juices with or without the addition of fruit, nuts, marshmallows, whipped cream, etc. Flavored gelatin may be used as the base. May also serve as salad when placed on greens.
Frozen—frozen fruit juices called ices; with beaten egg white or milk called sherbets.
Fruit tapioca.

PREPARATION OF CREAM SOUPS AND ACCOMPANIMENTS
AND SIMPLE FRUIT DESSERTS FOR LUNCHEON AND
SUPPER MENUS[5]

LUNCHEON OR SUPPER MENUS

	I	II	III	IV
Soup	Cream of corn	Cream of potato	Clam chowder	Cream of tomato
Accompaniment	Paprika crackers	Whole wheat crackers	Crisped crackers	Cheese crackers
Salad or relish		Relishes	Tossed salad	

---

[5] Where time or facilities do not permit preparation of complete menus, place proper dishes for the foods not prepared on the trays. Where no actual food preparation is possible, use food models.

LUNCHEON OR SUPPER MENUS

	I	II	III	IV
Dessert	Apple crisp	Prune souffle	Cherry cobbler	Jellied fruit
Beverage	Milk	Milk	Milk	Milk

Class Discussion of Luncheon or Supper Trays

LESSON 4. MILK, EGGS, CHEESE

Object: To study the nutritive value, preparation, and serving of milk, egg, and cheese dishes.

To prepare and serve simple luncheon or supper menus using milk, egg, and cheese dishes.

Discussion

A. **Milk.** Review pages 100–101.
B. **Cheese.** Review pages 101–102.
C. **Eggs.** Review pages 105–106.

Preparation and Use of Milk, Cheese, and Egg Dishes in Meals[6]

SUGGESTED DISHES

Milk Dishes

Junket

Starchy puddings

Cooked salad dressing

Rice pudding

Cream soups with vegetables

Beverages

Sauces   Chowders

Tapioca puddings

Cheese Dishes

Fondue

Souffle

Sauce

Rarebit

Toasted cheese sandwich

Grilled sandwich

Molded cottage cheese salad

Egg Dishes

Foamy omelet

Plain omelet

Baked omelet

Baked custard

Baked eggs

Shirred eggs

Scrambled eggs

Eggs a la Goldenrod

---

[6] Where time or facilities do not permit preparation of complete meals, place the proper dishes for the foods not prepared on the trays. Where no actual food preparation is possible, use food models.

Egg Dishes

Soft custard

Poached eggs

Coddled eggs

Sandwich filling

Egg salad

Egg cutlets

MENUS

I

Jelly omelet

Sliced tomatoes

Whole wheat bread and butter

Rice pudding

Milk

II

Creamed eggs on toast

Lettuce salad with boiled dressing

Junket

Milk

III

Toasted cheese sandwich

Carrot and celery sticks

Bread and butter

Fruit cup

Milk

IV

Cream tomato soup

Pear and cottage cheese salad

Saltines

Baked custard

Milk

Class Discussion of Meal Trays

Demonstration or student preparation: soft (stirred) custard baked custard Junket poached eggs scrambled eggs omelet egg cutlets.

LESSON 5. MEAT, POULTRY, AND FISH

Object: To study the nutritive value, preparation, and serving of meat, poultry, and fish dishes.

To prepare and serve dinner menus using meat, poultry, and fish dishes.

Discussion

Meat, poultry, fish. Review pages 102–105.

Exhibit. Commonly used cuts of meat (or models or posters) Commonly used fish: whole, steaks, fillets.[7]

Demonstration. Preparation of oven roast, pot roast, scraped beef, gravy making. Stuffing and roasting poultry, frying chicken, cooking fowl. Baked fish fillets or steaks. Oven-fried fish.

---

[7] A field trip to a supermarket where meat cuts and fish are sold could be substituted for this exhibit.

Preparation of Meat, Poultry, and Fish Dishes for Dinner Menus[7]

DINNER MENUS

I

Meat loaf or
Ham loaf
Baked potatoes
Buttered spinach
Bread and butter
Canned peaches
Cookies
Milk

II

Braised pork chop
    or
Pan broiled shoulder lamb chop
Scalloped tomatoes
Rolls and butter
Gingerbread and whipped cream
Milk

III

Pot roast (from demonstration) with
    browned potatoes, carrots, and
    onions or
Beef or lamb stew
Hard rolls and butter
Waldorf salad
Milk

IV

Broiled fish fillet
    or
Baked fish
Creamed potatoes
Buttered green beans
Cabbage salad
Bread and butter
Lemon pudding
Milk

Class Discussion of Dinner Menus

LESSON 6. VEGETABLES

Object: To study the nutritive value, preparation, and serving of vegetables. To prepare meals using vegetables.

Discussion

Vegetables.   Review pages 106–108. See boiling guide for vegetables, page 109.

Exhibit.   Less well-known vegetables and suggestions for use.[8]

Demonstration.   Vegetable garnishes and sauces.
Relish trays.
Pressure cooking vegetables.
"Waterless" cooking of vegetables.

---

[7] Where times or facilities do not permit preparation of complete meals, plaee the proper dishes for the foods not prepared on the trays., Where no actual food preparation is possible, use food models.

[8] A field trip to a supermarket may be substituted for this exhibit.

Preparation and Use of Vegetables in Meals[9]

MENUS

I

Baked potato
Buttered broccoli
Harvard beets
Whole wheat muffins and butter
Baked custard
Milk

II

Creamed asparagus on toast
Buttered carrots
Broiled tomato
Hard rolls and butter
Spanish cream
Milk

III

Scalloped tomatoes
Buttered spinach
Toasted cheese sandwich
Baked apple
Milk

IV

Scalloped peas, carrots, and celery
Parsleyed potatoes
Pear and cottage cheese salad
Oatmeal and raisin cookies
Milk

Class Discussion of Meal Trays

LESSON 7. SALADS AND SALAD DRESSINGS: SANDWICHES AND SIMPLE BAKED PRODUCTS

Object: To study the nutritive value, preparation, and serving of salads and relishes. To prepare meals in which salads are used as the main course, accompaniments to a meal, or as desserts.

To study the properties, preparation, and serving of sandwiches, and simple quick breads, cookies, cake, and pastry, and their use in meals.

Discussion

Salads. Review pages 110–112.

Exhibit. Unusual greens and raw vegetables used in salads.
Attractive relish tray.
Cheese and cracker tray to accompany salad service.

Demonstration. Preparation of lettuce for salads.
Prepration of garnishes—radish roses, carrot curls, etc.
Tossing a salad with oil, vinegar, and seasonings.
Peeling tomatoes; peeling and sectioning citrus fruits; cutting fresh pineapple.
Tomato aspic with cottage cheese
Fruit juice molded with fruit
Evaporated milk salad dressing

---

[9] Where time or facilities do not permit preparation of complete menus, place proper dishes on trays for the foods not prepared. Where no actual food preparation is possible, use food models.

Sandwiches. *Kinds:*

Hearty: serve as main dish of meal hot or cold, knife and fork or finger style, of meat, cheese, fish, poultry, eggs.

Less hearty: to serve with soup course, salad, tea.

Canapes: open sandwiches and specially garnished.

Tea: dainty sandwiches cut in various shapes and with bread crusts removed.

Sandwich fillings: sliced meat, chopped or grated vegetables, peanut butter, baked beans, tasty chopped mixtures of meat, fish, poultry, eggs, etc.

French toasted sandwiches; many types may be French toasted.

Preparation Points

Use day old bread except for rolled.

Slice thin for dainty tea sandwiches and canapes; thicker for main dish sandwiches.

Remove crusts for dainty sandwiches (plan to use crusts for croutons, crumbs, or in puddings).

Spread sandwiches with softened (not melted) butter.

Cut in different shapes for eye appeal.

Have fillings fresh and crsip.

Use variety of breads: white, whole wheat, rye, nut, raisin, fruited.

Use appropriate garnish for sandwich service when desired.

Quick breads : made with quick acting leavenings as baking powder, or soda and sour milk, or steam. Ratio of liquid to flour varies.

Types:

Pour batters: popovers, griddle cakes, waffles.

Drop batters: muffins, cakes.

Stiff doughs: pastry, cookies.

Oven-baked: biscuits, muffins, corn breads, quick loaf breads.

Griddle baked: griddle cakes, waffles.

Steamed: dumplings, brown bread.

Deep fat fried: doughnuts, fritters.

Commercial mixes.

Cakes. *Types:*

Shortened or butter cakes: contain shortening.

Unshortened cakes: sponge and angel food contain no fat and depend chiefly upon the air which is beaten into the egg whites to leaven the cake. The air expands during baking and causes the cake to rise.

Commercial mixes.

Building a menu around a salad, breadstuff, and dessert with milk as beverage

Main course	*Accompaniment*	*Dessert*
Fruit salad	Cheese and crackers	Gingerbread
Tossed vegetable salad	Bran muffins	Baked custard
Meat, fish, or egg salad	Baking powder biscuits	Apple sauce
	Currant jelly	
Vegetable soup	Pinapple and cottage cheese salad	Oatmeal cookies
Toasted cheese sandwich	Relishes	Salad fruit
Waffles	With honey or maple syrup	Frozen fruit salad

Preparation of salads, salad dressings, and quick breads.[10]

---

[10] Where time or facilities do not permit preparation of complete menus, place proper dishes for the foods not prepared on the trays. Where no actual food preparation is possible, use food models.

Use of Salads and Dressings, and Quick Breads in Meals

Menus to be planned by class.

Class Discussion of Meals

Demonstration (if desirable). Preparation of baking powder biscuits. Preparation and baking of yeast rolls, angel food cake, preparing pastry for pie tins. (Regular recipes or mixes may be used.)

LESSON 8. FAMILY MEALS: LOW COST FOODS; RACIAL FOODS

Object: To prepare and serve meals for a family group.
To prepare low cost foods, substitute dishes, and meals.
To learn dishes and meals typical of different nationality groups.

Discussion

Meal planning.   Review pages 127–130.
Low-cost meals.   Review pages 127–129.

Preparation of Low Cost Main Dishes and their Use in Family Meals[11]

MENUS[12]

I	II	III	IV
Cheese fondue	Scrambled eggs with luncheon meat	Kidney stew	Baked beans
Baked squash		Green or yellow vegetable	Hot cornbread
Green vegetable	Baked potato	Apple and raisin salad	Carrot and cabbage slaw
Apple and celery salad with nuts	Carrot and celery sticks	Cookies or cake	Baked custard
Cookies	Tomato aspic salad	Milk	Milk
Milk	Fruit dumplings		
	Milk		

V	VI	VII	VIII
Tomato juice	Chicken with dumplings	Rice with chicken	Brown beef stew
Ham and scalloped potatoes	Broccoli	Spinach with hard cooked egg	Green salad
Snap beans	Gelatin vegetable salad	Celery and carrot sticks	Baked pear
Cabbage salad	Date and nut pudding	Fruit pickle	Milk
Prune whip	Milk	Peach pie	
Milk		Milk	

Class Discussion of Meals

Preparation of Racial Dishes and Meals

Demonstration. Racial dishes prepared by class members who represent different racial backgrounds.

Field Trips. Visit to restaurant—for observing or eating a meal—where foreign dishes are prepared. Visit to a market in foreign section of city to observe some of the foods used by different racial groups.

LESSON 9. FOODS FOR THERAPEUTIC DIETS

Object: To become familiar with types of foods served on certain therapeutic diets.

Discussion, Demonstration, Exhibits, Food Preparation, or Food Models

Tube feedings
High protein, high calorie liquid feedings
Day's meals for 1200 to 1500 calorie diet
Day's meals for a fat restricted diet
Day's meals for a fat controlled diet
Low sodium foods available for sodium restricted diets
Preparation (and tasting) of vegetables for sodium restricted diets
Foods for the progressive four stage regimen for ulcer
Foods prepared for allergy diets: without milk; without eggs; without wheat

---

[11] Where time or facilities do not permit preparation of complete menus, place proper dishes for foods not prepared on the trays. Where no actual food preparation is possible, use food models.

[12] *Money-saving Main Dishes*, Home and Garden Bulletin No. 43, Washington, D. C., U.S. Department of Agriculture. adapted.

APPENDIX

GENERAL REFERENCES

Anderson, L., and J. H. Browe: *Nutrition and Family Health Service,* Philadelphia, W. B. Saunders Company, 1960.

Bogert, L. J., G. M. Briggs, and D. H. Calloway: *Nutrition and Physical Fitness,* 8th edition, Philadelphia, W. B. Saunders Company, 1966.

Fleck, H., and E. Munves: *Introduction to Nutrition,* 2nd edition, New York, The Macmillan Company, 1971.

Howe, P. S.: *Basic Nutrition in Health and Disease,* 5th edition, Philadelphia, W. B. Saunders Company, 1971.

*Krause, M. V.: *Food Nutrition and Diet Therapy,* 4th edition, Philadelphia, W. B. Saunders Company, 1966.

Leverton, R. M.: *Food Becomes You,* Revised 3rd edition, Ames, Iowa, Iowa State University Press, 1965.

Michelson, O: *Nutrition Science and You,* New York, Scholastic Book Services, 1964.

*Mitchell, H. S., H. J. Rynbergen, L. Anderson, and M. V. Dibble: *Cooper's Nutrition in Health and Disease,* 15th edition, Philadelphia, J. B. Lippincott Company, 1968.

Mowry, L. and Williams, S: *Basic Nutrition and Diet Therapy for Nurses,* 4th edition, Saint Louis, The C. V. Mosby Company, 1969.

Nutrition Foundation: *Present Knowledge in Nutrition,* 3rd edition, New York, The Nutrition Foundation, 1967.

Peyton, A. B.: *Practical Nutrition,* 2nd edition, Philadelphia, J. B. Lippincott Company, 1962.

Robinson, C. H.: *Basic Nutrition and Diet Therapy,* 2nd edition, New York, The Macmillan Company, 1970.

Robinson, C. H.: *Fundamentals of Normal Nutrition,* New York, The Macmillan Company, 1968.

*Robinson, C. H.: *Normal and Therapeutic Nutrition,* 14th edition, New York, The Macmillan Company, 1972.

Stare, F. J.: *Eating for Good Health,* New York, Doubleday & Company, 1964.

Vail, G. E., R. M. Griswold, M. M. Justin, and L. O. Rust: *Foods,* 5th edition, Boston, Houghton Mifflin Company, 1967.

White, P. L.: *Let's Talk About Food.* Chicago, American Medical Association, 1967.

Wilson, E. D., K. H. Fisher and M. E. Fuqua: *Principles of Nutrition,* 3rd edition, New York, John Wiley and Sons, 1972.

Yearbooks, U. S. Department of Agriculture, Washington.
 Food–1959
 Consumers All–1965
 Food for Us All–1969.

---

*Contain recipes suitable for class preparation or demonstration.

OTHER SOURCES OF NUTRITION INFORMATION

American Diabetes Association, 18 East 48th Street, New York 10017

American Dietetic Association, 620 North Michigan Avenue, Chicago, Illinois 60611

> *Journal of American Dietetic Association*
> List of publications available

American Heart Association, 44 East 23rd Street, New York, New York 10010

American Home Economics Association, 1600 Twentieth Street N. W., Washington, D. C. 20006

> *Journal of Home Economics*
> List of publications available

American Medical Association, 535 N. Dearborn Street, Chicago, Illinois 60610

> *Today's Health*
> List of publications of the Council on Foods and Nutrition available

American Public Health Association, 1790 Broadway, New York, New York 10019

> *American Journal of Public Health*
> List of publications of Food and Nutrition Section available

Food and Nutrition Board, National Research Council, 210 Constitution Avenue, Washington, D. C. 60625

Metropolitan Life Insurance Company, Health and Welfare Division, One Madison Avenue, New York, New York 10010

The Nutrition Foundation, Inc., 99 Park Avenue, New York, New York 10016

The Society for Nutrition Education, California, 119 Morgan Hall, University of California,

> *Journal of Nutrition Education*

U.S. Department of Agriculture, Washington, D. C.

> List of publications available from Office of Information.

U.S. Department of Health, Education, and Welfare, Washington, D. C.

> List of publications available from
>> Children's Bureau
>> Office of Education
>> Food and Drug Administration
>> Public Health Service

State departments of public health, state capital

State extension services, state college

Better Business Bureaus

> *Free Publications*

Dairy Council Digest

Dairy Council News and Recipes

Nutrition News

> National Dairy Council, Chicago, Illinois

Food and Nutrition News

Pamphlets and recipes

> National Live Stock and Meat Board, Chicago, Illinois

Nutrition Program News

Food and Home Notes

> U. S. Department of Agriculture, Washington, D. C.

DESIRABLE
WEIGHTS
FOR MEN
of ages 25
and over

Weight in Pounds According to Frame (In Indoor Clothing)

HEIGHT (with shoes on) 1-inch heels Feet Inches	SMALL FRAME	MEDIUM FRAME	LARGE FRAME
5 2	112–120	118–129	126–141
5 3	115–123	121–133	129–144
5 4	118–126	124–136	132–148
5 5	121–129	127–139	135–152
5 6	124–133	130–143	138–156
5 7	128–137	134–147	142–161
5 8	132–141	138–152	147–166
5 9	136–145	142–156	151–170
5 10	140–150	146–160	155–174
5 11	144–154	150–165	159–179
6 0	148–158	154–170	164–184
6 1	152–162	158–175	168–189
6 2	156–167	162–180	173–194
6 3	160–171	167–185	178–199
6 4	164–175	172–190	182–204

DESIRABLE
WEIGHTS
FOR WOMEN
of ages 25
and over

HEIGHT (with shoes on) 2-inch heels Feet Inches	SMALL FRAME	MEDIUM FRAME	LARGE FRAME
4 10	92– 98	96–107	104–119
4 11	94–101	98–110	106–122
5 0	96–104	101–113	109–125
5 1	99–107	104–116	112–128
5 2	102–110	107–119	115–131
5 3	105–113	110–122	118–134
5 4	108–116	113–126	121–138
5 5	111–119	116–130	125–142
5 6	114–123	120–135	129–146
5 7	118–127	124–139	133–150
5 8	122–131	128–143	137–154
5 9	126–135	132–147	141–158
5 10	130–140	136–151	145–163
5 11	134–144	140–155	149–168
6 0	138–148	144–159	153–173

For girls between 18 and 25, subtract 1 pound for each year under 25.

From Metropolitan Life Insurance Company, 1959

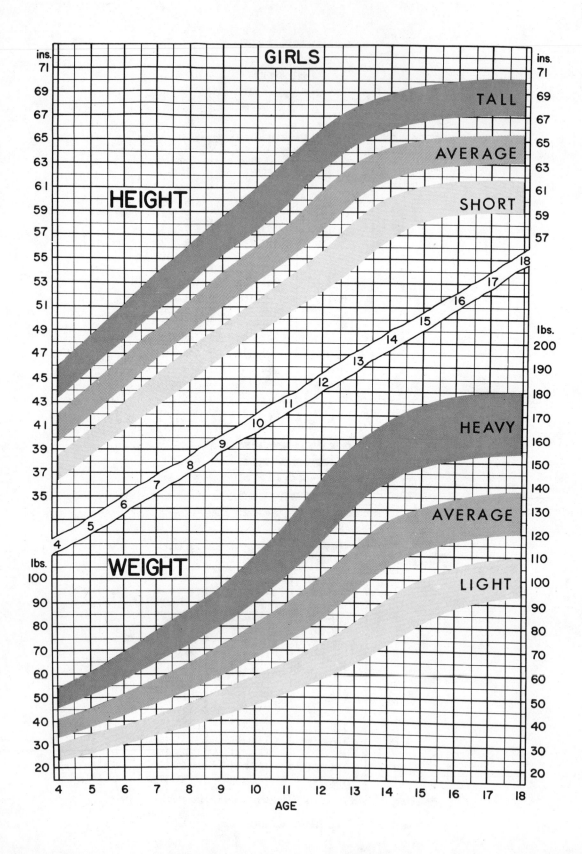

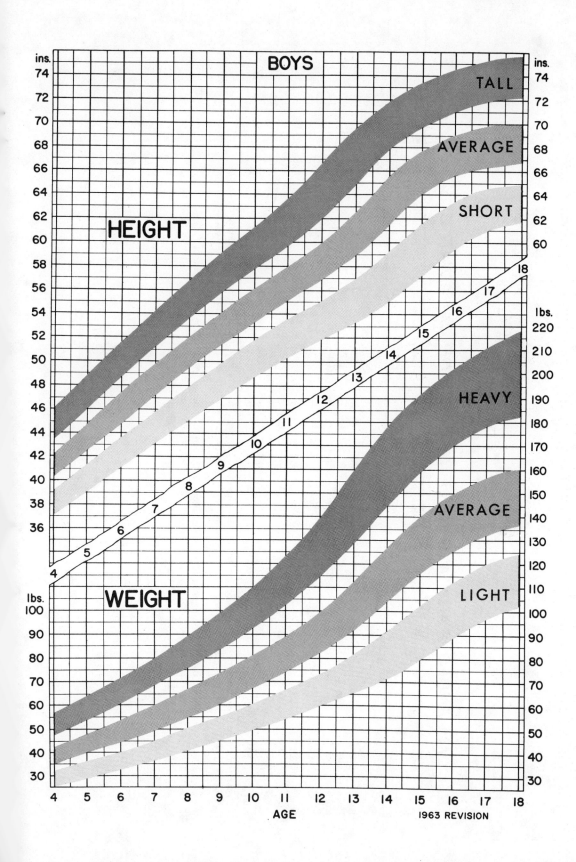

RECOMMENDED DAILY NUTRIENT INTAKES FOR CANADIAN BOYS AND GIRLS*

Sex	Age	Weight	Activity Category	Calories	Protein	Calcium	Iron	Vitamin A	Vitamin D	Ascorbic Acid	Thiamine	Riboflavin	Niacin
	yrs.	lbs.			g.(1)	g.	mg.	I.U.(2)	I.U.	mg.	mg.	mg.	mg.
Both	0-1	7-20	Usual	360-900	7-13	0.5	5	1000	400	20	0.3	0.5	3
Both	1-2	20-26	Usual	900-1200	12-16	0.7	5	1000	400	20	0.4	0.6	4
Both	2-3	31	Usual	1400	17	0.7	5	1000	400	20	0.4	0.7	4
Both	4-6	40	Usual	1700	20	0.7	5	1000	400	20	0.5	0.9	5
Both	7-9	57	Usual	2100	24	1.0	5	1500	400	30	0.7	1.1	7
Both	10-12	77	Usual	2500	30	1.2	12	2000	400	30	0.8	1.3	8
Boy	13-15	108	Usual	3100	40	1.2	12	2700	400	30	0.9	1.6	9
Girl	13-15	108	Usual	2600	39	1.2	12	2700	400	30	0.8	1.3	8
Boy	16-17	136	B(3)	3700	45	1.2	12	3200	400	30	1.1	1.9	11
Girl	16-17	120	A(4)	2400	41	1.2	12	3200	400	30	0.7	1.2	7
Boy	18-19	144	B(3)	3800	47	0.9	6	3200	400	30	1.1	1.9	11
Girl	18-19	124	A(4)	2450	41	0.9	10	3200	400	30	0.7	1.2	7

(1) Protein recommendation is based on normal mixed Canadian diet. Vegetarian diets may require a higher protein content.
(2) Vitamin A is based on the mixed Canadian diet supplying both Vitamin A and Carotene. As preformed Vitamin A the suggested intake would be about 2/3 of that indicated.
(3) Expenditure assessed as being 113% of that of a man of same weight and engaged in same degree of activity.
(4) Expenditure assessed as being 104% of that of a woman of the same weight and engaged in the same degree of activity.
* Dietary Standard for Canada. Canadian Council on Nutrition. Canadian Bulletin on Nutrition, Vol. 6, No. 1, 1964 (revised 1968).

NUTRIENT INTAKES RECOMMENDED FOR CANADIAN ADULTS OF DIFFERENT BODY SIZE AND DEGREE OF ACTIVITY*

Weight (lbs.)[1]	Activity[2]	Calories	Protein g.[3]	Calcium g.	Iron mg.	Vitamin A I.U.[4]	Vitamin D I.U.	Ascorbic Acid mg.	Thiamine mg.	Riboflavin mg.	Niacin mg.
Males:											
144	Maintenance	2150	44	0.5	6	3700	—	30	0.6	1.1	6
	A	2650	44	0.5	6	3700	—	30	0.8	1.3	8
	B	3400	44	0.5	6	3700	—	30	1.0	1.7	10
	C	4000	44	0.5	6	3700	—	30	1.2	2.0	12
	D	4600	44	0.5	6	3700	—	30	1.4	2.3	14
158	Maintenance	2300	48	0.5	6	3700	—	30	0.7	1.2	7
	A	2850	48	0.5	6	3700	—	30	0.9	1.4	9
	B	3650	48	0.5	6	3700	—	30	1.1	1.8	11
	C	4250	48	0.5	6	3700	—	30	1.3	2.1	13
	D	4900	48	0.5	6	3700	—	30	1.5	2.5	15
176	Maintenance	2500	54	0.5	6	3700	—	30	0.8	1.3	8
	A	3100	54	0.5	6	3700	—	30	0.9	1.5	9
	B	3950	54	0.5	6	3700	—	30	1.2	2.0	12
	C	4600	54	0.5	6	3700	—	30	1.4	2.3	14
	D	5350	54	0.5	6	3700	—	30	1.6	2.7	16
Females:											
111	Maintenance	1750	35	0.5	10	3700	—	30	0.5	0.9	5
	A	2200	35	0.5	10	3700	—	30	0.7	1.1	7
	B	2800	35	0.5	10	3700	—	30	0.8	1.4	8
	C	3300	35	0.5	10	3700	—	30	1.0	1.7	10
	D	3800	35	0.5	10	3700	—	30	1.2	1.9	12
124	Maintenance	1900	39	0.5	10	3700	—	30	0.6	1.0	6
	A	2400	39	0.5	10	3700	—	30	0.7	1.2	7
	B	3000	39	0.5	10	3700	—	30	0.9	1.5	9
	C	3550	39	0.5	10	3700	—	30	1.1	1.8	11
	D	4100	39	0.5	10	3700	—	30	1.2	2.0	12
136	Maintenance	2050	43	0.5	10	3700	—	30	0.6	1.0	6
	A	2550	43	0.5	10	3700	—	30	0.8	1.3	8
	B	3250	43	0.5	10	3700	—	30	1.0	1.6	10
	C	3800	43	0.5	10	3700	—	30	1.1	1.9	11
	D	4400	43	0.5	10	3700	—	30	1.3	2.2	13
Pregnancy-during 2nd & 3rd Trimesters add		up to 500	9	0.7	3	500	400	10	0.15	0.25	1.5
Lactation-add		500 to 1000	23	0.7	3	1500	400	20	0.3	0.5	3

(1) Weights include indoor clothing without shoes.
(2) A=Sedentary; B=Moderate; C=Heavy; D=Very Heavy.
(3) (4) See footnotes (1) and (2) to Table.
* Dietary Standard For Canada; Canadian Council on Nutrition. Canadian Bulletin Nutrition, Vol. 6, No. 1, 1964 (revised 1968).

Weights illustrated are the 25th, 50th, and 75th percentiles of the 25-29 year age group in the Canadian population.

FOOD COMPOSITION TABLE FOR SHORT METHOD OF

Food and Approximate Measure	Weight, gm.	Food Energy, Cal.	Protein, gm.
Milk, cheese, cream; related products			
Cheese: blue, cheddar (1 cu in., 17 gm),			
cheddar process (1 oz), Swiss (1 oz)	30	105	6
cottage (from skim) creamed (1/2c)	115	120	16
Cream: half-and-half (cream and milk) (2 tbsp)			
For light whipping add 1 pat butter	30	40	1
Milk: whole (3.5% fat) (1c)	245	160	9
fluid, nonfat (skim) and buttermilk (from skim)	245	90	9
milk beverages, (1 c) cocoa, chocolate drink made with skim milk. For malted milk add 4 tbsp half-and-half (270 gm)	245	210	8
milk desserts, custard (1c) 248 gm, ice cream (8 fl oz) 142 gm		290	8
cornstarch pudding (248 gm), ice milk (1 c) 187 gm		280	9
White sauce, med (1/2c)	130	215	5
Egg; 1 large	50	80	6
Meat, poultry, fish, shellfish, related products			
Beef, lamb, veal: lean and fat, cooked, inc. corned beef (3 oz) (all cuts)	85	245	22
lean only, cooked; dried beef (2 + oz) (all cuts)	65	140	20
Beef, relatively fat, such as steak and rib, cooked (3 oz)	85	350	18
Liver: beef, fried (2 oz)	55	130	15
Pork, lean & fat, cooked (3 oz) (all cuts)	85	325	20
lean only, cooked (2 + oz) (all cuts)	60	150	18
ham, light cure, lean & fat, roasted (3 oz)	85	245	18
Luncheon meats: bologna (2 sl), pork sausage, cooked (2 oz). frankfurter (1), bacon, brolied or fried crisp (3 sl)		185	9
Poultry			
chicken: flesh only, broiled (3 oz)	85	115	20
fried (2 + oz)	75	170	24
turkey, light & dark, roasted (3 oz)	85	160	27
Fish and shellfish			
salmon (3 oz) (canned)	85	130	17
fish sticks, breaded, cooked (3–4)	75	130	13
mackerel, halibut, cooked	85	175	19
blue fish, haddock, herring, perch, shad, cooked (tuna canned in oil, 20 gm)	85	160	19
clams, canned; crab meat, canned; lobster; oyster, raw; scallop; shrimp, canned	85	75	14
Mature dry beans and peas, nuts, peanuts, related products			
Beans: white with pork & tomato, canned (1c)	260	320	16
red (128 gm), Lima (96 gm), cowpeas (125 gm), cooked (1/2c)		125	8
Nuts: almonds (12), cashews (8), peanuts (1 tbsp), peanut butter (1 tbsp), pecans (12), English walnuts (2 tbsp), coconut (1/4c)	15	95	3
Vegetables and vegetable products			
Asparagus, cooked, cut spears (2/3c)	115	25	3
Beans; green (1/2c) cooked 60 gm; canned 120 gm		15	1
Lima, immature, cooked (1/2c)	80	90	6
Broccoli spears, cooked (2/3c)	100	25	3
Brussels sprouts, cooked (2/3c)	85	30	3
Cabbage (110 gm); cauliflower, cooked (80 gm); and sauerkraut, canned (150 gm) (reduce ascorbic acid value by one-third for kraut) (2/3c)		20	1
Carrots, cooked (2/3c)	95	30	1
Corn, 1 ear, cooked (140 gm); canned (130 gm) (1/2c)		75	2
Leafy greens: collards (125 gm), dandelions (120 gm), kale (75 gm), mustard (95 gm), spinach (120 gm), turnip (100 gm cooked, 150 gm canned) (2/3 cooked and canned) (reduce ascorbic acid one-half for canned)		30	3

Wilson, E.D., K. H. Fisher, and M. E. Fuqua, Principles of Nutrition, 2nd edition, New York, John Wiley and Sons, 1966.

DIETARY ANALYSIS (3RD REVISION)

Fat, gm.	Carbohy-drate, gm.	Calcium, mg.	Iron, mg.	Vitamin A Value, I.U.	Thiamine, mg.	Riboflavin, mg.	Niacin, mg.	Ascorbic Acid, mg.
9	1	165	0.2	345	0.01	0.12	trace	0
5	3	105	0.4	190	0.04	0.28	0.1	0
4	2	30	trace	145	0.01	0.04	trace	trace
9	12	285	0.1	350	0.08	0.42	0.1	2
trace	13	300	trace	—	0.10	0.44	0.2	2
8	26	280	0.6	300	0.09	0.43	0.3	trace
17	29	210	0.4	785	0.07	0.34	0.1	1
10	40	290	0.1	390	0.08	0.41	0.3	2
16	12	150	0.2	610	0.06	0.22	0.3	trace
6	trace	25	1.2	590	0.06	0.15	trace	0
16	0	10	2.9	25	0.06	0.19	4.2	0
5	0	10	2.4	10	0.05	0.16	3.4	0
30	0	10	2.4	60	0.05	0.14	3.5	0
6	3	5	5.0	30,280	0.15	2.37	9.4	15
24	0	10	2.6	0	0.62	0.20	4.2	0
8	0	5	2.2	0	0.57	0.19	3.2	0
19	0	10	2.2	0	0.40	0.16	3.1	0
16	—	5	1.3	—	0.21	0.12	1.7	0
3	0	10	1.4	80	0.05	0.16	7.4	0
6	1	10	1.6	85	0.05	0.23	8.3	0
5	0	—	1.5	—	0.03	0.15	6.5	0
5	0	165	0.7	60	0.03	0.16	6.8	0
7	5	10	0.3	—	0.03	0.05	1.2	0
10	0	10	0.8	515	0.08	0.15	6.8	0
8	2	20	1.0	60	0.06	0.11	4.4	0
1	2	65	2.5	65	0.10	0.08	1.5	0
7	50	140	4.7	340	0.20	0.08	1.5	5
—	25	35	2.5	5	0.13	0.06	0.7	—
8	4	15	0.5	5	0.05	0.04	0.9	—
trace	4	25	0.7	1,055	0.19	0.20	1.6	30
trace	3	30	0.4	340	0.04	0.06	0.3	8
1	16	40	2.0	225	0.14	0.08	1.0	14
trace	4	90	0.8	2,500	0.09	0.20	0.8	90
trace	5	30	1.0	450	0.07	0.12	0.7	75
trace	4	35	0.5	80	0.05	0.05	0.3	37
trace	7	30	0.6	10,145	0.05	0.05	0.5	6
trace	18	5	0.4	315	0.06	0.06	1.1	6
trace	5	175	1.8	8,570	0.11	0.18	0.8	45

FOOD COMPOSITION TABLE (CONTINUED)

Food and Approximate Measure	Weight, gm.	Food Energy, Cal.	Protein, gm.
Peas, green (1/2c)	80	60	4
Potatoes-baked, boiled (100 gm), 10 pc French fried (55 gm) (for fried, add 1 tbsp cooking oil)		85	3
Pumpkin, canned (1/2c)	115	40	1
Squash, winter, canned (1/2c)	100	65	2
Sweetpotato, canned (1/2c)	110	120	2
Tomato, 1 raw, 2/3c canned, 2/3 c juice	150	35	2
Tomato catsup (2 tbsp)	35	30	1
Other, cooked (beets, mushrooms, onions, turnips) (1/2c)	95	25	1
Others commonly served raw, cabbage (1/2c, 50 gm), celery (3 sm stalks, 40 gm), cucumber (1/4 med, 50 gm), green pepper (1/2, 30 gm), radishes (5, 40 gm)		10	trace
carrots, raw (1/2 carrot)	25	10	trace
lettuce leaves (2 lg)	50	10	1
Fruits and fruit products			
Cantaloup (1/2 med)	385	60	1
Citrus and strawberries: orange (1), grapefruit (1/2), juice (1/2c), strawberries (1/2c), lemon (1), tangerine (1)		50	1
Yellow, fresh: apricots (3), peach (2 med); canned fruit and juice (1/2c) or dried, cooked, unsweetened: apricot, peaches (1/2c)		85	—
Other, dried: dates, pitted (4), figs (2), raisins (1/4c)	40	120	1
Other, fresh: apple (1), banana (1), figs (3), pear (1)		80	—
Fruit pie: to 1 serving fruit add 1 tbsp flour, 2 tbsp sugar, 1 tbsp fat			
Grain products			
Enriched and whole grain: bread (1 sl, 23 gm), biscuit (1/2), cooked cereals (1/2c), prepared cereals (1 oz), Graham crackers (2 lg), macaroni, noodles, spaghetti (1/2c, cooked), pancake (1, 27 gm), roll (1/2), waffle (1/2, 38 gm)		65	2
Unenriched: bread (1 sl, 23 gm), cooked cereal (1/2 c), macaroni, noodles, spaghetti (1/2 c), popcorn (1/2 c), pretzel sticks, small (15), roll (1/2)		65	2
Desserts			
Cake, plain (1 pc), doughnut (1). For iced cake or doughnut add value for sugar (1 tbsp). For chocolate cake add chocolate (30 gm)	45	145	2
Cookies, plain (1)	25	120	1
Pie crust, single crust (1/7 shell)	20	95	1
Flour, white, enriched (1 tbsp)	7	25	1
Fats and Oils			
Butter, margarine (1 pat, 1/2 tbsp)	7	50	trace
Fats and oils, cooking (1 tbsp), French dressing (2 tbsp)	14	125	0
Salad dressing, mayonnaise type (1 tbsp)	15	80	trace
Sugars, sweets			
Candy, plain (1/2 oz), jam and jelly (1 tbsp), sirup (1 tbsp), gelatin dessert, plain (1/2 c), beverages, carbonated (1 c)		60	0
Chocolate fudge (1 oz), chocolate sirup (3 tbsp)		125	1
Molasses (1 tbsp), caramel (1/3 oz)		40	trace
Sugar (1 tbsp)	12	45	0
Miscellaneous			
Chocolate, bitter (1 oz)	30	145	3
Sherbet (1/2 c)	96	130	1
Soups: bean, pea (green) (1 c)		150	7
noodle, beef, chicken (1 c)		65	4
clam chowder, minestrone, tomato, vegetable (1 c)		90	3

The use of the short method of dietary analysis reduces the time required to compute the nutritive value of a diet. In the evaluation of a mixed dietary using this method the accuracy approximates that of computations using the conventional food table.

Fat, gm.	Carbohydrate, gm.	Calcium, mg.	Iron, mg.	Vitamin A Value, I.U.	Thiamine, mg.	Riboflavin, mg.	Niacin, mg.	Ascorbic Acid, mg.
1	10	20	1.4	430	0.22	0.09	1.8	16
trace	30	10	0.7	trace	0.08	0.04	1.5	16
1	9	30	0.5	7,295	0.03	0.06	0.6	6
1	16	30	0.8	4,305	0.05	0.14	0.7	14
—	27	25	0.8	8,500	0.05	0.05	0.7	15
trace	7	14	0.8	1,350	0.10	0.06	1.0	29
trace	8	10	0.2	480	0.04	0.02	0.6	6
—	5	20	0.5	15	0.02	0.10	0.7	7
trace	2	15	0.3	100	0.03	0.03	0.2	20
trace	2	10	0.2	2,750	0.02	0.02	0.2	2
trace	2	34	0.7	950	0.03	0.04	0.2	9
trace	14	25	0.8	6,540	0.08	0.06	1.2	63
—	13	25	0.4	165	0.08	0.03	0.3	55
—	22	10	1.1	1,005	0.01	0.05	1.0	5
—	31	35	1.4	20	0.04	0.04	0.5	—
—	21	15	0.5	140	0.04	0.03	0.2	6
1	16	20	0.6	10	0.09	0.05	0.7	—
1	16	10	0.3	5	0.02	0.02	0.3	—
5	24	30	0.4	65	0.02	0.05	0.2	—
5	18	10	0.2	20	0.01	0.01	0.1	—
6	8	3	0.3	0	0.04	0.03	0.3	—
trace	5	1	0.2	0	0.03	0.02	0.2	0
6	trace	1	0	230	—	—	—	—
14	0	0	0	0	0	0	0	0
9	1	2	0.1	45	trace	trace	trace	0
0	14	3	0.1	trace	trace	trace	trace	trace
2	30	15	0.6	10	trace	0.02	0.1	trace
trace	8	20	0.3	trace	trace	trace	trace	trace
0	12	0	trace	0	0	0	0	0
15	8	20	1.9	20	0.01	0.07	0.4	0
1	30	15	trace	55	0.01	0.03	trace	2
4	22	50	1.6	495	0.09	0.06	1.0	4
2	7	10	0.7	50	0.03	0.04	0.9	trace
2	14	25	0.9	1,880	0.05	0.04	1.1	3

The values in this Table were computed chiefly from the figures compiled by Watt and Merrill in Agriculture Handbook 8, *Composition of Foods–Raw, Processed, Prepared,* revised 1963.

Courtesy of Leichsenring and Wilson, *J. Am. Dietet. Assoc.* Nov., 1965.

ABBREVIATIONS AND EQUIVALENTS

t.   teaspoon (s)
T.   tablespoon (s)
c.   cup (s)
pt.   pint (s)
qt.   quart (s)
g.   gram (s)
mg.   milligram (s)
mcg.   microgram (s)
kg.   kilogram (s)
oz.   ounce (s)
lb.   pound (s)
I. U.   International Units
cal.   calorie (s)
carb.   carbohydrate (s)
Ca   calcium
Fe   iron
P   phosphorus
Na   sodium
vit.   vitamin (s)

5-1/3 T. = 1/3 c.
16 oz. = 1 lb.
1 oz. = approx. 30 gm.
1 lb. = 454 gm.
100 gm. = approx. 3/5 oz.
1 gm. = 1000 mg.
1 mg. = 1000 mcg.
1 kg. = 2.2 lb.
1 gm. carb. = 4 cal.
1 gm. fat = 9 cal.
1 gm. protein = 4 cal.

To convert grams to ounces, divide by 28.35 (For a rough estimate, divide by 30).

To convert ounces to grams, multiply by 28.35.

To convert pounds to kilograms, divide by 2.2.

To convert kilograms to pounds, multiply by 2.2.

To convert milligrams to grams, divide by 1000 by moving the decimal point three places to the left.

To convert micrograms to milligrams or grams to kilograms, divide by 1000 in the same way.

INDEX